Life OFF THE LABEL

This book contains the opinions and ideas of its author. It is intended to provide general information on the subjects it addresses. It is not in any way a substitute for the advice of the reader's own physician(s) or other medical professionals for individual conditions, symptoms, or concerns. Readers should seek further advice from a competent physician and/or other qualified health care professionals for personal medical, health, dietary, exercise or other assistance or advice. The author specifically disclaims all responsibility for injury, damage or loss that the reader may incur as a direct or indirect consequence of following any directions or suggestions given in this book by the author, or by participating in any programs or events described in the book, recommended or offered by the author.

Life Off the Label. Copyright ©2016 by Colleen Kachmann. All rights reserved. No part of this book may be reproduced, scanned or distributed in any printed or electronic form without permission. Please support author's rights. Do not participate in, or encourage piracy of copyrighted materials. Purchase only authorized editions.

Self-published by Colleen Kachmann. Printed in the United States of America by Walsworth Print Group, 306 N. Kansas Ave. Marlene, MO 64658.

Edited by Lori Parker of Lori Parker Editor Writer Poet, Chicago, IL.

Book design, graphic images and e-book by Heather Shively, Bodacious Girl Studio, Fort Wayne, IN.

ISBN 978-0-9977024-0-8 (print)

ISBN 978-0-9977024-1-5 (e-book)

The Library of Congress Cataloging-in-Publication Data is available upon request.

Life Off the Label may be purchased in bulk for promotional, educational or business use. Email ColleenKachmann@lifeoffthelabel.com for pricing and delivery.

First edition: September 2016

For my family. If we can't be normal, let's be healthy . . .

Welcome Readers . . .

Life Off the Label: A Handbook for Creating Your Own Brand of Health and Happiness includes far more than the book you are holding in your hand. You'll discover that the value of the resources now available to you far exceeds the cover price. This printed copy offers extra-wide margins for your notes, ideas and questions. The Normal vs Healthy sections at the end of each chapter include extra space for further reflection. If you don't wish to write in this book, or have borrowed it from a friend or the library, print fresh copies from the website. The recipes, info-graphs and other content labeled with the printer icon throughout the book, an audio mp4 file for each chapter and much more can be downloaded at colleenkachmann.com/members.

Use the password: LOL2017BonusMaterial

The bonus resources are designed to provide you with everything you'll need as you begin your journey. They serve as an immediate return on your investment. You are supported and in good company!

Thank you for joining the mission to make it normal to be healthy. Let's get started!

Contents

Preface:	The Back Story	vi
Chapter 1:	Awareness and Freedom	2
Chapter 2:	The Reality of Food Addiction	18
Chapter 3:	Food Imposters and Free-Fat Calories	30
Chapter 4:	A Culture of Chemicals	54
Chapter 5:	Dangerous AgVentures	78
Chapter 6:	Prescriptions for Pain	108
Chapter 7:	The Great Debate: Organic Food	138
Chapter 8:	The Dairy Dilemma	156
Chapter 9:	The Allegory of Asthma and Allergies	174
Chapter 10:	The Gut-Brain Connection	192
Chapter 11:	Western Diet Feeds Western Medicine	208
Chapter 12:	Seeds of Health	224
Chapter 13:	Kid Food Kills	240
Chapter 14:	Afford the Best on a Budget of Less	262
Chapter 14B:	Invest the Rest	290
Chapter 15:	Create Your Own Brand of Health and Happiness	310
Index		324
Endnotes		332
Acknowledgements		356

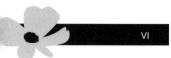

Preface

The
Back
Story

> *"The first step towards getting somewhere is to decide that you are not going to stay where you are."*
>
> J. P. MORGAN (1837-1913) AMERICAN FINANCIER, ENDED THE STOCK MARKET PANIC OF 1907

MUCH TO MY OWN SURPRISE...

On February 2, 2009, I decided to become a vegan.

Carrying a harmless looking copy of *The Kind Diet*, I naively boarded a plane for a weekend getaway. The author, actress Alicia Silverstone, had appeared on *Oprah!* to talk about her book. Despite having no desire to follow in her vegan footsteps, I was intrigued. She looked amazing. Plus, I needed something entertaining to read on the plane.

The first "ah-ha" moment happened before I finished the first chapter. *The Kind Diet* is not a set of rules that lead to an emaciated figure and a smug sense of superiority—though I confess that was what I was looking for. Instead, it illuminates the path to freedom. I had been a prisoner of my own mind for far too long. The book opened my eyes to the fact that I had been hurting myself. I could let go of my food issues whenever I was ready to let go of my fears. The ham sandwich I'd packed to eat on the plane went uneaten. I devoured the book instead.

I can remember skipping meals at the tender age of eight for fear of getting fat. I had knobby-knees and was affectionately referred to as "Colleen, the string bean," so my concerns were unfounded. My young adult life was essentially a never-ending diet. I assumed I would outgrow the food issues that consumed my energy and time. Unfortunately, they followed me into motherhood and midlife.

For twenty-five years, I was a meticulous calorie-counter. Every calorie consumed was balanced by exercise. Each day, the number on the scale determined my level of confidence and course of action. I'd swallow anything that promised to reduce my appetite or speed up my metabolism. If a binge got the best of me, I'd stick my finger down my throat. I did my best to keep the crazy hidden from those around me. But food was the enemy. My body was the battleground.

After a lifetime of daily struggles against cravings and appetite, I was open to the idea that I could no longer fight for peace and expect to win. Silverstone described freedom. The more I read, the more I realized that my own ignorance was holding me prisoner to self-defeating habits and beliefs. I was able to envision myself living an informed and conscious life.

The Kind Diet reveals that good food is kind to the body (and the mind). I had been operating with a lot of false assumptions as to what *good food* actually is. The book explains the benefits of eating living foods filled with micronutrients, i.e. antioxidants, enzymes, vitamins and minerals. I realized that I was overfed and severely under nourished. It made perfect sense. I was inspired to reject meat and dairy. The horrible conditions and hidden realities to which animals are subjected are shocking. The antibiotics and hormones given to livestock are making us sick. By the time the plane landed at my destination, I was a card-carrying vegan looking for my first meal.

I committed to a 40-day trial. Downtime that weekend was spent shopping on-line. The vegan staples and hard-to-find ingredients would be waiting back home. I even ordered a t-shirt, key chain and bumper sticker.

Game on. Vegan challenge accepted.

My motivation was not entirely pure. I had no frame of reference for what life would be like if (when) I was free to enjoy my food. We are taught from day one that life is supposed to be hard. Nothing worth doing is easy, right? In retrospect, the clear boundaries of the vegan diet provided me with a sense of control over my impulses. I had to test it before I could trust it. Regardless, I had unwittingly stumbled onto the path of real healing.

My all-or-nothing approach left no room for transitions or compromise. I just started wearing my vegan t-shirts and dealt with the details as they appeared. Withdrawal symptoms were a welcome sign that I was doing something right.

And as my body detoxed, cravings for problematic foods disappeared. The more I ate foods that did not come in a package, the less labels there were to feed my obsession. I forgot to worry about calories, portion sizes and protein/fat ratios. This was the mental freedom I had longed for. My focus shifted to learning new recipes, experimenting with flavors and textures, and enjoying the fruits of my labor. Food became my friend.

As I continued to research the vegan philosophies, my eyes were further opened to the poisons in the American food supply. Many are listed on the labels I've read my whole life (though many are not). I became more and more disillusioned. My 40-day trial seamlessly transitioned into a lifestyle and I knew I would never go back.

At first, my plant-based diet was a huge inconvenience to family and friends. Veggie broth must be used in place of chicken stock to make soup. Salads need to be more than just pale green lettuce and a handful of shredded carrots. When I refuse to join the conga line to the dessert table, it becomes clear that cheesecake is a choice, not an obligation. That is a party foul that makes people edgy. Especially if those people are your family and grandma made the cheesecake.

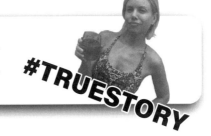

I'm not saying my diet is better than yours. It's just different. In a better way. #TRUESTORY

As a mother of four, I soon discovered that declaring our diets to be "vegan" is easier than making vague demands for "healthy" food. Most people think they eat "pretty well" and take offense at the notion that their choices won't meet my standards.

With raised eyebrows, they explain, "Oh, I eat healthy. I only "cheat" on special occasions like holidays, vacations, in restaurants and at parties. Of course, my birthday includes a once-a-year free pass."

Right. But it's *someone's* birthday every day. And aren't we all required to celebrate? Hence, the aforementioned plethora of special occasions.

Vegan t-shirts and bumper stickers put me in a protected class, similar to diets that are gluten-free, nut-free, or kosher. The vegan label allows my eating preferences to seem more than just a snobby statement of "healthier than thou."

Instead, my diet adds cultural diversity to the party population. "Wow!" people comment, "I've never met a real vegan! Where do you get your protein?"

This book leaves no stone unturned. I will dissect the vegan propaganda with the same tenacity as foods that claim "100 percent all natural ingredients." I will tell you why I am no longer 100 percent vegan, though I do follow a plant-based diet.

Food is medicine. The body has an innate ability to heal when properly nourished. In my research I have learned that many factors play into a person's nutritional requirements. There is no one-size-fits-all approach. The journey to wellness is unique for everyone.

Life off the label does not require extraordinary discipline or sacrifice. There is no agenda or dogmatic principles to which you must adhere. You do not need to become vegan or restrict all processed foods. You can decide what products to keep and what to avoid. No commitment forms are required. You will always have the freedom to choose and the ability to change as you see fit.

> There are no mistakes. There's *what you do,* what you *don't do,* and *what happens next.*
>
> Colleen Kachmann, Life off the Label

PREFACE

CHAPTER 1

AWARENESS AND FREEDOM

"None are so hopelessly enslaved than those who falsely believe they are free."

JOHANN WOLFGANG VON GOETHE (1739-1832)
GERMAN PHILOSOPHER, POET AND STATESMAN

BONDAGE BEGINS

My head was pounding. She would not stop screaming. I lifted my t-shirt and her tiny mouth devoured my breast. I scurried about the kitchen, collecting random ingredients for my signature "Whatever's-Left-in-the-Fridge Casserole." Damn. I needed to go to the grocery store. My boys had outgrown the shopping cart with the blue two-seater car that allowed them both to "drive." The ensuing meltdown was inevitable. But only the red, semi-truck style cart would accommodate the boys, my two-year-old daughter, the infant carrier seat, and maybe a few grocery items. The thing had the momentum and steering capacity of a freight train. I needed the patience of Job and the energy of a superhero to get to the store and back.

I checked the milk in the fridge. It was half full. A few quick calculations told me the trip to the grocery could wait another day. Sippy cups of chocolate Ovaltine and peanut butter-slathered toast would serve as tomorrow's breakfast. I topped the casserole with the last of the shredded cheese and set the oven timer. If the family doctor was on-schedule for my 4 o'clock appointment, we'd be eating dinner by 5:30 p.m.

Anna was sitting in the living room on her potty-chair, breastfeeding her baby doll. She was peaceful and quiet, captivated by her favorite characters on the television screen. Kyle was watching it from the balcony, straddling the bars and kicking his dirty bare feet against the sunbeams on the wall. Marlin and Dory had just escaped the sharks when I paused the DVD player.

"Mommy! It's not o-ber!"

I unlatched Kate and the screaming resumed. I laid her on a soft pink blanket and changed her diaper while I spoke to Anna in my calm-understanding-mommy-voice. "I know, precious. But I have to go see the doctor. You can finish *Finding Nemo* after dinner. Let's choose your big-girl panties. Do you want Dora the Explorer or The Little Mermaid?"

Distracted by the pleasure of making a choice, she began to layout her options.

I took the same approach with my next obstacle. "Kyle, do you want to go find your brother or help Anna with her shoes?" He immediately raced out the front door, leaving it wide open and allowing the two Labradors to escape. Exasperated, I watched them disappear on a joy-run.

After loading all four kids, I drove down the road to find the dogs visiting with neighbors. I invited them to go for a ride. Tails wagged as they hopped into the trunk of my SUV. The journey was brief. I pulled back into the garage, herded them into the house and shut the door on their disappointment.

Twenty minutes later, I unstrapped the girls from their car seats and loaded the double jog-stroller with a diaper bag full of books, toys, snacks and extra clothes. The boys raced ahead, propping open the tunnel of doors that lead to the doctor's waiting room. From five feet away I was blasted with frigid air and the smell of antiseptic. I angled my approach and negotiated my way through the tight space. I only scraped one knuckle that day.

Thirty minutes later, still in the waiting room, I washed down two Tylenol and shared a pretzel with Anna. I wondered when the mother of those two rowdy boys would get them under control. Kate was quiet because her head was up my shirt. She continued to suckle after my name was called. I rose to relocate my monkeys and my circus to exam room number five. My ability to breastfeed while simultaneously carrying a toddler, filling out forms and sheep-dogging two boys was impressive.

I set the baby down when the nurse asked me to step on the scale. There was a 30-second delay before the shock of denial registered in her brain. Her response rivaled a tornado alert siren. It had been six months since she was abruptly removed from my body via cesarean section; she'd been trying to get back in ever since. She had her mother's skill for strategy: did I want to listen to her scream or let her suck on my boob?

I got on the scale backwards. I did not want to see a number that would contradict my dedication to exercise, Diet Coke and fat-free foods.

The boys surveyed the contents of the cabinets while the nurse took my blood pressure. They were slamming the drawers when the doctor knocked and entered. He surveyed the situation with a look of empathy.

Tears fell as I described the severity of my headaches. Every day, I had chronic pain in my neck and lower back. I couldn't sleep. I was already taking citalopram for postpartum depression. Yet the sight of an over-flowing laundry basket still tripped my emotional circuit breakers. My doctor seemed to understand the problem. I left his office with prescriptions for Ativan to ease my anxiety, Ambien to help me sleep and pain pills to interrupt the cycle of suffering.

Normal versus Healthy

America is the land of the free and the home of the brave. It is also the land of the obese and home to the most medicated people on the planet. Nearly 70 percent of us qualify as overweight and take at least one prescription medication.[1]

Chronic disease and disorders are redefining normal American life. Our diets are filled with processed foods. Our medicine cabinets are filled with pain relievers, anti-inflammatories, antibiotics and allergy medications. We take our kids to the doctor as often as our elderly parents. Prescriptions ease the suffering but symptoms get worse each year. Additional, and often stronger, drugs are required.

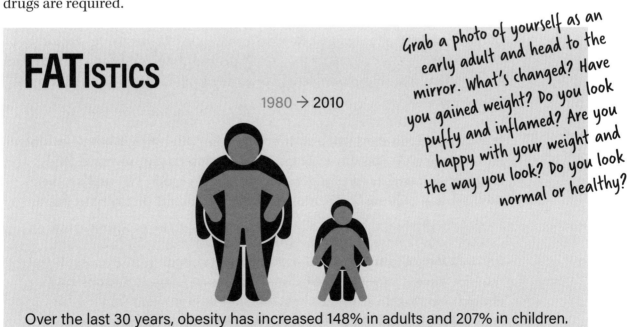

FATISTICS 1980 → 2010

Over the last 30 years, obesity has increased 148% in adults and 207% in children.

Grab a photo of yourself as an early adult and head to the mirror. What's changed? Have you gained weight? Do you look puffy and inflamed? Are you happy with your weight and the way you look? Do you look normal or healthy?

AWARENESS AND FREEDOM

Life has not always been this way. The trajectory of our fate is clear. It is obvious to anyone paying attention that "normal" is inversely proportional to healthy. As one goes up, the other goes down. Forty years ago, Americans spent 16 percent of their income on food and 8 percent on health care. Today, it's the exact opposite. We have the cheapest food on the planet and the most expensive health care in the world.[2] The consequences of this reality are abysmal.

Since 1950, celiac disease has risen by 400 percent.[3] Inflammatory bowel disease is up over 50 percent.[4] Since just 2001, asthma diagnosis have increased by 50 percent in both children and adults. Disease rates are on the rise. Many of us wonder if we have a thyroid condition or other autoimmune disease. We are all one lump away from a cancer diagnosis. Everyone is allergic to something. Depression and anxiety disorders are no longer dealt with in secret. Mental illness used to be considered shameful, so people suffered in silence. That has changed—and that is good. What is not good is so many of us are now affected that it's *abnormal* to meet someone who isn't.

PAIN IS PROFIT

A quick look around the world reveals that as other countries adopt our western lifestyle, they are waking up to the same realities. The consequences of replacing old-world habits with new and improved alternatives are clear and predictable. And disastrous.

Americans are consumers. We like to buy stuff. Our capitalistic society is based on the exchange of goods and services. We are supplied with endless products that promise convenience, health and happiness. We have been brainwashed by mass marketing campaigns. Need to lose weight? *There's a program for that.* Don't feel well? *There's a pill for that.* Got a problem? *There's an app for that.* And the company that sells the trifecta (a program, a pill and an app!) will lead the industry in profits.

In this book, I will show you that our role as the "consumer" has been mutated into the role of the "producer." Large corporations supply processed foods, pharmaceuticals, beauty products and disposable goods. We produce their profits. Our minds are bombarded with advertisements that keep us running to the store for everything we are told we "need."

An onslaught of toxic chemicals overburdens our bodies. Subsequent illness demands treatment. Medications suppress symptoms and obstruct the fact that we get sicker each year. The flow of supply and demand has reversed: supply now drives demand. As a result, addiction and disease fuel the economy.

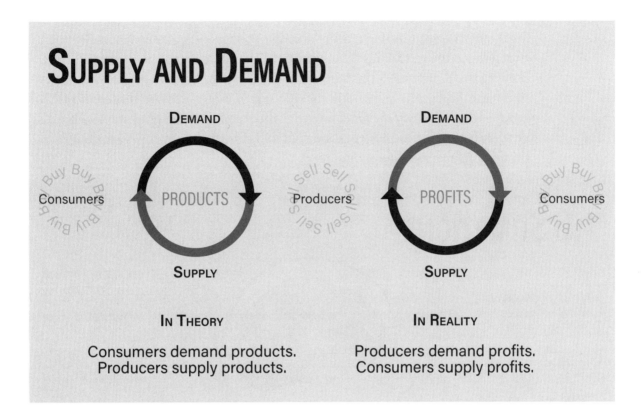

Sugar, salt, fat and scent have immediate effects on the pleasure centers of the brain. The ingredients of everything that comes in a package are chemically engineered to produce the biggest "hit" for the smallest buck. Thousands upon thousands of patented formulations are listed in databases. Computer models generate a precise combination that's most likely to attract customers. Trials are then conducted with paid participants using the same questions optometrists use to test our vision: "*better or worse*?" The appeal of flavor, texture, appearance, smell and packaging are carefully analyzed to maximize sensory satisfaction. Marketing teams then research the psychology of the targeted demographic and advertising campaigns are launched.[5]

Some brands advertise that their products are scientifically proven to make you happy.[6] This is not commercialized exaggeration. It's true. Chemical recipes are manipulated to illicit bliss. (So is heroin.) Extensive research and cunning strategies are used in manufacturing so that you will want to try and subsequently *need* to buy. The Supersized, New and Improved, All Natural junk is not designed to create health and happiness for you. It is designed to create profits for them.

The purpose of this book is to expose the truths that you don't even know that you don't know. Wellness isn't possible in the framework of our current culture. The bottom line is that no one profits unless you are sick or in need. If everyone were to choose a life off the label, Corporate America would collapse. But you are not obligated to sacrifice your health for the sake of the economy.

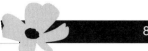

Throughout this book, I use terms like Big Tobacco, Big Pharma and Big Food to reference the industries that comprise Corporate America. Big Brands are holding their customers hostage. Awareness is your best weapon if you want to escape. Just as the concept of life *off the grid* is attractive to those who crave independence, life *off the label* provides the freedom to be (and stay) well. Each chapter includes vital information that will show you how to create your own brand of health and happiness.

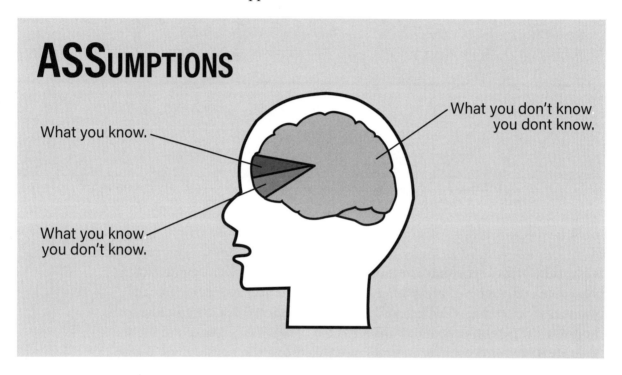

Chapter 1—Awareness and Freedom: Welcome! You are here,

Chapter 2—The Reality of Food Addiction: Cravings are a symptom of food addiction. Overeating is not an emotional malfunction. Synthetic chemicals stimulate an endorphin release. Artificial ingredients are not nutrients that support bodily functions. Consequently, they must be eliminated. Leftovers are stored in fat cells, making it very hard (close to impossible) to lose weight. We've been taught wrong. *A calorie is not a calorie.*

Chapter 3—Food Imposters and Free-Fat Calories: Sugar-free drinks and low-fat foods keep us thin, right? Wrong. Artificial sweeteners make us fat. Fake foods are toxic. Zero-calorie foods do not have zero-impact on the body. Just the opposite. The more chemicals we ingest, the more fat is required to protect us. Food is fuel, not fool's gold. Learn about the micronutrients (vitamins, minerals and antioxidants) that are essential to sustainable health. Say goodbye to weight issues. Real foods don't make you fat. You'll gain freedom as you lose weight. *You don't have to eat less. You just have to eat right.*

Chapter 4—A Culture of Chemicals: Every day we are bombarded by thousands of chemicals in food, medications, household goods and beauty supplies. We assume the products we buy are safe or they wouldn't be on the market. But studies aren't done on products. Single additives are isolated and tested in sterile laboratories free of contaminating variables. The problem? We don't live in sterile laboratories. And the many ingredients in food aren't isolated. Many legal additives are problematic but until a substance is proven harmful, proof of safety is assumed. We live in a toxic soup that is making us artificially fat and increasingly ill. *Synergy: the total impact is greater than the sum of isolated parts.*

Chapter 5 — Dangerous AgVentures: A look at history shows that Big Tobacco purposefully induced addiction to keep sales steady. When the whistle was blown, the tobacco industry took their playbooks into another arena with the acquisition of Big Food. The same conspiratorial strategies now generate billions of dollars as our addiction supplies the demand. In addition, increased use of genetically modified (GM) crops correlates to an alarming increase in chronic disease. Our food supply is completely different than it was twenty years ago. Corn is now a corn-pesticide hybrid. Altered DNA can't be washed off. *If a worm won't eat the corn, neither should you.*

Chapter 6—Prescriptions for Pain: Medications designed to suppress symptoms do not cure illness. Many aggravate the same symptoms they promise to alleviate. We've been conditioned to pop a pill to reduce pain, infection, inflammation and allergic reactions. This allows us to continue the behaviors that are irritating us, making the problems worse. Reducing symptoms does not reduce illness. The immune system grows stronger when it's relied upon — and weaker when it's not. *The more medication we take, the more healthcare we need.*

Chapter 7—The Great Debate: Organic Food: Organic food is not a designer label. Premium prices do not make the little farmers rich. Quite the contrary. Organic foods do not always contain superior nutrition (though often they do). What they *don't* contain is critical to being and staying healthy. We'll prioritize for the sake of our budget and look at when to spend the extra money on the organic label (and when it's safe to skip it). *Low-quality health is far more expensive than high-quality food.*

Chapter 8—The Dairy Dilemma: Dairy is everywhere in the American diet (even in whole grain bread). Symptoms of dairy intolerance are difficult to spot because they don't appear to be diet-related. We'll deconstruct the common misperceptions about the benefits of dairy and learn how to reduce intake with little effort. Not all dairy products are created equal; there is room for compromise. It's all about feeling your best. Got Symptoms? *To cure the disease, eliminate the cause.*

Chapter 9—The Allegory of Asthma and Allergies: Chronic allergies and asthma get worse every year. Symptoms are triggered by allergens. But when the immune system attacks otherwise benign substances, the allergen is not to blame. Taking medications to suppress inflammation is akin to disabling the fire alarm without investigating the smoke. Don't run to the drug store in preparation for allergy season; go to the produce section. *Thy food is thy medicine.*

Chapter 10—The Gut-Brain Connection: We all know what a "gut-wrenching" experience feels like. The brain and the digestive system are intimately connected. Each has a direct impact on the other. Emotions trigger biochemical reactions in the gut. In turn, tummy troubles can induce anxiety, stress and depression.[7] If you are struggling with either, both must be addressed to alleviate the symptoms. *The best advice is to go with your gut.*

Chapter 11—Western Diet Feeds Western Medicine: Medications can save lives. Nutritional deficiencies can devastate them. When illness strikes, support healing with micronutrients that strengthen the immune system. Western diseases (cancer, heart disease, diabetes, and more) can be reversed and eliminated with a plant-based diet. You don't have to commit to a vegan lifestyle. Just eat more vegetables! We'll dissect the vegan propaganda and contrast idealism with reality. We are what we eat. *Do you want to be colorful, alive and vibrant; or fat, sick and nearly dead?*

Chapter 12—Seeds of Health: We know that vegetables are healthy. But why? Vegetables have antioxidants, which disable free radicals. Understanding how and why will motivate you to increase your intake. Complete nutrition is never the prize at the bottom of a cardboard box. If fortified foods supplied what the package labels promise, our nation wouldn't be the sickest on the planet. Whole and unprocessed plant foods counteract the harmful effects of the toxins we eat, breathe and absorb. Consuming the maximum amounts of vitamins and antioxidants supports wellness and even allows for a few indulgences. *Good nutrition can subsidize bad decisions.*

Chapter 13—Kid Food Kills: Parenting is far more complicated than it used to be. The onslaught of advertisements brainwash us to believe that sugar frosted flakes are part of a nutritious breakfast. Food fights seem impossible to win when even congress qualifies ketchup and pizza sauce as vegetables. Develop strategies for getting more good food into those precious little bodies. *Don't buy the B-O-L-O-G-N-A.*

Chapter 14—Afford the Best on a Budget of Less: Time and money are limiting factors when it comes to lifestyle changes. We'll go through the products under the kitchen and bathroom sinks, in the laundry room and cleaning supply closet. Make room in your budget for organic and unprocessed food while simultaneously reducing exposure to chemicals. *[Spoiler Alert]* I haven't used shampoo in over a year, I make my own deodorant and laundry detergent. My skin care regime is not available in salons. I spend less money on healthy food than I once spent on normal food. *A rich man has money. A wealthy man has time.*

Chapter 14B — Invest the Rest: We spend a lot of time talking about our ailments. We spend a lot of money trying to fix them. Bad food makes us sick and medications keep us running on empty. Create wellness using the tools and strategies outlined in this chapter. A high quality life requires effort. Invest in yourself. You're worth it. *If you don't make time for wellness, you'll have to make time for illness.*

Chapter 15—Create Your Own Brand of Health and Happiness: Being healthy is not normal. But illness and disability aren't fun. There are many social and emotional challenges that interfere with the desire to act in your own best interest. Learn how to maneuver the obstacles. Fight the buffet bullies without being a party pooper. Identify the subconscious thoughts that limit your potential. Rewire the emotional circuits of bad habits. Set firm goals with flexible strategies. *Change requires change, whether you like it or not.*

Freedom Found

The prescriptions I carried as I left the family doctor that day did not make life easier or less painful. They precipitated a downhill slide (not the fun kind). Healing would not begin until I accidentally woke up vegan five years later. That pivotal decision changed the course of my life. I was a strict vegan for over five years. I've since discovered there are a few vegan rules that don't work for my body. Sustainable wellness requires awareness. Action plans may vary, but the end goal is the same.

Americans pay more attention to the quality of fuel in their cars than the quality of food in their bodies. It's time to rearrange our priorities. Cars run on gas. Humans run on food. Low quality food breaks down the body. High quality food keeps the body running on all cylinders. Nutritional bonus points can even sponsor an upgrade from a base-model vehicle to a high performance race car. In this race, what kind of body do you want to drive?

I'll take the sexy Ferrari, thank you very much.

Processed foods and conventional meat and dairy are loaded with chemicals that are of no use to our bodies. The countless additives are toxic and destructive. Consequently our bodies are in a constant state of stress: filtering, storing and repairing damage done by all the incoming trash.

It's normal to believe that you can't live without cheese, dairy or meat and that low quality food is essential to a high quality life. That's why it's not normal to be healthy. But we can live without cheese, dairy, meat and low quality foods. People do it all the time. Unchallenged beliefs limit us.

Freedom is the ability to separate fact from opinion. Parents, educators and respected authoritites shape our conclusions. Our conscious beliefs are often the product of subconscious assumptions. Realizing that who we are is separate from what we think is the key to independence.

> "Most people are *other people*. Their thoughts are *someone else's opinions*, their lives *a mimicry*, their passions *a quotation*."
>
> Oscar Wilde (1854-1900) 19th Century Playwright

THE ALLEGORY OF THE COIN

An ambitious pharaoh wanted majestic stone pyramids built in his honor. He had many slaves to move the stones. The potential problem was that the slaves far out-numbered the guards.

Worried about an uprising, he decided to dress, sleep, eat and work among his slaves. He listened to their convrsations. Indeed, a revolt was imminent.

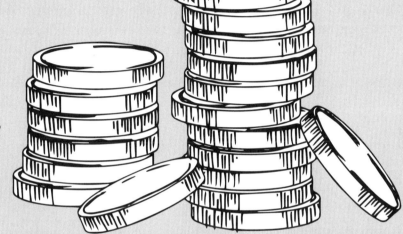

The pharaoh returned to his throne and pondered his dilemma. How could he indenture these men without worry of rebellion? How might he compel them to offer their own children for the sake of his empire?

The answer came to him. It was so simple! He would take off the shackles and tell each slave he was free. He would then offer a coin for each delivered stone. The free men could exchange the coins for the shelter, food and clothes he provided for them.

The pharaoh was honored as a legendary hero. The free men no longer plotted to escape. They worked harder than before. Soon, they began to cheat, steal and swindle each other for coins.

The pyramids were built. The empire prospered. Eventually the pharaoh organized an army to fight for the release of slaves everywhere so they too could be free.

What is the difference between slavery and freedom?

AWARENESS AND FREEDOM

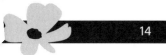

SHOP FOR SUCCESS

The information in this book takes time to digest. The challenge to change is daunting if you don't know how to start. Here's a shopping list. These ingredients will prepare you for the recipes and ideas in later chapters. Most items are available on Amazon (except for the fresh produce).

Go for the rainbow with every meal. Colorful produce is nutrient-dense (high in micronutrients and low in calories). Energy-dense foods are just the opposite (high in calories and low in micronutrients). Skip added sugars and oils. Minimize bread and pastas, even whole and multi-grain. Avoid processed foods with ingredients you don't recognize. Choose organic, local and sustainable brands. The bulk of your grocery cart should be full before you leave the produce section.

RECIPE INGREDIENTS:
- Nutritional yeast flakes
- Garlic Expressions Vinaigrette
- Balsamic vinegar
- Maple syrup (pure, grade A or B)
- Olive oil
- Coconut oil
- Raw cashews
- Raw apple cider vinegar
- Organic Ranch flavor packets
- Ground mustard, cayenne pepper, ginger, turmeric and garlic salt (or powder)

DETOX ESSENTIALS:
- Lemons
- Miso Paste
- Diluted oil of oregano
- Cruciferous vegetables such as broccoli, brussel sprouts, cauliflower, bok choy
- Dark, leafy greens such as spinach, kale, watercress, mustard, turnip and collard greens
- Oranges, apples, berries, fresh pineapple
- Green tea

CLEANING AND BEAUTY PRODUCTS:
- White vinegar
- Hydrogen peroxide
- Baking soda
- Borax
- Arm and Hammer SuperWashing Soda
- Fels Naptha or Kirk's Castille bar soap
- Dr. Bronner's 18-in-1 Pure-Castille Soap

GENERAL ITEMS:
- **VEGETABLES**: Get outside of your comfort zone. Spaghetti squash can be used in lieu of pasta. Butternut and acorn squash can serve as the base to "cheesy" cream sauce. Grill (or smoke) broccoli, cauliflower, mushrooms, onions and garlic. Roast beets, carrots, sweet potatoes and other root vegetables. Stuff sweet peppers, zucchini and tomatoes with quinoa, diced vegetables and seasonings. Kale, watercress, mustard and collard greens are soft and flavorful when lightly sautéd. Top any and all with cashew cream.

- **GRAINS**: Whole and unprocessed grains are key. White, processed carbohydrates are broken down into sugar and stored as fat. Remember this rhyme: *The whiter the bread the sooner you're dead.*
  » Uncommon grains such as quinoa, barley, bulgur, farro, teff, and buckwheat have many health benefits. Try one at a time, follow preparation directions and decide what you like. Quinoa qualifies as a complete protein as it contains the nine essential amino acids.
  » Rice comes in many colors and flavors. Avoid white, refined or polished varieties. Texamati mix contains long-grain, basmati and wild rice. Blends are family-friendly and a great way to get used to new textures.
  » Organic brown rice, quinoa, edemame and black bean pastas are gluten-free and high in protein. Each has unique texture and flavor. The biggest caveat is overcooking them. Reduce the rate carbohydrates are absorbed by serving them al dente.

- **PANTRY**:
  » Organic, dairy-free broths can be used as starters and flavor in a stir-fry, chili and soups.
  » Prepared organic soups are great for lunches and quick meals.
  » Lentils and beans: black, red, kidney, northern, pinto, garbanzo and more.
  » Organic seasoning packets and spices
  » Dairy-free mayonnaise, organic soy sauce (Tamari is a gluten-free substitute), ketchup, mustard
  » Plant milk: Non-GMO soy, almond, hemp, rice and coconut
  » Organic canned tomatoes; jars of marinara and salsa
  » Nuts (cashews, almonds, walnuts, pecan, macadamia) and seeds (sunflower, pumpkin, sesame, chia, flax)

- **OILS**: Cold-pressed varieties provide the highest nutrient content. Expeller-pressed yields a light toasted taste. Avoid refined and hydrogenated oils (most vegetable oil blends). Various oils offer a variety of flavors. Experiment with avocado, coconut, and olive oils as well as all nut and seed oils such as hazelnut, walnut and sesame. If the oil doesn't explicitly state how it is processed, assume it was heat-extracted using chemicals, like bleach.

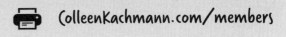 ColleenKachmann.com/members

Normal vs Healthy

Where do your beliefs come from? Are they based on your own experiences or the commercialized messages of Big Business? Do the products you buy really make your life easier? Do the medications you take actually eliminate illness? Do the foods you eat strengthen immunity and sustain wellness?

Are you ready to exchange normal for healthy?

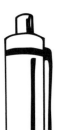

What processed foods do you consume? Why? What benefits do they offer you?

What will wellness look and feel like for you?

What symptoms do you manage with medications?

What life goals will you pursue when food addictions and illnesses no longer hold you back?

ColleenKachmann.com/members

LIFE OFF THE LABEL

PS I left this facing page blank for you.
Fill it with whatever you like. Questions, comments, to-do's, thoughts, etc.
You're welcome . . .

CHAPTER 2

THE REALITY OF FOOD ADDICTION

> *"[Addiction is] when you can stop but you don't,
> and when you want to stop but you can't."*
>
> LUKE DAVIES
> AUTHOR OF CANDY: A NOVEL OF LOVE AND ADDICTION

FOOD ADDICTION IS NOT AN EMOTIONAL MALFUNCTION

Addictions can hide in plain sight when everyone has the same problem. Seventy percent of us are overweight and on medication. Twenty percent of us take more than five prescription medications.[1] This is the new version of normal. "Typical American" camouflages the poor health of our nation.

We fork over $40 billion to the diet industry because no one wants to be fat.[2] We spend $3.8 trillion a year on healthcare because no one wants to stay sick.[3] And the last thing the government wants to do is to blame the trillion-dollar industrial food system.

Election campaigns are funded with lobby money donated by the owners and operators of Big Industry.[4] Public health initiatives (funded by Big Food) encourage the "normals" to exercise and use portion control. Eat less. Move more. Get your free pedometers at the nearest drive-thru! The advice is bad but the food tastes too good. We keep going back for more—unwitting victims of addiction.

Addiction is a scary concept because it indicates a loss of control. When we can't resist an urge that we know can cause harm, we lose our sense of power and thus our self-respect. We take bad behaviors underground. We don't want to be judged. This fear feeds our addictions. Secrets have power. We feel ashamed of our weakness. Pain, pleasure and guilt create a viscous cycle.

We struggle to hide our addictions from friends and families. That is why the word is taboo. An occasional indulgence or much needed relief can quickly take on a life of its own. Judgy McJudgers wag their tongues and point fingers. Being labeled an "addict" is a sobering experience (or not so much). Shame is an obstacle to freedom.

I can admit that I have an addictive personality. And no, that doesn't mean that everyone around me can't get enough of my witty commentary and peppy personality. I prefer to over-do everything with a Go-Big-or-Go-Home approach to life. Obsessive-compulsive habits have gotten me into trouble more than once. I've been cited for addiction in numerous areas (most of them legal).

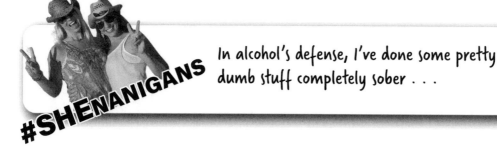

#SHENANIGANS In alcohol's defense, I've done some pretty dumb stuff completely sober . . .

Most of my addictions are cured when the dependence loses appeal. Whether it's a buzz, a short cut or a comfort measure, the honeymoon of addiction is short-lived. For example, extended-wear contacts make my eyes dry. Visine eliminates the itching. But daily use has a rebound effect. Chronically blood shot eyes are not hot.

In another instance, I was prescribed narcotics after a back injury. The mild sense of euphoria was a nice distraction from the pain. However, tolerance develops fast. Soon, I needed more for the same effect. My doctor didn't agree. The refill on addiction was denied.

There is a fine line between habit and addiction. I've experienced psychological and physical cravings. I know the pain of withdrawal. I've smoked cigarettes, drank too much wine, popped energy pills and swallowed laxatives. I've had to detox from pharmaceuticals prescribed for depression, anxiety, sleep disorders and migraines. But thankfully, I am blessed with a healthy case of ADD to compliment the OCD. I get bored with my own neuroses. Licking self-inflicted wounds and applying cucumbers to teary, swollen eyes is not fun for long. Once I remember that I can let go of the chains that bind, I skip off in search of a new bad habit that promises to be more fun.

Everyone is working hard to solve the obesity-diabetes crisis (now termed *diabesity*[5,6]). Subway sponsors the Olympics with an "Eat Fresh" campaign and Burger King provides playgrounds. McDonalds passes out pedometers to encourage movement and raise awareness to reduce portion sizes.[7] Our PTAs collect Box Tops[8] for health classes, promote processed foods from Market Day,[9] and sell candy bars to raise money for physical education.

But if everyone is working so hard, why are we still the most obese people on the planet? Could it be that ordering salads and mini portions at fast food joints isn't realistic for an addict? Are the Box Tops of sugary cereals and processed foods the problem and not the solution? Do candy sales support athletics or exemplify the term *oxymoron* for language arts?

In the end, it's the fat people that carry not only the extra weight but also all of the blame. Overweight children and adults are not the problem. No one wants to be unhealthy. They are merely symptoms of the epidemic. Our national crisis is a direct result of the Corporate Kool-Aid we are drinking 24/7. Health and happiness are severely compromised because our freedoms to pursue both are being undermined. What shackles us to this cycle of self-destruction? The answer is simple. Addiction.

Food addiction is not an emotional malfunction. It is a biological reality. After a lifetime of fighting cravings, I have experienced the truth. Eating real (unprocessed) food is the only way to conquer the addiction to fake food.

Big Food is the New Cigarette

Food addiction is an anomaly. Most addictions can be attributed to a single substance or behavior. Addictions are beaten when the desire for freedom is stronger than the temptation. An alcoholic can't get sober by exchanging whiskey for gin and tonics. An alcoholic must stop drinking. But no one can stop eating.

The good news is that it is not the basic elements of food (natural sugars, starches, proteins and fats) that cause addiction. Artificial ingredients, identified on the labels by words we cannot pronounce, stimulate the pleasure centers of the brain. Innocent consumers do not have the option of saying no if they are unaware they've even said yes.

When Big Tobacco added extra nicotine to cigarettes, they did so for the sole purpose of creating addiction. People smoke every few hours because they experience withdrawal if they don't. The pleasure of smoking is really only relief from pain. It's like wearing your belt too tight because it's such a relief to take it off.

Big Food is doing the same thing. Seriously. Think about it. Krispy Kreme Doughnuts deep-fried dough can stimulate cravings from a mile away. The aroma triggers an almost painful pulling sensation in the saliva glands. Dr. Ivan Pavlov (1849-1936) proved that dogs drool in response to the sound of a bell they've learned to associate with mealtime. The bell stimulates appetite in anticipation of the food. Likewise, the smell of donuts stimulates appetite because we associate it with mouth-watering pleasure. The reflex to recapture it is hard-wired into the brain. You recall the feathery glaze that lingers on the lips and the sweet, buttery cream that clings to your tongue. Perfection melts in your mouth. You've died and gone to heaven! Memories of the sugar crash and heaviness in your gut are banished. The craving is overwhelming. The Hot Light is on. You know you should run the opposite direction, but you can't. The lure is too strong. The high is pure bliss.

Well played, Krispy Kreme. Well played.

You want to know how to tell if a food is addictive? It's easy. If it stimulates your appetite or makes your mouth water when you are not hungry, it's addictive. Case closed.

Sugar lights up the pleasure center in the brain and releases dopamine, the "feel-good" chemical. Eating, or even seeing pictures of processed food lights up the brain the same way a shot of heroin would. And if you are one of those people who feel like you gain weight just by looking at a doughnut, don't dismiss that concept as paranoia. The addictive centers of the brain respond to the mere suggestion of sugar. Remember Pavlov's dogs? The body pumps out insulin in preparation of foods the brain remembers as pleasurable. Sight, smell and, yes, even thoughts can cause a hormone (insulin) release in anticipation. Insulin triggers fat storage. Therefore, so too can the smell of a doughnut.[10]

Though the truth resonates in your saliva glands, it might help to see the proof.

A recent study showed that high sugar, high-glycemic foods are addictive in the same way as narcotics.[11] Addiction is measured by how hard an animal will work to get a fix.[12] Concentrated sugars like high fructose corn syrup (HFCS) are eight times more addictive than cocaine.[13] What does that mean? A rat will work eight times harder for sugar than for cocaine (pushing levers and running through mazes.) This has startling implications for humans. Big Food has made it so cheap and easy to obtain the processed sugars that we must work harder to *avoid* the fix. This is why so many of us succumb to addiction.

A test was done with 12 overweight men, ages 18-35 years, using two indistinguishable milkshakes. The flavor, texture and calorie count of the shakes were the same. The only difference was in the sugar content; one shake had a low glycemic (sugar) index of 37 percent and the other a whopping 84. (A low glycemic index is anything under fifty-five; seventy or more is high.) Researchers compared brain response, blood sugar and subsequent hunger levels.

Without exception, the high-sugar shakes caused spikes in blood sugar and insulin levels and yielded reports of increased hunger and cravings within four hours. Even more telling was that the addiction response center in the brain lit up like a Vegas casino. The brain did not respond to the low glycemic shakes. The men couldn't differentiate the subtle differences but the truth was obvious to the brain.

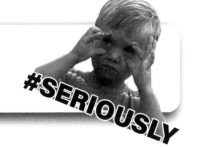

Whoever put the "b" in subtle deserves a pat on the back.

Big Tobacco hooked their customers with nicotine. Big Food has done the same with sugar and other addictive additives. Processed foods have little to no nutritional value, yet intense cravings coerce us to eat them until we are fat and sick. Alcoholics must stop drinking. Junk-food-aholics must stop eating junk food. Complete elimination will break the cycle and alleviate temptation. Freedom from addiction feels great.

THE GLYCEMIC INDEX (GI)

The Glycemic Index (GI) ranks the effect of various carbohydrates on blood sugar levels. Sugar levels are measured every 15 minutes over a two-hour period. High GI foods are digested rapidly. This results in dramatic fluctuations in blood sugar and insulin levels. High glycemic foods correlate with type 2 diabetes, obesity and coronary heart disease. Low GI foods reduce insulin levels and resistance, control appetite and delay hunger.

There are Glycemic Index values for every food out there, including processed and junk foods. Do your homework. The next two pages will help you understand and use the glycemic index to your advantage.

Understanding the Glycemic Index

The GLYCEMIC INDEX (GI) ranks carbohydrates on a scale of 1-100 based on how fast they are converted to sugar (glucose) in the blood. The higher the number, the more quickly blood sugar rises. Insulin is released to collect excess sugar.

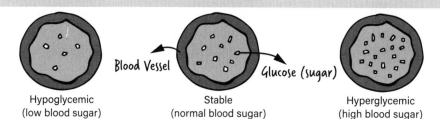

Hypoglycemic (low blood sugar) — Stable (normal blood sugar) — Hyperglycemic (high blood sugar)

BLOOD GLUCOSE is the level of free-floating sugar in the blood. Excess is converted to glycogen in the liver. Small amounts of glycogen can be stored in the muscles. Unlimited amounts can be stored in fat.

HIGH BLOOD SUGAR feels like a bad hangover, with or without the headache.

INABILITY TO CONCENTRATE *LACK OF FOCUS* **SENSE OF HEAVINESS**
WEIGHT GAIN *SLUGGISHNESS* EXCESSIVE HUNGER
LOW ENERGY NO MOTIVATION *LOW LIBIDO*

The GLYCEMIC RESPONSE is dependent on the type and amount of carbohydrate consumed. The more you eat, the higher your blood sugar. The glycemic index accounts for only one serving. Average the GI when combining foods for a (very) rough estimate.

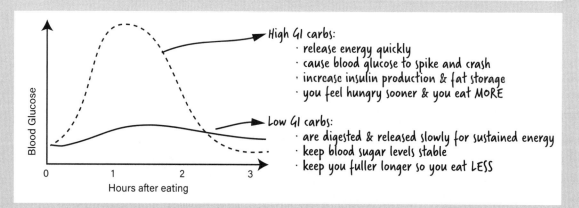

High GI carbs:
- release energy quickly
- cause blood glucose to spike and crash
- increase insulin production & fat storage
- you feel hungry sooner & you eat MORE

Low GI carbs:
- are digested & released slowly for sustained energy
- keep blood sugar levels stable
- keep you fuller longer so you eat LESS

Choose your carbs wisely... Carbs break down into glucose which your body needs to provide fuel to organs, cells, your brain and muscles. Use the chart and tips on the next page and use the Glycemic Index to your benefit.

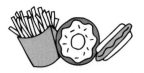 VS.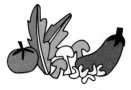

Using the Glycemic Index

Tips for Reducing a Food's Glycemic Index

Reduce Cooking Time: Starches and grains cooked at high temperatures are easier to digest and get into the bloodstream faster.

Reduce Cooking Temperature: Heat breaks down grains and starches. Cooking at high temperatures increases the GI by making carbohydrates easier to digest.

Avoid Over-Processing: Juicing removes fiber. Mashing breaks down starches. Removing the outer hull and bran from grains and rice also removes the fiber, vitamins and minerals.

Combine with Other Foods: Adding oil or other fat, and pairing with high fiber and protein-rich foods will slow the digestion and absorption of carbohydrates.

Vary Preparation Techniques: Boil versus bake potatoes and cook pasta al dente.

The Glycemic Index of some Common Foods

LOW GI (<50)	MEDIUM GI (50-69)	HIGH GI (70-100)
Prunes and dried apricots (29)	Apricots and kiwis (58)	Watermelon (72)
Apples and pears (39)	Raisins (56)	Pumpkin (75)
Oranges, peaches, and strawberries (≈41)	Figs (61)	Dates (103)
	Bananas and grapes (≈60)	
	Pineapple and cantaloupe (≈65)	Short-grain white rice (72)
Broccoli, cabbage, lettuce, cucumbers, mushroom, onions, spinach, asparagus, tomato, and red peppers (10)		Instant rice (87)
	Green peas (51)	Baked sweet potato (94)
	Yam (54)	Baked potato (111)
	Corn (60)	Boiled potato (82)
Carrots (35)	Beets (64)	
Boiled sweet potato (46)		Whole wheat bread (71)
	White spaghetti boiled 20 min (58)	White bread (71)
Fettuccini (32)	Udon noodles (54)	Bagel (72)
Ezekial Bread (35)	Couscous (65)	French baguette (95)
Multi-grain bread (45)	Brown rice (51)	Parmesan cheese pizza (80)
Al dente spaghetti (46)	Long-grain white rice (56)	Cheerios (72)
Steel-cut oats (46)	Quinoa (53)	Corn Flakes (83)
	Rolled oats (55)	Waffle (109)
Almonds, pecans, and walnuts (0)	Sour dough bread (52)	Instant oatmeal (83)
Peanuts (7)	Whole grain bread (53)	
Cashews (27)	Pumpernickel bread (56)	Popcorn (72)
Hummus (6)	Corn tortilla (52)	Pretzels (83)
Soy beans (15)		Average cookie (114)
Pearled barley (28)	Honey (61)	Graham crackers (77)
Kidney beans and lentils (≈29)	Table sugar (65)	Gatorade (78)
Black beans (30)		
	Potato chips (51)	
Corn chips (42)	Snickers (51)	
Peanut M&Ms (33)		
Tomato juice (38)	Orange juice (50)	
	Cranberry juice (68)	

Don't go hungry! You don't have to cut carbs, just make simple swaps from HIGH GI foods to LOW GI foods.

ColleenKachmann.com/members

The Reality of Food Addiction

A Calorie is Not a Calorie

Despite what the United States Department of Agriculture (USDA), clinical dietitians and Weight Watchers drill into our heads, a calorie is not a calorie. Different foods trigger different responses in the brain, blood, digestive tract and immune system. We know the truth because we experience it. Mountain Dew is a pick-me-up. Thanksgiving turkey puts everyone to sleep. Sugar-highs are not just for kindergarteners and the lethargy of a sugar coma can be reversed with more sugar.

Ask any small child if a 180-calorie pack of M&M'S is as healthy as 180 calories of vegetables. Hmm. They'll ponder and search for the answer that will reward them with a "treat." They crave the brightly colored rainbow of sugar-filled morsels.

We experience pleasure when we eat foods that spike our blood sugar. Sugar goes straight to the brain. We feel good after we get a hit but deprived once it fades. This is why we have cravings, eat more than we should, and go back to the store for more.

Occasionally I hit a wall and reach for the promise of energy in a can. I know better, but I am human. Maybe it works one day, so I have another the next. Or two. But soon enough, I feel like crap and remember that Red Bull is the problem, not the solution. I might spend a few hours battling the cravings but it's pain well spent. Water, rest and reducing the stress that sends me in search of a pick-me-up will restore balance to my mind and body.

Recovery Rewards

You can heal your body of food addictions without going to rehab or completing a 12-step program. Unfortunately, you cannot reduce your sugar intake by replacing it with artificial sweeteners. Fake sugars are even worse than real sugars. Sugar substitutes are not the answer they are advertised to be.

Diet drinks and low calorie substitutes work *against* your body's ability to lose weight. Fat cells store the toxins contained in these products, which helps to protect us from their harmful effects. Fat-free foods should be properly labeled as free-fat foods. (I'll explain why in the next chapter.) To lose weight, fat must be used for energy. As toxins in the fat cells are released back into the bloodstream, sugar cravings increase and immunity is reduced. Learn the facts so you can make an informed decision. Feel free to sip on a Diet Mountain Dew while you read. It may be the last one you ever drink.

A Healthy Perspective on Normal

Enhanced Water Improves Life: Radioactive drinks were marketed to the public in the early 1900s. They improved vitality. Also, they hastened death. This epic fail was a sad day for health seekers (and providers). Next, manufacturers tried using cocaine as an additive. Everyone felt great again. The euphoria was problematic and thus short-lived. But the demand was clear and lucrative. Cocaine was replaced by sugar and caffeine. One hundred years later, high rates of obesity, diabetes and high blood pressure call for yet another adjustment. These days, "healthy" people are embracing vitamin water. A normal bottle includes 33 grams of sugar.

Bloodletting Cures All: Bloodletting was the standard treatment for many conditions. It was believed that purging the blood eliminated the toxins that caused disease. Doctors felt that any treatment was better than no treatment, if only for the placebo effect. Bloodletting was at the forefront of healthcare for nearly 3,000 years. These days, normal people embrace modern remedies that scientists have proven as "healthy."

Tapeworms Make You Skinny: Tapeworms are parasites that feed on the same foods we eat. What better way to lose weight than to outsource digestion? It makes perfect sense. Unfortunate side effects include vitamin deficiencies, constipation and diarrhea, not to mention migration to other areas of the body, including the brain. These days, normal dieters have "healthy" alternatives like bariatric surgery.

Lobotomies Restore Mental Health: Lobotomies were a mainstream procedure in the United States for over twenty years, despite recognition of frequent and serious side effects (catatonia and death). But treating mental illness has always been controversial. Highly educated and informed people can look at the same symptoms and form vastly different conclusions. Luckily, the introduction of antipsychotic medications in the 1950s demoted the lobotomy from medical science to historical peculiarities. These days, pills provide "healthy" treatment options for people that aren't normal.

Slavery is Ethical: Only 150 years ago, it was normal for black people to be slaves. White people who "owned" black people were considered smart businessmen. The health of the Southern economy depended on the slavery of human beings. These days, "healthy" economies depend on the addictions of normal people.

Healthy people would be wise to challenge "normal" every time and every place they encounter it.

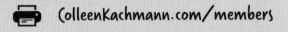
ColleenKachmann.com/members

Normal vs Healthy

List the foods that you love to eat but wish you didn't. How long are you happy after you eat them? At what point do you feel regret? What does this tell you about these foods?

When you eat, regardless of what you choose, observe how you feel. Evaluate from both a physical and emotional perspective. Compare sensations of pleasure before, during, and for several hours after, you eat.

What food habits do you have that qualify as normal but not healthy?

You don't have to eat less. You have to eat right. Plan regular meals and snacks that will nourish your body and reduce cravings.

ColleenKachmann.com/members

LIFE OFF THE LABEL

PS I left this facing page blank for you.
Fill it with whatever you like. Questions, comments, to-do's, thoughts, etc.
You're welcome . . .

CHAPTER 3

FOOD IMPOSTERS AND FREE-FAT CALORIES

"Honesty is, for the most part, less profitable than dishonesty."

PLATO (428-348 BC)

ARTIFICIAL SWEETENERS MAKE YOU FAT

If the fake sugars available on the market actually delivered on the zero-calorie promise, the diet industry would be out of business. According to a fourteen-year study of over 66,000 women, drinking just 20 ounces of diet soda a week increases the risk of diabetes by a whopping 66 percent. Those who drink diet sodas consume twice the amount of those that drink regular.[1] Sugar substitutes are even more addictive than sugar despite assumptions that zero-calories have zero-effect on the body.

Artificial sweeteners stimulate appetite and increase cravings for carbs. Taste buds alert the brain there is sugar (energy) on the way. When the sugar is not delivered, hormones signal for more. A study that followed 5,000 adults for seven years found diet soda drinkers were more likely to become obese. The more diet soda they drank, the greater their weight gain.[2]

Remember this 1980s jingle? Sing along...

Great Pepsi Taste.
But Diet Pepsi won't go to your waist.
Oh Diet Pepsi, just one calorie.
Now you see it, now you don't!

Great song. Amazing promise. Complete lie.

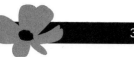

In the mid-eighties, reduced calorie, low-fat, lite and fat-free versions became standard offerings and a necessary compromise for anyone conscious of their weight. We were told we could have our cake and eat it too—and wash it down with a soda pop. Sugar alcohols, saccharin, aspartame and other artificial sweeteners replaced the evil originals. Skinny was guaranteed to those smart enough to buy diet products.

Awesome. I want a refund.

Diet to Insanity

As a teenager, I read the magazines, watched the commercials and bought into the concept of "dieting." My strategy was to drink Diet Coke and trade regular sour cream for the nasty fat-free version. It was the price of being thin and vanity trumped my taste buds.

I still drank too much beer in college and thought Outback Steakhouse's Bloomin' Onion™ qualified as a vegetable. I countered these rookie errors with exercise, which allowed me to keep shopping in the juniors department. Still, there was an obvious conspiracy by Levi's to ensure jeans shrank in summer storage. Refusing to buy a larger size, I'd up my intake of Diet Coke and starve myself until Christmas.

As food companies cashed in on their promise that diet products were the key to super-model skinny, consumer demand exploded. The War on Fat was next in the battle of the bulge.

With the introduction of Olestra, potato chips were put back on the low-calorie menu. Best. Day. Ever! Thanks Pringles! Advances in science made the jingle "*Once you pop you just can't stop!*" an invitation instead of a threat.

But the fat-substitute Olestra developed a crappy reputation due to the unfortunate side effects of diarrhea and headaches. The next solution was a fat-blocker. This time the manufacturers were upfront about the side effects of the product named Ally: "May cause anal seepage."

Undaunted, I dropped $60 on a bottle of these little pills and bought panty liners. I swallowed the miracle appetizers and ordered a pizza. The greasy orange discharge was problematic, but the trade-off was acceptable. I stocked up on this latest drug in case some weakling couldn't manage their end of the bargain and complained to the Federal Drug Administration. A wise decision given the lesson I'd learned after they banned ephedrine for use in appetite suppressants. You may remember ephedrine; it killed a few people.

It's quite a letdown to finally find something that works only to lose it when haters over-emphasize the negative side effects. I imagine this must be how my parent's generation felt when smoking was considered cooler than eating, only to have the government disagree. A few people got lung cancer and suddenly there were "no smoking" signs on the plane. Even worse, those that quit gained weight.

Speaking of smoking, I was 15 when I asked my mom to buy me a pack. I had read in Glamour that cigarettes raise metabolism by 25 percent. The article warned that the healthy choice to quit might have the unfortunate side effect of weight gain. Consequently, I didn't want to quit . . . I wanted to start! I told my mom I'd be happy to smoke outside. She rolled her eyes. Evidently, this was the stupidest thing she'd ever heard. She shared my desire to be thin, however. She admonished me for being willing to sacrifice my health for the sake of vanity. But compromised by giving me Slimfast Shakes and free-fat Twizzlers from her secret stash.

Do you see the irony there? She was drinking a chemical meal and eating diet candy to maintain her own figure. My idea wasn't stupid, just behind the times.

I went to college at age 18. I was not an official smoker on surveys or insurance forms. I was, however, a "social smoker." I lit up to burn off the deep fried chicken wings when I didn't feel like running the calories off the hard way. Sometimes I'd bum cigs from the ballerinas who lived in my dorm. They were very thin. Smoke was all they seemed to eat. Plus, I enjoyed their melodramatic feigns of deprivation and educational tips on bulimia. I soon mastered the art of sticking my finger down my throat so I could party with the boys. Only a frat guy can carry a beer gut with confidence.

After college, I cleaned up my act and tried to be healthy in a more natural way. Babies kept me busy. When I learned that breastfeeding burns 500 calories a day, I decided I would pump for the rest of my life. I wanted to keep the big nursing boobs and reap the caloric benefits.

I considered myself a nutritional genius because I knew better than to finish my kids' Happy Meals. I bought snacks for my toddlers that didn't tempt me. I joined a fitness center and worked out for two hours a day. That was the maximum time childcare was available. I was a fitness and parenting genius as well.

I spent so much time at the gym that the owner offered me a job. He sponsored my group exercise and personal training certifications. I was grateful for the opportunity. As a gym employee I not only had to show up, I was required to lead the class whether I felt like it or not. No more back-row shenanigans for me! Another benefit? The 2-hour childcare limit no longer applied.

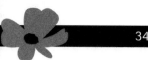

My genius has no boundaries.

Regardless, four pregnancies threatened to expand my mid-thirties mid-section. My search continued for effective strategies to stay ahead of the curves.

I saw the movie *Bounce*. In one scene, Gwyneth Paltrow explains to Ben Affleck that the only reason she is smoking cigarettes is to "get off the gum."

Eureka! My ten-year hiatus from nicotine was over. What a great concept! I immediately adopted an expensive habit of smoking cessation products, self-prescribed for off-label use as metabolic enhancers. I preferred the mints, as the patch was itchy and the gum made my jaws ache (as it had for Paltrow's character). Smoke-free nicotine became my new and improved addiction.

At first my friends rolled their eyes at my silly logic. But the desire to eat more and weigh less tempted several to try it. To the uninitiated, however, nicotine induces vomiting. No one ever wanted a second mint.

Really? You quit before you start because your tummy got upset?
Ha! Amateurs.

Two years later, a routine dental visit exposed the fatal flaw in my unconventional wisdom. After 35 years of bragging rights to a perfect record of no cavities, my dentist announced, "You need four fillings."

We discussed my flossing habits and brand of toothpaste but found nothing. There was no reason at all for this sudden change.

I argued and lamented with the man. "I'm a strict vegan," I pleaded, "I don't eat candy or drink regular soda pop. I eat more vegetables than anyone I know—green ones, lots of them."

But it did no good. The cavities did not disappear. We were both stumped. Then, he brightened.

"Colleen, do you chew sugar-free gum? Artificial sweeteners change the pH balance in a person's saliva."

"No, that's not it either, doctor. I don't chew gum. It gives me a headache. But I do use nicotine mints. Not to quit smoking, just to boost my metabolism. Do you think that could be the problem?"

He stared at me in silence for a long second. I have a talent for astonishing those around me with shocking revelations, but this was exceptional, even for me. As the seconds ticked by, I wondered if, being a fellow fitness fanatic, he was contemplating my ingenuity or my insanity.

The silence ended with a conspiratorial grin. He asked, "Does that work?"

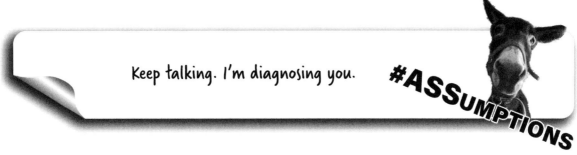

Keep talking. I'm diagnosing you. #ASSUMPTIONS

Ha! I am a genius.

"Heck yeah, doctor. But I can't recommend it now. Evidently, it causes cavities."

It was a sad moment for both of us.

So, I had to give up the mints. Undaunted, I kept searching for the next new trick—whatever it would take to keep those ~~Levi's~~ Rock Revivals from shrinking. Subconsciously programed from early adolescence, I believed outside assistance was necessary to stay thin and look beautiful.

SEGUE TO SANITY

When I decided to go vegan, I went cold tofu. My new diet still contained some processed foods like "not-dogs" and "soy-sauges." But the effects on my body were noticeable, positive and thankfully sustainable. As I continued my journey, I unconsciously let go of those transition products. I did not crave them anymore. As I learned more about the toxic chemicals added to processed foods (vegan or not) I did not *want* them anymore.

I focused on the new foods I wanted to try and let go of self-limiting convictions. The old mantras of "I can't live without cheese," "my body craves meat," and "I don't have time to cook" were replaced with the philosophies and nutritional bonuses of a vegan lifestyle.

I did, however, keep one belief with the tenacity of stubborn 2-year-old who will not relinquish the stolen sucker.

I announced to the world, "The day I give up Diet Coke is the day they pry it out of my cold, dead hands." Not negotiable. Even when *Skinny Bitch* (author Kim Barnouin) explained that Diet Coke is a toxic poison, I did not consider

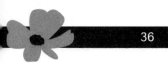

my options. I savored a Diet Coke as I read that acidic soft drinks clean a toilet bowl as well as bleach.

"Whatever, Skinny Bitch." A vice is a vice by definition.

I encourage you to do the same with whatever it is you're not willing to give up (yet). Keep the vices you hold sacred for as long as you need them. Just educate yourself so that the decisions you make are informed. Addiction is a self-imposed prison sentence. Don't fall prey to chemicals disguised as food. I suffered for years with eating disorders and food addictions. I found life-long freedom via short-term withdrawal pains. I'll never relinquish my independence again.

When the whistle was blown on Big Tobacco for using additives to ensure steady sales, the government finally acknowledged that smoking is addictive. Their remedy was to demand labels on the packages to warn people of the health risks.

People who smoke can no longer deny that there are consequences. The "right to smoke" has been defeated by the "right to breathe." It's taken a lot of education and time but freedom demands the right to choose.

Diet sodas are poison. Aspartame breaks down into formaldehyde, which accumulates in the brain. This deadly neurotoxin causes frontal lobe inflammation, migraines, neurological and cognitive problems and increases the risk of cancer. Some airlines prohibit pilots from drinking diet colas because they can cause visual apparitions.[3]

As I ate more veggies and unprocessed foods, chemical flavors lost their appeal. I was finally ready to give up Diet Coke. I poured the rest of my stash into the toilet.

Once you see and feel the benefits of choosing foods that make you healthy, you'll develop an aversion to the food imposters that once made your mouth water. The best strategy for choosing a vice is to give it up until the cravings disappear. This may take a while but stay with it. Small victories will keep you motivated. Soon you will be able to reassess from a place of freedom instead of addiction.

Drop the Pop

If you drink soda, you really don't need to worry about all the other bad stuff you put into your body. Regular consumption of this highly corrosive chemical will ensure declining health and disease. This is the number one action item for improving your health. Repeat after me. Pop is poison. Switch to coffee, tea or non-carbonated natural energy drinks if you are dependent on caffeine. Make the decision, don't make exceptions and you'll be feeling much better in about a week. Use leftover soda to clean your toilet. It's just as corrosive as bleach.

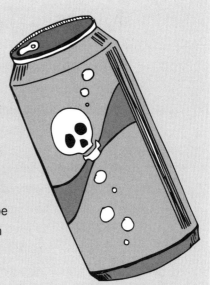

Freedom from Fraud

By declaring myself vegan, I stumbled onto the path of real nourishment and true wellness. My obsessive micromanagement of fat grams and carb-to-protein ratios was no longer possible without package labels to "educate" my brain. As I ate more whole foods, I was able to go for days without the compulsive calorie counts. As my body detoxed, so did my emotional attachment to the concept of dieting.

I have learned a few things from my years of mental and physical self-torture. From this side of 40, I know that if I am hungry when I shouldn't be, something I am eating is working against me. Sweet tooth and carbohydrate cravings are signs of biological addiction to artificial ingredients. The chemicals in processed foods are designed to enhance pleasure and create withdrawal so that we buy more.

Freedom feels great. I no longer berate myself for cravings that I cannot conquer. I don't waste time thinking about what I should or shouldn't eat, how much to eat or when I can eat again. I just eat when I'm hungry. I stop when I'm full. Who knew eating was so simple?

If you are struggling with weight or food issues, it is essential to develop a mind-body-health connection. Shift focus from what you *want* to eat to what you *did* eat and how it made you feel. Addictive foods have a negative impact on both physical and mental wellbeing. You will gain time, energy and vitality when you eat nourishing foods. Feeling awesome is just as addictive as junk food. When you take an off-the-label approach, a better version of you will emerge.

Muffin Tops and Beer Guts

Muffin tops and beer guts come and go throughout life. My first experience with weight gain was the cliché Freshman-15. They really should disclose on the glossy college brochure that the average freshman gains fifteen pounds in the first year.[4] Dorm food, beer and freedom are fun but also fattening.

We've all welcomed the first warm day of spring only to be saddened that last year's shorts are out of style (too tight). We might blame the extra fluff on a long winter and seasonal affective disorder, but happiness leads to over-indulgence too. The love hormones of romance drive us to procreate, eat and repeat as often as possible.

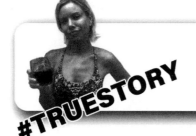

How did we get here? Booze and bad decisions, my friends. That's how we got here.

If biology wins that round we are soon "eating-for-two" and painting the nursery. We worry about unprocessed cheese and listeria on lunchmeat. We are hyper-vigilant and scour labels for the known no-no's. But if French fries dipped in ice cream suppress prenatal nausea, midnight runs to the nearest drive-thru are physician-approved and delivered on-demand.

When expectant parents collectively gain sixty pounds, yet the new bundle of joy accounts for only 7.3, post-partum depression can set in fast. Unfortunately, weight loss is not a common side effect of depression.

Later, when children have stolen all personal time, space and money, eating on-the-go becomes a sacrifice of love. Dads pat their beer guts and moms complain of muffin tops. Yet, everyone cheering from the bench will celebrate either success or failure with a post-game party at Pizza Hut. Because that's where the kids want to go.

Damn kids.

At some point we surrender to a size we'd swore to never wear, and a New Year's resolution is made. Enter the personal trainer.

Exercise professionals are trained to believe that weight loss can only happen if more calories are burned than consumed. They recommend regular protein-rich meals and frequent snacks to keep metabolism running on high. Then they prescribe circuit and interval training to increase muscle mass and burn fat.

This approach leads to short term results that often fade when members cannot pay $60 an hour for motivational sessions. This keeps the fitness industry in business. Members continue to pay for the gym membership because when "things get back to normal" they intend to "get back on track." The problem is that normal doesn't include free weights, stationary bikes and a track.

Well played, fitness industry. Well played.

Why Are We Fat?

"How do I maintain a healthy weight?"

The answer will not be revealed until you ask the question, "Why am I fat?" That's the mystery.

As discussed in Chapter 2, a calorie is not a calorie. A 100-calorie Fun-Sized Snicker is not the same as 100 calories of organic kale. It's a fact that regular consumption of zero-calorie Diet Coke leads to weight gain. Artificial ingredients provoke a far different biological response than micronutrients and antioxidants.

Metabolism cannot be manipulated. The belief that small, frequent meals leads to weight loss because "hunger sends the body into starvation mode" (i.e. fat-storing mode) is out of context.

> "Your life *does not get better* by chance, it gets better by *change*."
>
> Jim Rohn (1930-2009) motivational speaker

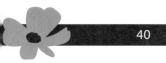

All processed foods have labels—even organic ones. Energy bars, diet drinks and 100-calorie snack packs are keeping you on the hamster wheel of habits that are making you fat. Get off the label. Food without fuel serves no purpose. If you can read the label, you are too close.

Not going anywhere? Put down the Snickers bar.

Hate Exercise? You'll Love This!

Sedentary activities that engage the mind but neglect the body leave us feeling lethargic and fatigued. We revert to shallow chest breathing and even forget to breathe, which is why we yawn.

Deep breathing is a high-quality aerobic exercise that improves circulation, immune response and functions of the lungs and brain. It decreases heart rate, blood pressure, pain and tension. It even promotes weight loss.

Most of us use about 15 percent of our lung capacity as we move throughout our busy day. Inhaling deeply so the abdomen inflates delivers six times more oxygen, stimulates endorphins and promotes emotional wellbeing. It increases metabolism, improves digestion and reduces stress.

Exhaling rids the body of carbon dioxide. High levels foster cancer, infections, hormonal imbalances and fatigue. A complete exhale lifts the diaphragm and creates a vacuum effect that stimulates the flow of lymph through the body. The deeper the breath, the more impact it has on the lymphatic system's detoxification processes.[5]

The next time you can't find the motivation to exercise, give your lungs a workout with three sets of ten. Take breathing breaks throughout the day (set reminders on your phone). It's the only exercise that you won't avoid and may actually tip the scales for motivation to do more.

 ColleenKachmann.com/members

Metabolism Mistakes

Metabolism is not complicated. You are either metabolizing food or you are not. When there is no food to digest, stored fat is the energy source used for tissue repair, building muscle, and generating new cells.

If you are in a constant state of digestion, your body is not building muscle, renewing cells or detoxifying. Increasing time between completing digestion and the next meal is essential to both healing and weight loss.

It's all about balance. Learning to feel what's going on in your body instead of thinking about what you're going to eat next doesn't require willpower. It requires a shift in focus. Doing, eating and go-go-going must be countered with being, feeling and stay-stay-staying. Tune into what you *need* to avoid the things you don't want.

If you are struggling with your weight, stop looking for external interventions. Turn your focus inward. Distinguish between hunger and cravings by *feeling* them instead of thinking about them. Take deep breaths while you assess. Where in your body do the sensations occur? What triggers them? Don't assume the urge to eat is a biological message of survival.

Cravings for sugar and processed carbohydrates are a sign of addiction. The high of the feel-good endorphins precedes a dramatic drop in energy. This leaves you lethargic and hungry again. The next time you eat something you know you shouldn't, take the opportunity to observe this process. Feel the blood sugar spike and subsequent drop. Notice that low blood sugar feels like hunger. But it's not. It's a cycle that will be broken when problem foods are avoided.

When you get an urge to eat, give it a minute. Or twenty. Experience the desire without reacting to it. Put time and space between urge and action. Become aware of the difference between hunger and appetite. Observe how they are alike. Feel how they are different. Continue these observation exercises until you can identify the difference.

Relax. You won't starve.

Drinking water between meals aids in weight loss and detoxification. Shift your focus from the memories of pleasure that provoke the craving to the sensations of need and denial. Observe the back and forth as you struggle to feel instead of think. It takes practice.

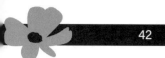

Pretend you are babysitting someone else's body. When your inner child wants a cookie, witness the sensations without participating, judging or reacting. Love yourself enough to comfort your body without harmful foods.

> ## "You don't have to eat *less*, you have to *eat right*."
>
> Author unknown

But she's brilliant.

SUGAR SETBACKS

Processed foods and sweets disrupt the balance in gut flora. Microbes have a reputation for causing disease, but millions of beneficial microbes live in the intestines and are essential to good health. Foods that feed problematic bacteria and fungus disrupt the gut and interfere with bodily functions. Foods that nourish a healthy microbial population in our gut strengthen our immune system and slow the aging process.

Imbalances in gut flora often go undetected and lead to health issues that mimic other illnesses. It is estimated that over 70 percent of Americans have too much Candida in their bodies.[6] (Is it coincidence that 70 percent of us are also overweight?) Candida (yeast) infection, in particular, makes weight loss difficult, if not impossible.

Yeast is a fungus that feeds on sugar. Cravings for sugar intensify when yeast multiply unchecked. The dilemma is a Catch-22. A diet high in sugar perpetuates yeast overgrowth. The overgrowth perpetuates the cravings for sugar. The cycle cannot be broken until yeast populations are balanced.

Yeast occurs naturally in the mouth, skin and intestinal tract. When it gets into the blood stream, however, systemic infection causes inflammation. Yeast creates and releases over 70 different toxins.[7] These toxins disrupt the function of otherwise healthy organs and systems. Symptoms of yeast overgrowth are subtle and difficult to diagnose. It's very confusing to look healthy, yet feel sick.

Vaginal yeast infection and thrush are obvious signs of overgrowth. But hormone imbalance, thyroid problems, reduced liver function and digestive issues lead doctors to treat symptoms that seem unrelated. Yeast overgrowth is the root cause of many chronic diseases.[8] Treating the symptoms and ignoring the cause does not lead to wellness.

Yeast infections compromise nutrient absorption and can lead to malnourishment. This stimulates an autoimmune response, which creates intestinal inflammation. Subsequently, undigested food escapes into the bloodstream, triggering autoimmune reactions such as allergies, arthritis, endometriosis and eczema.

Doctors prescribe anti-fungal medications when yeast gets into the bloodstream. Systemic infections are life threatening to immune-suppressed patients. Yeast mutates easily. Stronger strains withstand the medications and breed further infections. This is why otherwise healthy people should think twice about using anti-fungal medications. The long-term risks of the drugs may outweigh the short-term gains.

Do you have Yeast Overgrowth?

Symptoms include:[9]

- skin and nail fungal infections.
- feeling tired, worn down, chronic fatigue and fibromyalgia.
- digestive issues such as acid reflux, bloating, constipation, and/or diarrhea.
- autoimmune diseases such as Hashimoto's, rheumatoid arthritis, Lupus, psoriasis, scleroderma or multiple sclerosis.
- poor memory and concentration, brain fog, lack of focus, ADD and ADHD.
- skin issues—rashes, hives, psoriasis, and eczema.
- irritability, mood swings, brain fog, anxiety and depression.
- vaginal and urinary tract infection; rectal or vaginal itching.
- seasonal allergies or itchy ears.
- cravings for sugar, alcohol, cheese, bread, pickles and refined carbohydrates.

ColleenKachmann.com/members

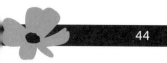

The most effective way to counteract yeast overgrowth is to starve it. Fill up on nutrient-dense whole foods. Eliminate sugar, alcohol, processed and high glycemic foods. Remember that artificial sugars increase the cravings and toxic load on your body. Don't be tempted to use them as a substitute. If you need something sweet, eat a piece of fruit. Fermented foods, cultured vegetables and yeast-inhibiting probiotics promote beneficial microbes that compete with yeast's food supply. Natural healing takes time—up to six months. But self-sustaining wellness requires a balanced gut flora. Allow your cravings for life to free you from cravings for sugar. Take it one day at a time and celebrate each improvement. Enjoy the journey.

Think Less. Feel More. Become Aware.

The *only* way to become fat is to eat foods of little to no nutritional value. Unnecessary weight gain is not a side effect in any stage of life. Being overweight is a symptom of being undernourished. Processed foods do not provide the living enzymes and antioxidants we need to thrive. They do, however, pollute the body with artificial toxins that are subsequently stored in fat cells.

People look at my diet and the evolution of my lifestyle over the past seven years and shake their heads. "You must be so disciplined!" they say.

It doesn't take discipline to feel good. It takes desire.

Oh, and detox. Detoxifying the body of poisons consumed in ignorance and addiction is the key. You read it here first: Detox is the new rehab.

The reward for cleaning out the body is freedom from fat, frumpiness and internal food fights. When detox is complete, the only discipline you'll need is to not go ballistic when someone offers you—or worse, your children—a poisonous treat wrapped in plastic. They might look offended when you politely decline but keep smiling.

You'll need to get comfortable with being uncomfortable. Welcome to my life.

There is only one way to lose weight and feel better. You must accept the short-term discomfort that leads to long-term health. So breathe. Relax. Have empathy for your body when it's suffering. Give it what it needs. The only person that can bring wellness to your life is you.

LIFE OFF THE LABEL

Win the Hunger Games

When you find yourself heading for the snacks or feeling tempted by a drive thru, interrupt your impulse with awareness.

Neurological science has discovered that impulses are electrical. The more a circuit pathway is used in our brain, the more unconscious it becomes. Thought patterns and behaviors that are repeated become habitual. Just like a reflex, we react to pictures, sounds, smells, emotions and even memories without realizing there are other options. When we see, hear, smell, or feel something that triggers a craving, our behavior is predictable. The cycle can only be interrupted with awareness.

Identifying triggers that stimulate appetite is easy. Food can make us feel good, especially when we are eating with others. Food brings us comfort; it gives us a high. Commercials for pizza and the mouth-watering smells of smoking meat are designed to make us hungry. But appetite is psychological. Advertisements and roadside barbeque's dramatically improve sales by appealing to emotional memory.

Hunger for nourishment does not lead to self-defeating eating habits. Compulsive eating happens in response to social pressure, the desire to feel good and images and smells that trigger pleasant memories. If past experiences with a certain food have been pleasurable, then temptation can feel overwhelming. You can counter that Pavlovian response by removing yourself from the temptation or, at the very least, focusing your attention on something else.

Resistance is hard. But is it actually painful? Take a few minutes to find out. You must believe that you have the power to say "yes" to wellness in order to exercise the freedom to say "no" to illness.

Shift your awareness from the mental agitation in your mind to your physical body. Locate the sensation of the craving. Where do you feel it? On a scale of one to ten, how much intensity does it create? What kind? How long does it last?

Do you have the ability to say, "No?" If not, doesn't that kind of piss you off? Why must you fight for control over your own body? Reclaim your power. The cravings will disappear after you stop eating the poisons that generate them.

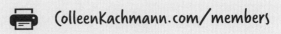 ColleenKachmann.com/members

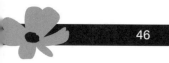

Juicing: Pure Power

A few years ago, I was pressured into doing a shot of wheatgrass at my yoga studio. The viscous milk-of-mulch goes down like pungent muck. It can repulse even extreme health nuts. A yogi bullied me into trying this "nectar of the gods." I bravely took the challenge, contorting my face with a suppressed gag. She offered condolences with a humble, "Namaste."

"Nope. That was nama-nasty," I retorted.

Regardless of the health benefits, wheatgrass tastes like grass. And wheat. I didn't want to try it again. But when I watched the documentary *Fat, Sick and Nearly Dead*, I saw how a 60-day juice fast prevented death and restored a man's life. Juicing greens and other produce removes the fiber. This delivers a concentrated shot of micronutrients directly to the bloodstream, and allows the digestive tract to rest.

The documentary did a fantastic job detailing the profound rewards of juicing. Still, I hesitated. My digestive system doesn't get "tired" very often. Actually it prefers to eat food several times a day. And the taste of wheatgrass is not easy to forget. I begrudgingly bought a juicer and stashed it on the floor of my pantry. It remained, unopened, for three months.

One day, I woke up with a tickle in my throat. A case of impending doom threatened to take me down. The words "concentrated shot of micronutrients" cut through the fog of congestion that had already ruined my appetite.

I raced to the pantry in search of a miracle. I opened the box and put the appliance together. Well, not on the first try. I didn't read the directions. Step one for me is always, "how hard can this be?" Twenty minutes later, the green snot pouring out of my nose matched the colorful language spewing from my mouth.

With my throat swelling, I raided my refrigerator for every piece of produce I could find. Kale, carrots, spinach and an apple juiced into about a cup of hope. I couldn't smell so I couldn't taste. I would not have cared. It was medicine. I drank every last drop, licked the sides of the glass and crawled up the stairs to my bed.

Three hours later I walked back into the kitchen and was confused by what appeared to be a crime scene. A huge knife lay in the middle of the floor surrounded by gouged cardboard and plastic. The brand new juicer was covered in sticky green blood. Shredded and pulpous produce littered the counters. But when I remembered that the guilty party had been panicked and sick, I happily cleaned up on her behalf.

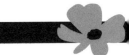

> *Take care* of the Body.
> It's the ONLY place
> you have to *live.*
>
> Jim Rohn (1930-2009) motivational speaker

THE MISSING INGREDIENTS

Chapter 4 will cover the effects of various chemical ingredients on the body. But the *missing* ingredients in fake food are equally important. To produce a food with a stable shelf life, certain changes must take place. The tempting flavors, colors and natural aromas of real food attract mold and bacteria. Thus, manufacturers remove them—almost all of them. This refining process leaves the food nutritionally worthless (pick a snack, any snack) and unappetizing. The final stage of the process is to add artificial ingredients. These entice human taste buds and repulse the microbes that spoil the fun.

Our bodies need what are called *macronutrients*: protein, fat and carbohydrates. But *micronutrients* are just as crucial. Micronutrients are the vitamins and minerals in real food, producing the flavors, colors and aromas that entice you to eat them. They are vital to the healthy functioning of all the body's systems, from bone growth to brain function. They don't just strengthen the immune system; they are the immune system.

This is why the majority of Americans are overweight yet undernourished. Processed foods contain protein, carbohydrates and fat. But artificial ingredients that replace micronutrients 1) burden the body with toxins 2) deprive the body of tools that aid in digestion and 3) compromise the immune system.

It's like buying a cheap desk. The oak veneer looks like wood, but polish can't restore it from wear and tear. The weak metal framing inevitably bends and screws come loose as threads crumble. The desk looks great when it's new. But the more it's used, the quicker it falls apart. This analogy shows why it seems that kids can eat about anything. Their bodies are new. But keep feeding them low quality junk food and their health will deteriorate in time.

In the old days, if you wanted a desk, you found an ax and built it yourself. If

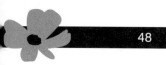

you expected to eat, you planted a garden or grabbed a gun and went hunting. Creating something of lasting quality required an investment. Now, we rely on corporations to tell us what we need and how to use what we buy. We read the labels, expect instant gratification and believe that satisfaction can be guaranteed.

The function of food is not simply to gratify. Its essential purpose is to deliver nutrients that fuel the body. The following is a glossary of the basic requirements.

There are three types of **macronutrients**:

- **Proteins** are made up of amino acids. They are the building blocks for muscle and cell structures. Enzymes that catalyze thousands of chemical reactions are proteins. Antibodies that bind to foreign particles like viruses and bacteria are proteins. Proteins "read" our DNA, transport hormones and allow the body to move.
- **Fat** cushions and insulates the skeleton. Fat provides the "skin" for every cell membrane. (Oil doesn't mix with water; without fat, structures in our body would simply dissolve.) Fats sheathe nerve cells, synthesize hormones and absorb fat-soluble nutrients. Our brain is more than 60 percent fat.
- **Carbohydrates** are classified as simple or complex. Sugars and starches are simple carbohydrates that cells use for energy. Complex carbohydrates push food through the digestive system. Fiber keeps the intestines and colon clean and healthy.

Micronutrients are the molecular tools required in millions of anatomical processes. They catalyze reactions and support the repair of DNA and cellular structures. The aging process slows when the body has what it needs to function. The body cannot make its own micronutrients. They must be obtained from food.

Antioxidant is an umbrella term that can be used to describe any and all of the vitamins, minerals and phytochemicals (living nutrients from plants). The word *antioxidant* indicates the ability to neutralize free radicals. **Free radicals** are electrically unstable molecules generated from pollution, radiation and processed foods. Think of them as little fireballs. Antioxidants extinguish their flame and protect cell structures from damage. More information about antioxidants and free radicals can be found in Chapter 12.

Vitamins participate in every bodily process. For example, the eyes need vitamin A to produce the retinal that allows us to see light. Bone, muscle and connective tissues (tendons, ligaments and skin) need vitamin C to form collagen.

Vitamins are fragile and break down easily in heat, air and acid. This is why:

- vegetables and fruits begin to lose nutrient value the moment they are picked.
- microwaves and cooking with high heat reduce nutritional value.
- acidic, artificial foods and drinks interfere with the absorption of vitamins.

There are 13 vitamins. Vitamins A, D, E and K are fat-soluble (which is why fortified skim milk can't deliver as promised). Vitamin C and the B vitamins are water-soluble.

Minerals are the inorganic elements. Muscles need potassium, sodium, and chlorine (referred to as **electrolytes**) to contract. Calcium, phosphorus and magnesium form bone, cartilage and teeth. Trace minerals such as iron, cobalt, copper, zinc, manganese and selenium are essential for nutrient transport and enzyme formation throughout the body.

Phytonutrients are found only in plants (and fungi such as mushrooms). These active chemicals neutralize free radicals and support health in many ways. They are classified by color and function. *Carotenoids* are orange and red in color. They promote eye health, digestive function and blood flow. *Flavonoids* are yellow, red and purple. They inhibit inflammation, viruses and cancer. *Lignins* are fibrous. They help to keep cholesterol levels low by inhibiting the formation of arterial plaque, and disrupt the growth of hormonal cancers.

Bacteria outnumber human cells in the body by ten to one. Bacteria known as *gut flora* or *microflora* provide key support to the digestive and immune systems. Consuming and maintaining the "good' bacteria to boost population and ensure they out-number harmful bacteria.

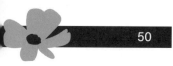

Cashew Cream Sauce

Cashews can be transformed into creamy Alfredo sauce, ranch dressing and even cheesecake. They are essential in the "real" food budget. There are 5 lb. bags of organic, raw cashews available on Amazon at less than half the cost of the grocery store. They freeze well and are cheapest when purchased in bulk.

Soak raw cashews for four to eight hours and rinse well. Water activates the sprouting enzymes, maximizes nutritional benefits and removes the bitter flavor. Divide into one-cup portions and freeze.

Put one cup of thawed cashews in a blender. Add enough water to cover the cashews. The amount of water determines the consistency. Use less (or none) if you want a thick paste similar to ricotta cheese. Use more for salad dressings and cream sauces.

Blend on high. A high-powered machine gives the best results. Add about ½ cup yeast flakes (more for a cheesy pungent tang) a dash of ground mustard, a splash of apple cider vinegar and ¼ packet of organic ranch seasoning. A bit of garlic salt will create a simple Alfredo that goes great over pasta and/or sautéed vegetables. Add Italian, Mexican or Asian spices to further enhance flavor. A packet of organic ranch seasoning with a dash of cumin makes the perfect Southwest cream sauce.

For a delicious, all veggie meal, serve over spaghetti squash in lieu of pasta. Be careful not to overcook the squash. The fibrous strands are a great substitute for al dente pasta.

 ColleenKachmann.com/members

Low to No-Calorie Sweet Tooth Solutions

Buy a stevia plant for your garden or purchase pure dried leaves online and grind them into powder. When purchasing products already sweetened with stevia, look for "whole leaf stevia."

Steer clear of processed products that list stevia extract, rebaudioside and other ingredients. These are manufactured from chemicals like acetone and isopropanol in brands like "Stevia in the Raw" and Truvia. And the first ingredient listed in those brands is not stevia, but rather GMO-corn based dextrose and erythritol.

Got Vodka?

To make your own liquid stevia extract, dry one cup of stevia leaves in the sun for 12 hours. Place dried leaves in a glass jar and cover with vodka. Allow the mixture to steep for 24 hours. Use a strainer to filter out the leaves. Heat the extract for 20 minutes on low (do not boil). Store in the refrigerator for up to 90 days.

Sugar alcohols (ethyritol, xylitol, mannitol, sorbitol) occur naturally in plants. Despite the name, they contain neither sugar nor alcohol. Some have antioxidant and antibacterial properties. Sugar alcohols are sweet, yet they don't affect blood sugar or insulin levels. They are not as sweet as other low-calorie options. Avoid them when they are used in combination with artificial sugars.

Sugar alcohols are not completely absorbed by the body, and can upset the digestive system. Symptoms of gas, bloating and diarrhea are usually dose related and vary from person to person. Ethyritol and xylitol are better tolerated, while mannitol and sorbitol sometimes carry warning labels that "excess consumption may have a laxative effect." Sugar alcohols are safe if you can tolerate them. Consume them in small quantities and listen to your body.

 ColleenKachmann.com/members

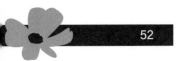

Normal vs Healthy

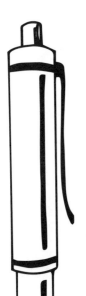

When and where do you consume processed foods? Why?

Don't think about hunger, feel it. Can you identify the triggers (other than hunger) that stimulate your appetite? How will you change your response?

How do you manage your intake of macronutrients? Has decreasing (or increasing) ratios of protein, carbohydrates and fat improved your health?

There is no need to restrict calories when you maximize consumption of real food. Calories and grams of protein, sugar and fat are of no concern when you eat foods that have no labels. Obsessive micromanagement of foods will fade and make time for new pleasures. How will you make use of the extra space in your life?

 ColleenKachmann.com/members

PS I left this facing page blank for you.
Fill it with whatever you like. Questions, comments, to-do's, thoughts, etc.
You're welcome . . .

CHAPTER 4

A CULTURE OF CHEMICALS

"Drive-thrus kill more people than drive-bys."

Ron Findley, Guerrilla gardener in South Central, Los Angeles

Fake Food. Real Disease.

Something is wrong in our modern world. Our children are just as sick as our parents. Despite all the money and research devoted to prevention, treatment, pharmaceuticals and education, rates of disease are increasing exponentially.

Packaged food-like widgets are produced on assembly lines fueled by profit. These branded flavors stimulate the economy just as much as they do your taste buds. Food that comes in a package is not food.

Even if you are not overweight, processed foods are a roller coaster ride to poor health: Hormonal imbalances, irritable bowel, acid reflux, headaches, brain fog, depression and emotional distress, just to name a few. Artificial foods cause inflammation, which is widely considered the root of all disease.

If you use fake foods and beverages to manage your mood and energy levels, you are not as healthy as you could be. Furthermore, unless you live off the grid, your children are also being given foods that will make a hot mess of their health—if they aren't already suffering.

Today's cure is tomorrow's scam. I'm not a doctor (though I do own a pair of scrubs and a blood pressure cuff), but it doesn't take a medical degree to see the difference between profit-generating, pseudo-scientific claims and legitimate research. If a study doubles as a sales pitch, it's biased.

A Culture of Chemicals

THE STATISTICS OF SYMPTOMS

When I started my website in 2010, the dramatic increase of diseases in the last two decades was alarming.

Houston, we have a problem.

When I began the grueling task of citing statistics for this book, I was horrified to discover how much worse things were five years later.

Houston, we're on fire!

Consider:

- Asthma rates have increased over 50 percent since 2001.[1] One in nine children[2] and one in eight adults have asthma.[3]
- Attention Deficit Hyperactivity Disorder (ADHD) has increased 21.8 percent in just four years![4]
- Autism rates of children under eight years have increased by 124 percent since 2000.[5]
- Food allergies have increased 18 percent in the last ten years.[6]
- Celiac disease has increased over 400 percent. Inflammatory bowel disease (IBD) has increased almost 5,000 percent in the last 50 years.[7]

#ASSUMPTIONS

Sicktistics: The science that proves being told you're one in a million isn't ALWAYS a compliment.

Most of us suspect our environment plays a significant role in these trends. As good people, we cheer environmental ideals for a cleaner planet. We support anti-pollution campaigns and stricter quality standards for our air, water and soil. We recycle when it's convenient. Some of us bicycle to work and use public transportation. Because that's good for the environment. Yet we fail to understand that every time we eat, we cast a vote with our dollars in support for or against the corporations polluting our internal and external world.

One in three kids born after 2000 will develop diabetes by adulthood.[8] We must intervene for their sake, if not our own. Even if everyone in your household has a government approved BMI (Body Mass Index), the threshold of toxicity will be crossed at some point. A thin frame is no guarantee of wellness. There is no free pass when it comes to eating processed foods.

The body has two ways of defending itself against the onslaught of the unnatural substances we ingest. One is to produce mucus to buffer the chemicals, which is why so many of us suffer from chronic congestion. The other is to encapsulate unprocessed toxins and store them long-term. Many chemicals are lipophilic, meaning they dissolve in oil but not water. Thus, they are stored in fat cells. Fat protects us from the harmful substances that would otherwise do damage. Continuing to ingest unnatural substances keeps the body in a constant state of defense.

It is extremely difficult to lose weight if your diet includes artificial ingredients. Fat cells store all of the trash that accumulates in the body. When fat is used as fuel, toxins are released back into the blood stream. Weight loss triggers detoxification. As fat reserves dissolve, you'll feel tired and get sick easier. It doesn't feel good (until it's over). Dieters who aren't prepared for this fall back on addictive foods in attempt to feel normal again. This stops the detox (and weight loss) process. Processed foods spike blood sugar and stimulate insulin production. Insulin is a fat-storing hormone. This is why most people who try to lose weight using fake foods end up heavier a year later.[9]

Most of us do not worry about the long lists of artificial ingredients we see on labels. We assume rigorous studies have proven the products we buy are safe. Nothing could be further from the truth. In fact, no studies are done on any product.

The controversial findings that make headlines are of studies that isolate single additives. The approach is severely flawed. Single-variable, double-blind studies investigate only one chemical at a time. We need studies that measure the *synergistic effects* of all the artificial ingredients as they are combined.

Think about it. Vinegar is a mild acid. Baking soda is fairly inert. But mix the two together and there is a volcanic eruption worthy of a science fair award. Add bright red food coloring and you get permanently stained carpet.

Chemicals react when they are mixed together. The results are not always predictable or desirable. The FDA has approved over 3,000 chemicals for use in our food supply.[10] Add pharmaceuticals, household goods and environmental contaminates to the mix and the potential for the unknown is infinite.

What are the effects of living in a toxic soup? Look around and observe for yourself. In the meantime, let's look at the more problematic ingredients. We'll start with the shot of controversy.

A CULTURE OF CHEMICALS

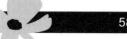

8 Tips for Surviving Detox

1. Take a probiotic supplement and include fermented foods like sauerkraut in your diet.
2. Eat sulfur-rich foods like garlic, onions, and cruciferous vegetables like broccoli, kale, collards, cabbage, cauliflower and watercress.
3. Take a supplement that provides liver and kidney support such as L-glutamine, N-acetyl-cysteine, Alpha lipoic acid or SamE.
4. Take a multi-vitamin that includes selenium, vitamins C, E, B_{12}, B_6, and folate (not the same as folic acid, the synthetic version added to fortified foods.) Folic acid is safe, though excessive amounts can be harmful to the malnourished.[11]
5. Eat fresh, detoxifying herbs like cilantro, parsley, dandelion greens, turmeric, and ginger.
6. Drink green tea. Add a lemon to maximize the absorption of antioxidants three to five times over.[12] Look for detox formulas that contain chamomile, milk thistle, stinging nettle and/or fenugreek.
7. Juice greens and vegetables like cucumbers, celery, beets, carrots, wheatgrass and fennel. Consume on an empty stomach for immediate absorption.
8. Use calcium bentonite clay. It can be dissolved in water to drink or made into a paste and applied externally to dark under-eye circles and skin irritations. (See Detox with Bentonite Clay in on page 281.)

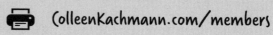

ColleenKachmann.com/members

The Vaccine Against Social Suicide

Never discuss religion or politics at a party unless you're at church or Campaign Headquarters. Or vaccines. Do. Not. Ever. Debate. Vaccines. Discussions are polarized. It appears to be a life or death decision. Anti-vaccine opinions are labeled as pro-plague. As we all know that guns don't kill people, people kill people, attempts to discuss the 50 shades of gray on this issue are immediate social suicide.

In truth, vaccines are not all good or all bad. They are not a simple concept that can be supported or rejected as a group. They are drugs, much like antibiotics, steroids and pain-relievers. Every drug has a unique set of risks and benefits. There are no sides to take, only possibilities to consider. Each vaccine has the potential to help and to harm. Individual reactions cannot be predicted, only observed after the fact.

Here are some basic facts to consider:

- The smallpox vaccine eliminated that fatal disease. The polio vaccine appears to be the second global success. Other vaccines have drastically cut many diseases that once killed or disabled millions of people. Diphtheria, hepatitis A, rubella, and tetanus, to name but a few.
- In 1950, the United States administered thirteen doses of four vaccines before the age of two, and never more than three per visit.[13] Today, children receive 37 doses of 14 vaccines by the age of two and as many as eight in a single visit.[14] That's 52 doses in 1950 compared to 518 doses today, a tenfold increase.

NOTE: To be fair, improvements in design have reduced the total number of potentially harmful ingredients per vaccine. But that's still a 900% increase in dosages per child.[15]

- Vaccines contain controversial ingredients. Mercury (thimerosal) and aluminum are used as preservatives. Both are neurotoxins. DNA from multiple species is spliced into bacterial strains and viruses to weaken them. Injection triggers an autoimmune response. The purpose is to create immunity in future exposures, but effectiveness varies as influencing factors lead to complications.
- Currently there is no evidence of a *direct* correlation between vaccines and the rampant rise in autoimmune disorders.
- Vaccines are Big Money. The flu vaccine alone generates $10-$15 billion per year. In 2015, total revenues for the global vaccine market are projected to reach $41 billion.[16]
- There are documented cases of bad outcomes. It is acknowledged that vaccines are not perfectly safe or equally effective. Studies show a percentage of people will be injured as a result. Because all 50 states legally require several vaccinations prior to entering kindergarten, the National Vaccine Injury Compensation Program was established in 1986 to compensate those who suffer adverse side effects.[17]

Vaccine protocols issued by the CDC (Centers for Disease Control) are largely the result of lobbying efforts by pharmaceutical companies. As there are 145 new vaccines in development,[18] the number of recommendations will increase. Health campaigns and public service announcements advertise the serious threats of disease. Pharmaceutical sales soar in response.

Big Pharma spent $41 million dollars on advertisements between January and September of 2009.[19] That's quite the marketing budget. But as vaccine revenues totaled $23 billion that year,[20] the campaigns are a strategic investment.

> "An opinion based on incomplete or *inaccurate information* should be used for *entertainment purposes only.*"
>
> Colleen Kachmann, author of *Life off the Label*

THE PENIS PREDICAMENT

When I took my oldest son for his 9th grade back-to-school sports physical, I got an unsolicited lecture from the pediatrician. His tirade about the harmful effects of a vegan diet on a young man's growth didn't last long. Once he realized I had an educated response for each of his uneducated concerns, he quickly changed the subject.

The doctor said, "Everything looks good. So the only two shots he needs today are the rotavirus and Gardasil."

I was confused. "Why? Isn't Gardasil to prevent the human papillomavirus from causing cervical cancer?"

"Yes," said the doctor.

"But he's a 13-year-old boy. He doesn't have a cervix."

"Right. Just think of it as a gift to his future wife," was the coached response.

I dismissed this with sarcasm. "I'd prefer the traditional approach where they register for gifts at Williams and Sonoma. So, no, thanks. And why do we need the rotavirus vaccine?"

"It's just a stomach bug. Worst case scenario is diarrhea and feeling bad for a few days."

"Ok, and what are the side effects of the vaccine?" I asked.

"Worst case scenario is diarrhea and feeling bad for a few days."

I shit you not.

"Hmm." I pretended to weigh the pros and cons. "I think we'll pass."

CIVILIZED BRUTALITY

Fortunately, I had the option of saying "no" to vaccinations I don't agree with. Many are not optional. Laws vary, but all 50 states require some vaccinations in order to enter kindergarten. The Supreme Court has provided states with *police power* to enforce individual compliance.

In June 2014, a New York court ruled against a family who refused a second dose of the DPT vaccination for their daughter. The little girl had a bad outcome after the first shot. Her doctor went on record that further exposure would likely result in serious injury.[21]

In the state of New York, exemptions are granted only for sincere religious reasons. The judge used the Catholic mother's own testimony against her. "She did not adopt her views opposing vaccination until she believed that immunization jeopardized her daughter's health."[22] The exemption was denied and the court insisted the child receive the vaccination.

The little girl had gone into anaphylactic shock after the first shot. Another shot might kill or severely disable her. A core tenant of the Catholic faith is the right to life. A core instinct of all parents is to keep their child from harm. The realities of this story are terrifying. Parents can refuse a vaccine for religious reasons, but not because it's likely to be life threatening.

Federal law states that if existing medical conditions increase an individual's risk of adverse effects, they can opt out of vaccinations. If that little girl's life-threatening reaction did not qualify her for an exemption, then what does? As of this writing, the case is pending appeal.

The dark side of the National Vaccine Injury Compensation Program is that it shields manufacturers and medical professionals who make and administer the drugs from liability. The USDA must substantiate a vaccine-related injury. To receive compensation, victims must forfeit the right to seek further damages.[23] It is illegal for individuals to sue manufactures or healthcare providers in court.

Vaccine makers are expanding their markets without the cost or threat of liability. In 2000, the CDC advised that only individuals over 65, women in the second and third trimesters of pregnancy, and immune-compromised people receive a flu shot.[24] In 2010, the CDC updated the protocols for the flu vaccine to include everyone over six months.[25] Additional vaccines are recommended to increasing segments of the population each year.

It appears that little (if any) good comes from the flu shot. And risks of negative side effects cannot be ignored. The Cochrane Collaboration is an international, non-profit network of scientists, researchers and medical professionals from over 120 countries. The group examines the validity of studies used to influence the recommendations of doctors and policy makers. They look at who pays for the research, how trials are conducted and if the resulting data supports the conclusions. An audit of 75 flu vaccine studies using over 300,000 children led them to a startling conclusion: only one case of influenza is prevented per 28 vaccinations.[26]

They also found evidence of wide spread manipulation of industry-funded data that conflicted with publicly funded research. They discovered a CDC employee who testified and submitted deceptive reports. The physician covered up a 4,250 percent increase in fetal deaths that corresponded to the double-dose vaccine administered during the 2009/10 H1N1 pandemic. Doctors were advised that the flu shot was safe and recommended for pregnant women. It wasn't. An estimated 590 fetal deaths occurred per one million pregnancies due to excessive levels of mercury.[27]

It is impossible to estimate the long-range impact for the babies that survived (to become customers for additional vaccinations). Vaccine studies only look at symptom onset in relation to the delivery date. The standard time frame for correlation is one to four weeks. But if researchers admittedly can't pinpoint the source of chronic diseases, how can they establish a relevant time frame?

Diseases can lay dormant for years. Yet, safety studies invalidate any correlation to disease that isn't full-blown within a month of a vaccination. There are no statutes of limitation for disease! And what about the cumulative effects of multiple vaccinations over a lifetime? How many milligrams of mercury need a person accumulate before the threshold of disease is crossed?

No one has a clue. Besides, the answer is different for everyone.

Aluminum is replacing mercury (thimersol) as a preservative in vaccines. That sounds harmless as aluminum is used in a lot of products. But tin foil and beer cans are not injected directly into our blood stream. Aluminum is toxic to the central nervous system and the brain. Affects are age and accumulation related.[28] The same question applies to aluminum as to mercury: How many milligrams of aluminum need a person accumulate before the threshold of disease is crossed?

Again, no one has a clue and the answer is different for everyone.

It's critical to acknowledge that some vaccines are very beneficial to both individuals and the population as a whole. But it's unreasonable to dismiss the side effects and cumulative consequences of the ever-increasing amount of immunizations. Vaccines are not an ethical concept and do not deserve immunity from scrutiny. They are a profitable product made by corporations and should be held to the same standards as all other drugs.

Unfortunately, the CDC and FDA standards benefit the manufacturers, not individuals. Subsequently, the herd of producers is protected at the expense of the herd of consumers.

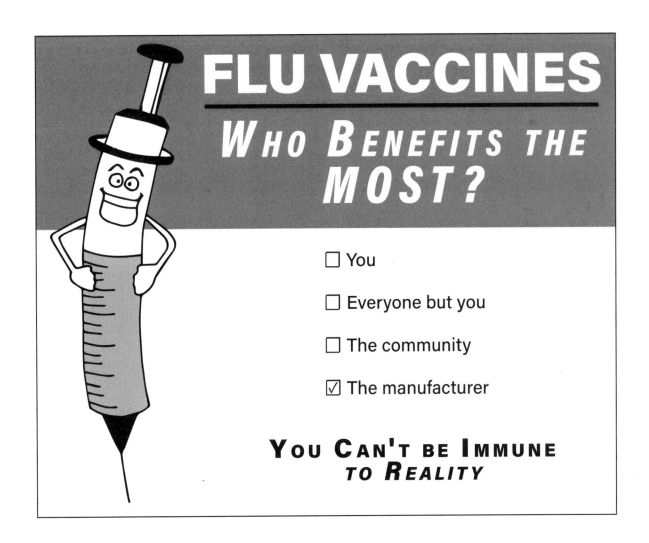

Nature's Flu Shot

Use this recipe to prevent and/or treat cold and flu symptoms.

- Juice of 6 fresh lemons
- 1 bulb of garlic
- 2 tsp. ginger powder
- 1 Tbsp. honey
- 3 cups pineapple juice
- ¼ tsp. cayenne pepper

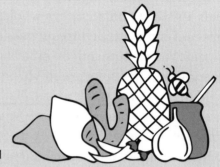

Blend all ingredients thoroughly. Store in a glass jar. Take 1 cup 4 times a day until the symptoms resolve.

 ColleenKachmann.com/members

Chemical Culprits

The biggest offenders found in the majority of the foods packed are listed on the label. Harmful ingredients are common additives used in schools, cafeterias, bakeries and restaurants. Eliminate (at least reduce) exposure to these normal toxins and improve your health.

Monosodium Glutamate (MSG)

MSG enhances the flavor in 80 percent of all processed foods. Listed on the next page are the names that can disguise its presence on a label. As you replace processed food with real food, you will not need to memorize anything for a test.

MSG stimulates the addiction centers of the brain and causes cravings for foods you otherwise wouldn't eat. That's why it's added to almost everything that you buy. It also stimulates the pancreas to produce three-times as much insulin as normal. This insulin supercharge converts the sugar in your blood to fat which, in turn, leads to a crash in blood sugar. The crash interferes with the brain's perception of fullness and often leads to uncontrollable hunger and over-eating.

Interesting fact: Scientists use MSG in food studies to induce obesity in mice.[29] Mice don't get fat eating the normal mouse diet. It's not like they sit down in front of a *Law and Order* marathon with a bag of chips and eat their way into an emotional funk. Google, "MSG obesity induced mice" and discover how scientists make fat rats.

MSG is a neurotoxin. It over-stimulates the brain and causes neurons to misfire, diminishing everything from hormone control to behavior and intelligence.[30] It can take a lifetime for subtle symptoms to cross the threshold of disease. Studies show that infant mice are fairly resilient. Diminished physical and mental capacities and obesity increase over time, masquerading as part of the aging process.[31]

Studies and consumer complaints have linked MSG to severe and chronic headaches, migraines, nausea, depression and anxiety. MSG has been shown to damage eyesight and promote degeneration of nerve cells in the brain.[32] It is a contributing factor in early brain disease, and intensifies symptoms of Alzheimer's, ALS (Lou Gehrig's disease), multiple sclerosis, strokes and Parkinson's disease.[33] Yet corporate food manufacturers have the right to use multiple names for this ingredient. The only purpose this serves is to confuse customers who wish to avoid it.

Industry scientists identify the threshold dose of MSG as the highest amount of additive that can be consumed (on average) with no adverse reactions. Manufacturers are catering to the below-average crowd. The rest of us need to stop buying and consuming products with MSG.

MSG IN DISGUISE

MSG can be legally labeled with over 50 names including the simple four-letter word salt. Avoid everything that contains the following most common words:

- "glutamate" or "hydrolyzed"
- gelatin
- yeast extract or autolyzed yeast
- yeast food or nutrient
- vegetable protein extract
- carrageenan
- anything "enzyme modified" or "enzymes"
- maltodextrin
- malt extract

- citric acid
- textured protein
- autolyzed plant protein
- glutamic acid
- protease
- bouillon, broth or stock
- "flavors" or "flavoring"
- barley malt
- natural seasonings

ColleenKachmann.com/members

High Fructose Corn Syrup (HFCS)

The three most common natural sugars are glucose, fructose and sucrose. The primary simple sugar, glucose, does not need to be broken down and can be immediately used for energy. Fructose is the sweetest of the simple sugars. It can be used as an immediate source of energy or converted to fat as an energy reserve. Sucrose (table sugar) is a compound molecule of glucose and fructose.

When glucose enters the bloodstream, insulin is released. The hormone allows the sugar to be processed at a controlled rate. When glucose and insulin are in the bloodstream, you do not feel hungry. If energy is available, there is no reason to eat.

Fructose does not cause an insulin response, however. High intake is associated with obesity, as insulin regulates appetite and excess fructose is stored as fat.

Fruits contain fructose and glucose. Fiber and multiple micronutrients slow the bloodstream's absorption of the sugars. Moderate fruit consumption does not cause a spike in blood sugar.[34]

> **Statistics:** The only science that *enables* **different experts** using the same figures to draw *different conclusions.*
>
> Evan Esar (1899-1995) American humorist

There is nothing natural about high fructose corn syrup (HFCS). It is highly concentrated and has an immediate negative effect on blood and brain chemistry. Because fructose does not trigger an insulin response, the body is defenseless. Excess fructose binds with proteins that act like little shards of glass, ripping through the inner lining of our blood vessels. This damages tissues, organs and limbs and accelerates the aging processes.[35] The fructose-protein molecules tear holes in the body's intestinal lining and trigger inflammation.[36]

Excess fructose feeds sugar-loving bacteria in the gut and interferes with our ability to fight infections. It is processed and stored as adipose fat in the liver. This causes inflammation and leads to non-alcoholic fatty liver disease. Adipose fat is recognized as an independent endocrine organ because it releases hormones like estrogen.[37] This compounds the harmful effects of being overweight.

Consumption of HFCS is now proclaimed to be the most significant influence for diabetes and obesity. HFCS increases blood pressure, metabolic disorders and insulin resistance, arthritis symptoms and the risk of cancer. It is a sad fact that the life expectancy of the next generation is expected to be shorter than ours.[38]

HFCS is extracted from corn (subsidized by our government and therefore unnaturally cheap) and highly concentrated to maximize sweetness. It is eight times more addictive than cocaine.[39] The effect of the fructose in an apple compared to HFCS-sweetened apple juice is comparable to a coca tea leaf versus crack cocaine.

HFCS is everywhere our kids are. It's in baby food, sport and fruit drinks, soda pop, salad dressings, ketchup, yogurt, candy, muffins, breakfast cereal and even whole wheat bread. The cheaper the food, the more HFCS it contains. Following the business model of Big Tobacco, Big Food is doing everything possible to turn kids into lifelong customers (addicts).

Thanks to lobbying efforts that conceal this ingredient, HFCS can be listed on labels under innocent-sounding pseudonyms. Look for "corn sugar," "corn sweetener," "corn syrup," and "corn syrup solids." The latest loophole simply identifies HFCS as "sugars," making it indecipherable from "sugar" to those not wearing bifocals.[40]

Sound familiar? Remember MSG?

Don't be fooled. Food Giants, Addiction Designers and Lying Lobbyists profit from products that make people sick. The only way to protect your health is to stop buying the crap.

Organic Junk Food

What do you think "100% All Natural" should mean?

Look for organic or Non-GMO certified packaged products. Corn, wheat and soy are found in nearly all processed foods, including snacks, soups, condiments and drinks. Organic products do not contain MSG, HFCS, preservatives, artificial colors or GMOs. Yes, you will pay more. Perfect. The less junk food you eat, the better. You won't want more than you need when cravings for addictive chemicals go away.

Sodium Nitrates and Nitrites

Nitrates enhance the flavor and color of meat by inhibiting the growth of bacteria. Nitrates are common additives in hot dogs, bacon, ham, smoked fish and lunchmeat. When heated, they form a carcinogen that damages DNA and promotes cellular degeneration. They deactivate the hemoglobin that carries oxygen in our blood. Regular consumption leads to lung disease; stomach, colorectal and prostate cancers; and increases pancreatic cancer risk by 68 percent.[41] Nitrates are also associated with Parkinson's, diabetes and Alzheimer's disease.

The USDA tried to ban nitrites in the 1970's. Big Food protested with expensive lobbying efforts. Nitrates make meat more appealing to consumers. A ban would undoubtedly diminish sales. They won. Their success is further evidence that the government treasures Corporate Profits far more than your health.

Partially Hydrogenated Oils and Trans Fat

The Harvard School of Public Health has labeled trans fat as one of the most harmful ingredients in our food supply. They are far worse for the heart and body than even low quality saturated alternatives.[42] The FDA says trans fat are "generally recognized as safe." Overwhelming research shows they are "generally recognized as dangerous." Many countries and communities have taken it upon themselves to ban them completely.

Trans fats increase bad cholesterol, decrease good cholesterol and inflame the linings of our blood vessels. They cause chronic medical problems when consumed regularly.[43]

Food makers use partially hydrogenated oils (trans fats) to increase shelf life and enhance flavor. The hydrogenation process converts healthy liquid oils to unhealthy solid fats. You can avoid trans fats by carefully reading food labels at the grocery. You cannot avoid them in bakeries, cafeterias, schools and restaurants. Steer clear and cook at home.

4 Tips for Lowering Trans Fat Intake

1. Read labels. Liquid vegetable oils and soft tub margarines contain little or no trans fats. Brands may look identical and be priced the same.
2. Avoid commercially prepared snack foods, baked goods (cookies, pies, donuts, etc.) processed foods and fast foods. Assume all products you don't make at home contain trans fats unless the menu or label says otherwise.
3. Avoid fried foods and desserts unless you cook them yourself. Frying foods in your own kitchen is time-consuming and messy, though the results can be delicious. This is a benefit. Minimal consumption of fried food is best.
4. Ask your favorite restaurants to use only trans-free oils and food. A pleasant request goes a long way. If asked often enough, business owners will comply (or lose business to the competition). Allow supply and demand to work in your favor.

BHA and *BHT*
(Butylated Hydroxyanisole and Hydroxytoluene)

BHA and BHT are petroleum-based preservatives that reduce the rate at which food spoils. They are found in bags of chips, boxes of cereal, cookies and crackers, butter, beer, chewing gum and flavor packets. Various studies associate them with allergic reactions, intestinal problems, neurological disorders, hormone dysfunction, and disorders in the liver and kidneys.[44]

BHA and BHT are in many cosmetics and skincare products. Skin is the largest organ of the body. When a product promises that skin will absorb the antioxidants, read the label. What other ingredients will be absorbed as well? BHA causes cancer (papilloma and squamous cell carcinomas) in both rats and hamsters.[45]

Check labels in your bathroom for these BHA ingredients: antioxyne B; antrancine 12; EEC #E320; embanox; nipantiox 1-F; protex; sustane 1-F; tenox BHA.

Chapter 14—*Afford the Best on a Budget of Less* contains many natural and effective alternatives to high-priced drugstore miracles that deliver more (and less) than labels guarantee.

CANCER CERTIFIED LUNCH MEAT

The Harvard School of Public Health has determined that it only takes an average of 1.8 ounces of processed meat per day to increase the proliferation of cancer by 50 percent, heart disease by 42 percent and diabetes by 19 percent.[46] In a week's time, that's a few cold-cut sandwiches and a couple of pieces of bacon.

The World Cancer Research Fund (WCRF) reviewed more than 7,000 clinical studies exploring the links between diet and cancer. Their recommendation leaves room for no compromise: processed meats are not safe for human consumption. Even small amounts consumed on a regular basis are unsafe. Consumers should stop buying and eating all processed meat products for the rest of their lives.[47]

A close look at Subway exposes the brainwashing effects of mass marketing. Deceptive slogans fool people into believing their "fresh" food is real food. Subway evades the stigma of fast food by branding stores "quick serve restaurants." What's the difference? The average Subway purchase has 784 calories. The average for McDonalds is 582 calories.[48] An average Subway purchase has 2,149 mg of sodium, compared to McDonalds 1,829 mg. So technically, fast food is the healthier option.

Subway's "all natural" breads contain over 40 artificial ingredients. They are negative for fiber and nutrients and high on the glycemic index. Fresh Fit® meats and dairy are not organic. They contain nitrates, MSG, genetically modified ingredients, preservatives and color dyes. The bottom line? Real food is expensive. Food sold at low prices is low quality. Unless the price of a $5 Footlong doubles because it's certified organic, the best way to "Eat Fresh" at Subway is to carry-in a lunch made at home.

Subway® is a registered trademark of a privately owned corporation named Doctors Associates Inc.© The name of the parent company supports the franchise's image. The not-so "Fresh Alternative" earned the American Heart Association's prestigious Heart-Check Meal Certification.[49] America's most recognized and trusted authority on heart health has placed its seal of approval on food that at the very least is not healthy, and at worse causes cancer.

It's clear there is only thing money can't buy. Integrity.

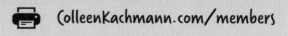

ColleenKachmann.com/members

Artificial Color and Food Dyes

We instinctively seek out foods with color. Vibrant green will always be more appealing than wilted brown. Antioxidants are the color we see in fruits and vegetables. Eating a wide-array of color is the best way to ensure balanced nutrition. Don't be fooled by fake foods. Ruby-red juice, bright yellow yogurts, outrageously-orange mac and cheese and berry-blue muffins are not the rainbow of wellness Mother Nature has hard-wired us to seek.

Food dyes are derived from coal tar. Studies confirm there is a definite link between synthetic colors and hyperactivity in children, migraines, anxiety, allergic reactions, asthma and cancer.[50]

The British government and European Union have banned food dyes common in American foods, including Red 40 and 3, Orange B, Yellow 5 and 6, Green 3, and Blue 1 and 2.[51] Meanwhile, the FDA does not argue that artificial colors have adverse side effects. But they regulate labels, not products. Disclosing ingredients on the label transfers responsibility to the consumer. The manufacturers and the government are absolved of blame. This approach began with Big Tobacco. Hey, if a product makes you sick, it's your fault for buying it.

But kids don't read labels or care. Many adults don't either. The overwhelming lists of additives might as well be written in another language. We see them so often that we don't notice them anymore. Toxins hide in plain sight and are irrelevant to the general population. The innocent may be ignorant, but the perpetrators are guilty.

Synergistic Effects

As scientists investigate the epidemic of chronic conditions, they are not finding singular causes for most diseases. Health is synergistic. Synergy occurs when multiple variables combine to produce an effect that is greater than the sum of single effects. In this way, multiple factors co-create disease. The most influential factors include:

- stress
- lack of exercise
- environmental toxins
- genetic susceptibility
- immune system dysfunction
- emotional and mental disturbances
- processed foods in the SAD (Standard American Diet)

False Advertising

Marketers stay ahead of the game by using consumer-appealing green and brown packaging and false promises of "100% All Natural Ingredients." The words "all-natural" have no legal definition. Other eye-catching terms are also meaningless. There are no certifications for "vegetarian fed," "no added hormones," and "antibiotic-free."[52] Unless you see the word "organic," there is no accountability. Manufacturers can say what they want.

Don't be fooled by labels that lie. Artificial ingredients, by definition, are *not* natural.

We are vulnerable to disease when our bodies are overwhelmed. There are limits to what any system can handle. Sometimes the bathroom circuit breaker trips when I am blow drying my hair. This only happens if I use a space heater to keep warm as I shower. It would be naive to blame the blow dryer for the overload. The energy required to power everything plugged into the circuit exceeds capacity.

The human capacity for all the chemicals that beset us daily is severely overestimated. The simmering toxic soup we all live in is a blend of:

- medications and vaccinations
- genetically modified foods
- artificial flavors, colors and preservatives in processed foods
- synthetic plastics and chemical-coated packaging
- pesticides and pollution

Aspartame is a legal additive, one of many dangerous chemicals common in our food supply. Sixty-seven percent of female rates develop tumors when aspartame is added to their drinking water.[53] Why is aspartame a legal ingredient? Because the FDA is more focused on the threshold of toxicity than the toxin itself. (The threshold of toxicity is how much the average person can ingest without immediate symptoms of illness.) Far worse, they are ignoring the cumulative threshold of multiple carcinogens.

Consider the potential synergistic effects of a normal American meal. The average purchase in a café includes a sandwich, side, dessert and drink. Lunch meat and cheese contain nitrates, growth hormones and antibiotics. A bag of tortilla chips adds genetically modified corn and MSGs. The dessert contains high fructose corn syrup and trans fat. A diet soda includes aspartame, acidic carbonated water and artificial colors derived from petroleum and coal tar.[54]

If it's packaged in a plastic bottle it may be contaminated with BPA (bisphenol A is an industrial chemical known to interfere with thyroid and hormone function). And there is no fiber and little (if any) micronutrients to give the body a fighting chance of blunting the effects of the chemical assault.

Where's the study that takes synergy into account? There isn't one.

We are all guinea pigs in an unofficial experiment. There is no way to measure the infinite interactions of the thousands of chemicals we are exposed to every day. Scientists suspect that weak carcinogens from multiple sources (food, air, soil, water, consumer products) have the same potential to cause disease as a single strong carcinogen.[55] Unfortunately, the synergies of addiction and profit are more powerful than the desire to prevent disease.

> **"It's easier to fool people than to convince people *they've been fooled.*"**
>
> Mark Twain (Samuel L. Clemens, 1835-1910) American author and humorist

How to Order in a Restaurant

When traveling, I prefer cuisine that comes from the produce section of a grocery store. I stock the hotel room mini-fridge with a small selection of fresh fruit and salad fixings. But as restaurants are venues for many social and business gatherings, learning to read between the menu lines is a basic skill in survival.

Local, single-chef establishments are the most likely to carry high-quality ingredients and accommodate dietary restrictions. If you can't talk to the cook, that's a bad sign. The best (and most polite) approach is to call ahead and discuss options before you arrive. This gives the staff time to prepare something that suits your needs.

Ironically, vegan and plant-based meals are often easy to order in a steakhouse. Meat and potatoes always include an obligatory side of vegetables. Asian and Mediterranean restaurants are usually veggie-friendly. Stay away from chain restaurants unless they advertise hormone and antibiotic-free meat and dairy. Remember, words like "all-natural," "fresh" and "real" have no legal criteria and mean nothing.

Most large cities have high quality, plant-based and organic restaurants. Be wary of vegan café's and diners. Unless they boast organic and GMO-free homemade ingredients (many do, but some don't), the fare is the vegan version of McDonalds. Imitation meats are filled with non-organic soy, texturized vegetable protein (TVP) and MSG. These options are better than animal-based fast food, but not much.

Peruse a menu for whole ingredients as opposed to entrées. Focus on the side offerings and the vegetables paired with entrées. Order a stir-fry. For example, broccoli, cauliflower, mushroom and onion can be flavored with Asian, Thai or marinara. An olive oil, lemon juice and pepper preparation is universal. Be aware that requesting "a little oil" does not always translate. Be specific. "No more than 1-2 tablespoons of oil, please." Also be clear if you include pasta or rice. "No more than ½ cup of pasta" will eliminate a bowl full of noodles garnished with a few spinach leaves. Inquire about the price of a customized dish when you order.

Celiacs and strict vegans need to be very specific. Sauces, condiments and even vegetable soup can contain hidden wheat and animal products. To ensure there are no unwanted ingredients, tell the server you have an allergy. The word "allergy" alerts the staff to take your request seriously.

Above all, be polite. Small restaurants may not have the resources to train inexperienced staff to service limited diets. If your meal is unfavorable, ask the manager to call you during off-hours for feedback. Those that appreciate your business want to improve. Restaurants willing and able to accommodate special requests will thrive. If your communication is pleasant and supportive, the world becomes a better place.

DIY Dressings, Seasonings & Dips
Quick and Easy Recipes to Make at Home

It's counter-productive to clean up your diet with healthy and whole foods only to flavor your meals with chemical condiments. Make your own seasoning packets with dried organic spices. Prepare in bulk. Label and store in resealable, BPA free containers.

Ranch: 2 Tbsp. parsley, 2 tsp. each of garlic powder, onion powder and dill weed, 1 tsp. each of ground mustard, celery salt and black pepper.

Southwestern ranch: Add 1 tsp. each of cumin, paprika and chili powder to the ranch recipe.

Caribbean jerk: ¼ cup onion powder, 2 Tbsp. each sea salt and thyme, 1 Tbsp. cinnamon, 2 tsp. allspice, 1 tsp. cayenne powder (optional).

Taco seasoning: 2 Tbsp. each of chili powder, cumin and sea salt (optional) ½ Tbsp. each garlic powder, onion powder, ½ tsp. oregano, thyme and black pepper.

Curry: ¼ cup paprika, 2 Tbsp. each of cumin and turmeric, 1 Tbsp. each of fenugreek, ground mustard and coriander. Optional ingredients include: ½ Tbsp. red pepper (for spiciness), cardamom (optional), ½ tsp. cinnamon, ¼ tsp. cloves.

Italian seasoning: 2 Tbsp. each of basil, marjoram, oregano, 1 Tbsp. each rosemary, thyme, ½ Tbsp. garlic salt.

Seasoning salt: 2 Tbsp. each of onion powder, garlic powder, black pepper, 1 Tbsp. each of chili powder, paprika, parsley, ¼ tsp. ground red pepper (optional).

Pumpkin pie spice: 2 Tbsp. cinnamon, 1 tsp. each nutmeg and allspice, ½ tsp. ginger, ¼ tsp. clove.

Mix seasonings with organic sour cream, plain Greek yogurt, cashew cream, hummus, avocado, or miso paste. Experiment with combinations. Tenderize meat or mix with olive oil and/or vinegar for veggie marinade.

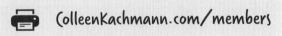
ColleenKachmann.com/members

Normal vs Healthy

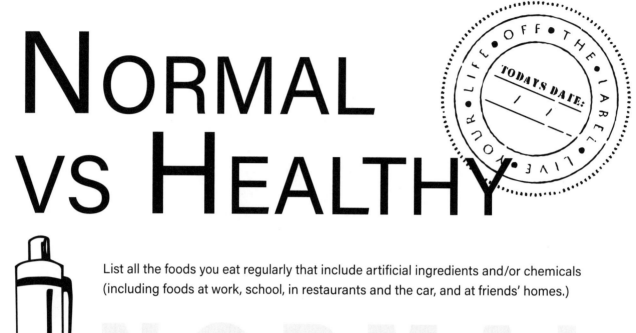

TODAYS DATE: ___/___/___

List all the foods you eat regularly that include artificial ingredients and/or chemicals (including foods at work, school, in restaurants and the car, and at friends' homes.)

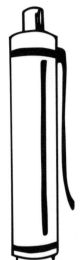

As you reduce your exposure to fake foods, you will experience withdrawal. How will you manage the symptoms of detox?

What symptoms do you experience that might be caused or aggravated by processed foods?

What processed foods will you eliminate and which will you keep? Why? When might you make exceptions? Why?

 ColleenKachmann.com/members

LIFE OFF THE LABEL

PS I left this facing page blank for you.
Fill it with whatever you like. Questions, comments, to-do's, thoughts, etc.
You're welcome . . .

CHAPTER 5

DANGEROUS AGVENTURES

> *"Make the lie big. Make it simple.
> Keep saying it and eventually everyone will believe it."*
>
> ADOLPH HITLER

CASH CROPS

The crimes of Big Tobacco created a blueprint for successful sales of unhealthy products. The profits have funded strategic expansion into an even larger market—the supermarket. In 1985, Philip Morris acquired General Mills for $5.6 billion. It was the largest non-oil acquisition of its time.[1] That same year, R. J. Reynolds purchased Nabisco for $4.9 billion, forming the largest U.S.-based consumer products company in the world.[2] Philip Morris later purchased Kraft Foods for $13.1 billion in 1988.[3]

And so goes the cliché: history repeats itself. Once again, public health officials scrutinize the rising disease rates and scratch their heads in confusion. Meanwhile, industry experts worm their way into government appointments to craft protective policies. The Surgeon General is thanking Big Food for their efforts to offer healthier foods and encourage kids to get more active.[4] Industry scientists conclude that obesity is an inherited, genetic disorder involving energy balance.[5] Nonprofit groups such as the American Heart Association certify lunchmeat and processed cheese as heart-healthy.[6] Corporate websites provide free online games to teach kids how to help the fat avatar lose weight.[7] Brand loyalty is rewarded with cash for schools.

The new generation of debates that pit aspartame against saccharine are reminiscent of those that once proclaimed low-tar Camel Lights healthier than Marlboro Reds. Which ingredient is responsible for the modern health crisis? Pick one. And then add the rest. Genetically modified seeds, agricultural chemicals, synthetic additives and shelf stable products are the new cigarette. In time, the creators and profiteers of artificial salts, sugars and fats will be held responsible for the healthcare problems associated with processed foods. And the tobacco/food industry is prepared for what they already know: liability suits are just a necessary cost of doing business.[8]

PSEUDO SAMARITANS TO THE RESCUE

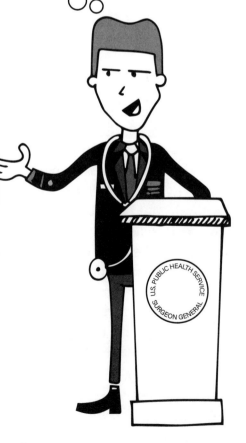

THE OBESITY CRISIS IS THE FASTEST-GROWING CAUSE OF DISEASE AND DEATH IN AMERICA. AND IT IS COMPLETELY PREVENTABLE.

AMERICA'S CHILDREN ARE ALREADY SEEING THE INITIAL CONSEQUENCES OF A LACK OF PHYSICAL ACTIVITY AND UNHEALTHY EATING HABITS.

I'M PLEASED THAT BUSINESSES LIKE KRAFT FOODS, COCA COLA AND NIKE ARE SUPPORTING MAJOR EFFORTS AND MAKING SIGNIFICANT CHANGES TO HELP KIDS MAKE HEALTHIER CHOICES.

SOME PEOPLE WANT TO BLAME THE FOOD INDUSTRY FOR OUR GROWING WAISTLINES. THE REALITY IS THAT RESTAURANTS, INCLUDING MANY FAST FOOD RESTAURANTS, NOW OFFER LOW-FAT, HEALTHY CHOICES.

TO MAKE HEALTHY CHOICES, PARENTS AND CHILDREN NEED EASY-TO-UNDERSTAND INFORMATION THAT FITS THEIR BUSY LIFESTYLES.

WE'VE GOT A LOT OF FAT AND LAZY KIDS. PARENTS ARE TOO BUSY TO CARE. LET'S THANK KRAFT FOODS, COCA COLA AND FAST FOOD RESTAURANTS FOR COMING TO THE RESCUE OF THESE PATHETIC FAILING FAMILIES. OH, AND PLEASE BUY SOME GYM SHOES FROM NIKE. JUST DO IT.

In 2013, the Surgeon General addressed the United States House of Representatives about the Obesity Crisis in America.

What he said and what he meant were two very different things.

GREED WEEDS

Most people want what's best for the greater good. Often, we ferociously disagree as to what that is. Even well-meaning people can (and do) inflict harm on others. But there are deviant masterminds who manipulate ideas, emotions, figures and the facts. Vulnerable people can be tricked into believing that bad behavior will serve a good cause.

That's Brainwashing 101.

From Watergate to Wall Street, history is filled with cover-ups that have required the cooperation of normal people. Pillow talk, political shenanigans and spyware technology confirm that the "government" is human. Government employees have strengths, vulnerabilities, and ethical beliefs just like the rest of us. They are everyday folk who go to work, do their jobs, and go home to their families. They aren't getting rich serving the public.

Conspiracy theorists would do well to note there is a basic flaw in the belief that Big Government is the Big Brother they fear. The government is not the mastermind, just a tool for those with power and influence. The large print on legislative policies diverts attention from the fine print that funds predatory practices disguised as free-market capitalism. Infotainers analyze the issues with red and blue crayons. We the people argue over gay marriage and gun control. Meanwhile, the rights of the American people are being exploited with a smoke screen of social discord.

Ideological extremists are easy to spot because money can't buy their silence. Their motivations may be revenge, religious beliefs, or political power. They are willing to interfere with commerce, chain themselves to a tree, and even strap on a bomb to promote their beliefs. They may take innocent lives and go out in a blaze of glory, but the tragedy rarely promotes their cause.

Unlike the obvious extremists, the most influential terrorists act professionally, speak intelligently and appear to play by the rules. They do not seek attention. They hide in plain sight. Alliances are strategic; loyalty is a liability. The love of money may be the root of all evils but in business it's the bottom line.

Contrary to what we are taught in high school government, politicians have little to do with the policies that shape our lives. Our leaders spend their days shaking hands, kissing babies and campaigning for the next election. It's the individuals appointed to write the legalese that have real control. And there is no shortage of specialists willing to offer their expertise in service to the public.

The 24/7 news channels would lose their sponsors if they exposed the enormous loopholes that keep corporate America profitable. Regardless, no one has the attention span or legal expertise to wade through the fine print in the 1,000-page bills presented to our congress each year. This includes the very lawmakers who sponsor legislation. Cliff Notes provided to the media highlight the social issues that grab our attention. Heated discussions stoke our emotions. Meanwhile, the unscrupulous details hidden in the deregulatory agendas go unnoticed.

One hundred years too late, we learned that the behind-the-scenes cooperation of corporate rivals was quite lucrative for Big Tobacco. Fair trade capitalism relies on competition. But selling dangerous and addictive products in the public marketplace requires clandestine politics. These strategies are still in play today. Later in this chapter, we'll meet a lawyer who infiltrated both the FDA and the USDA. His service to the public proved quite beneficial to private interests. Unfortunately, the policies enacted on his watch have proven to be harmful to the public's health.

The Guile of Denial

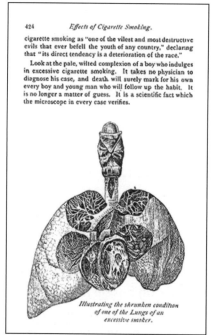

Figure courtesy US National Library of Medicine

In 1902 Philip Morris launched the Marlboro brand. By 1920, four million cigarettes were produced every day. Parallel to rising sales was an alarming increase in lung cancer and heart disease. Doctors and public health officials smoked cigarettes as they debated the perplexing conundrum.

In 1894, *Searchlights on Health* published evidence of the damaging effects of smoking. The book included detailed autopsy diagrams.[9] Yet 60 years passed before the connection between smoking and lung cancer was publicly acknowledged. The tobacco industry funded bogus non-profit organizations to ensure the evidence was branded inconclusive, despite the fact that it was not. In 1944, the American Cancer Society's official stance was still, "no definite evidence exists between smoking and lung cancer."[10]

An unchallenged lie obscures the truth. Thankfully, the truth can no longer be denied. Nearly one billion people have died over the last century as a direct result of smoking.[11]

> **There are two ways to be fooled.** *One is to BELIEVE what isn't true.* **The other is to *refuse to accept* what is true.**
>
> Søren Kierkegaard (1813-1855) Danish poet, existentialist philospher

GROWN-UP GAMES

I was 13 when I smoked my first cigarette. A friend had pilfered a few before a slumber party. Naive parents granted permission to three giggly, innocent girls to take a late evening walk. And so the shenanigans began.

My first attempt to inhale produced spastic coughing that made everyone laugh. "Whatever," I thought. I was determined to complete this essential rite of passage. I tried again and instantly came down with food poisoning. My friends were gracious enough to admit they too felt bad and held back my hair as I vomited. After surveying the contents my stomach had rejected, we collectively agreed to blame excessive Oreo consumption. Cigarettes may cause cancer in old people but they don't make *Kool* kids sick.

I made a second attempt when I was fifteen. A "good girl" friend invited me to take a stroll on a crisp, cool autumn night. The stars were bright as we twirled on the swings of an empty school playground, digging our toes into the chalky pebbles on the ground.

I was surprised when she pulled a pack of Camels from the depths of her purse. The flame of the lighter highlighted her pretty skin and large eyes. She did not draw the smoke into her lungs with the first drag. Instead, she collected it in her mouth and inhaled through her nose. The visual effect was that of swirling dry ice. She tilted her head and gazed thoughtfully into the darkness as her cigarette dangled loosely between her fingers. The performance continued. She took another drag, formed an "o" with her lips and used the tip of her tongue to press expertly rounded rings into the air. We watched the expanding wafts of haze fade into the twilight.

"Wow," I said, mesmerized.

I tried to look casual as I held out my hand. She flicked the ash and passed me the cigarette. We were just two girls sharing a smoke. With a little coaching, the French inhale was easy enough, but the smoke rings would need to be practiced in a mirror.

I did not throw up until I got home.

Of course I knew that smoking was unhealthy. But one cigarette doesn't kill you. Addiction did not seem to be a threat. Smokers stink. Non-smokers smoke for entertainment purposes only and brush their teeth when finished. Smokers spend money on cigarettes. Non-smokers do not. Bumming (versus buying) cigarettes is the loophole to lung cancer. And teenagers are immortal anyway.

Youthful rebellion requires risk. I experimented with smoking because it was fun to get away with it. In those days, secondhand smoke was not yet a recognized concern. When the smell of guilt clung to my hair, it was easy to breeze through parental security. A simple, "ugh, we were seated in the smoking section at Pizza Hut" was all it took to escape detection.

My mother had three teenagers worth of experience before she invented the "finger-sniff" test. My younger brother used denial to counter suspicion. "I don't smoke mom, I was holding it for a friend."

My sister's approach was far more brazen and now legendary among our family stories. "Yes, I was smoking. But at least it wasn't pot. Just relax! I'm not going to smoke when I grow up. Parents that smoke are gross. I love that you and dad don't smoke. Our home smells clean and fresh. I love my awesome parents."

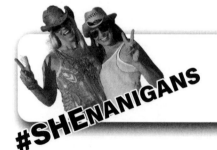

Relax. We're all crazy. It's not a competition.

My parents soon gave up. They focused on helping us get into college in hopes that we would all grow up and move out. "Just go 'not smoke' outside. Whatever."

I was a college graduate with a real 50-hour a week job when I invited my family to my new apartment for a 4th of July celebration. The evening was muggy and warm, but the enthusiasm of the holiday was infectious. My siblings were still teenagers; I was the first official grown up. As a legal adult, I was free and clear to make my own decisions. Somehow, this diminished the appeal of smoking. Still, I craved a sneaky cig for 'ole time's sake. I discreetly bummed a cigarette from my brother and walked outside.

A dense line of evergreens grew 10 feet from my patio. It was just getting dark as I retreated to the pine-scented hideout with my contraband. The field beyond was filled with children waving fiery sparklers. Bursts of brightly colored lights popped, whistled and spun. Music, laughter and the savory scents of grilled food floated in the air.

The sulfurous smell of the match served as tantalizing appetizer; the first inhale delivered a euphoric rush of pleasure. Unfortunately, the buzz was short lived. I felt the blood drain from my face when I realized that I was not the only secret smoker.

"Dad?"

"Colleen?"

My father and I were too stunned to claim that we were just holding a cigarette for one of my brother's friends. My sister was not around to cheerily remind us that at least we weren't smoking pot. We made small talk, avoided eye contact and acted as though the awkward situation was completely normal.

When we snuffed out the butts, I held out my hand. He placed the evidence into my palm. We walked back inside together with a casual air of innocence. I set the mouthwash on the bathroom counter and left out an old toothbrush so he could scrub his fingers. Mom's finger-sniff tests are hard to pass.

We never discussed that awkward event. Neither of us are smokers, so it never happened.

Lingering Legacy

Despite the warning labels and health education mandated by Congress, most people have smoked a cigarette. This speaks to the powerful influence of advertising on generations of people. Slogans from the 1940s-'70s made no attempt to be subtle.

Here's a sample from the archives:

- According to a nationwide survey, more doctors smoke Camels than any other cigarette.
- Vintage tobacco makes Phillip Morris naturally gentle and mild.
- Smoke Old Golds for a treat instead of a treatment.
- Camel is first in service to men in the Army, Navy, Marine Corps and Coast Guard.
- Farewell to the ugly cigarette. Smoke pretty. Eve.
- Science discovered it. You can prove it. ABC Cigarettes.
- Women began to smoke, so they tell me, just about the time they began to vote. Chesterfield.

The Surgeon General's labels warning us that smoking causes cancer cannot compete with the perception that doctors promote smoking. These treats are recommended over treatments? Sold. Women can celebrate their right to vote with a sexy inhale? Light me up. The brand favored by the troops is packed with patriotism? Sir! Yes, Sir! The best cigarettes are natural and safe, thanks to advances in science? Oh, the marvels of modern life!

By 1965, the Surgeon General decided he could no longer deny the link between smoking and lung cancer.[13] That year, half of Americans were addicted to cigarettes. Congress passed the Cigarette Labeling and Advertising Act. Public service announcements were issued on television and radio. The Tobacco Industry launched a counterattack.

Industry titans pooled their resources to form the Tobacco Industry Research Committee (TIRC). This non-profit group provided grants to tobacco-friendly scientists. The group's sole purpose was to challenge the conclusions of independent research and present their own contradictory evidence.[14] The mission of the TIRC was to examine the "alleged" association between tobacco and lung cancer and ensure the public was given "factual" information. In 1954, *The Frank Statement* was published in 448 newspapers.

The message to 43 million people worldwide was: [15]

- medical research indicates there are many possible causes of lung cancer.
- there is no agreement among the authorities as to the cause of lung cancer.
- there is no proof that cigarette smoking is one of the causes of lung cancer.
- statistics that link smoking with cancer can be applied with equal force to many other aspects of modern life.

Big Tobacco also recruited the film industry. Hollywood producers, writers and directors earned big bucks to feature stars lighting up on-screen.[16]

This lead to a new generation of "freedom fighters." Smoking was identified as a "right." Regulations and restrictions were vilified as Big Brother's infringement on personal liberty. "Give me liberty or give me death?" Ironically, tobacco addiction offers both.

It wasn't until February 4, 1996 that whistle-blower Dr. Jeffery Wigand finally exposed Big Tobacco's deceitful practices. At the time, he was the vice president of research and development at Brown & Williamson, manufacturers of several top brands of cigarettes. Wigand provided solid evidence of massive scandal. The industry had deliberately increased the levels of nicotine to make cigarettes more addictive. Industry insiders had wormed their way into government appointments to craft cunning public policies that provided protection and suppressed information. And the non-profit Tobacco Industry Research Committee was exposed as a fraud.

In 1998, the largest legal settlement in U.S. history delivered $206 million to 46 states. Yet today's global revenues for Big Tobacco are close to half a trillion dollars. Meanwhile, six million people die every year from smoking.[17] Tobacco companies have accepted liability suits as a necessary cost of doing business.[18]

Smoking causes cancer. The habit is now socially unacceptable. Consequently, modern debates on the new health crisis take place in non-smoking facilities, catered by Subway, Pizza Hut and Chic-Fil-A.

> "In real life, it is always *the anvil* that breaks the hammer."
>
> George Orwell (1903-1950) English novelist and political writer

The Seed Exchange

Genetically modified (GM) foods were introduced into our food supply in the mid-1990s. Grandiose commitments to eliminate world hunger struck emotional chords among policy makers. Approval was granted to the "seeds of hope" before any proof of safety was offered. Consumers were not notified that fundamental changes had been made to the food they purchased for their families. The entire planet has become the target market.

Genetically engineered (GE) crops are supposed to thrive regardless of soil conditions, drought, flood or pestilent plague.

The miraculous seeds promise:

- higher yields, increased production and less land use.
- less use of pesticides.
- higher nutritional quality.
- lower water requirements.

Biotechnology companies invest millions in research to design crops that can defy all environmental threats. Manufacturers patent the inventions (often referred to as "frankenseeds"), giving them exclusive right to make and sell their products. Some seeds have "terminator" genes implanted into their DNA that disable the plant's reproductive system. This is done to prevent non-paying customers from benefiting when the birds play with the bees. Seed designers make the errant assumption that farmers want to cross breed their crops with unknown contaminants. If unintentional pollination is discovered, insult adds to injury when the neighboring farms (who have refused the strong-armed sales tactics) are sued for trademark violations.

Genetically engineered crops are not grown with sustainable farming practices. The ancient arts of seed saving and cultivating next year's crop with the strongest survivors have been replaced by seasonal contracts. Seeds are re-designed each year in the laboratory to fine-tune field performance. Patented seeds are disposable products. New seeds must be purchased every year. Saving seeds is illegal, and violators are prosecuted to the full extent of the law.

GM crops do one of three things:

- **Produce pesticides** (Plants produce hormones, proteins and antibodies just like humans. So why not enable crops to be "naturally" poisonous to threatening pests? Well, the word "pest" is relative. Poison doesn't discriminate.)

- **Survive heavy exposure to herbicides and pesticides** (GM plants must thrive despite the onslaught of chemicals that kill surrounding foliage (weeds, wildflowers and grasses). Significant modifications are made to a plant's immune system to make this possible.)
- **Contain "promoter" genes that turn other genes "on" and "off"** (Theoretically, this allows for the selection of desired color, size, shape and even immunity to specific infections. But promoter genes can accelerate unnatural mutations that lead to unpredictable results.)

Just as people used to smoke without worry of consequence, Americans today are eating foods that are just as dangerous as cigarettes. Genetically modified foods produce destructive chemicals and over-stimulate the immune system. Crops are engineered to grow larger and mature faster than nature intended. There are alarming parallels between the manipulations of plant DNA and the subsequent manifestation of human diseases and disorders.

Paranoid theorists worry that Big Brother is monitoring cell phone conversations. Meanwhile, our food supply has been hijacked and no one seems to have noticed. We continue to eat as we did growing up, and allow our kids to do the same. Our habits haven't changed, but the food has. The consequences of our ignorance are deadly.

> **The devil doesn't *come dressed* in a red cape and pointy horns. *He comes as everything* you ever wished for.**
>
> Tucker Max, American author

THE GATE KEEPER

After graduating law school in 1976, Michael Taylor worked for the Commissioner of the FDA (Federal Drug Administration).[19] His significant expertise in food policy landed him a position with a private legal firm in 1981. One of the firm's largest clients was a company called Monsanto. Monsanto is the largest manufacturer of genetically engineered seeds, producing 90 percent of the global supply.[20] (Details of their role in this story are explained in the next section.)

On behalf of his clients, Taylor challenged the 1958 law that established a zero tolerance policy for *all* carcinogens in the food supply. He proposed a "minimum threshold" policy to replace it. Taylor reasoned the law should respect ever-evolving technological advancements. He pointed out that science is now able to detect minuscule levels of toxins that were not previously identified. Food producers were being restricted from using additives with no proof of threat to public health (there was no proof of safety).

Taylor won. The legal battle was a game-changer. Zero-tolerance was abolished. Regulations were updated. Food producers were now free to create the foods that Americans demanded without concern for the details no one cares about. The success catapulted Taylor's career.

He left private practice in 1991 and returned to the FDA as Deputy Commissioner of Policy. Under his leadership, more leeway was given to Big Food. BGH (Bovine Growth Hormone) was approved to increase milk production for dairy farmers. Most of our nation's major crops became genetically modified.

Neither BGH nor GMOs are regulated or identified on food labels. Manufacturers are responsible for the safety of their ingredients. Products are not subjected to the scrutiny of third party science.

In 1994, Taylor left the FDA for the USDA (U.S. Department of Agriculture). He was charged with updating standards for meat and poultry production. In 1996, he took a break from public service for the ultimate gig. Monsanto hired him to serve as Vice President of Public Policy. (Where is the alarm bell when a private corporation sees the need to hire an executive in charge of *public* policy?)

Taylor joined a non-profit think tank in 2000. In a joint effort with the Bill Gates Foundation, he cleared the way for Monsanto's philanthropic donation of drought-resistant seeds to South Africa. This back door attempt to enter a new market failed, however, when insects annihilated the crops. Monsanto responded by donating massive amounts of pesticides to eliminate the problem.[21]

Thanks, Monsanto.

In 2009, Taylor returned to government service as the Senior Advisor to the FDA Commissioner under the Bush administration. In 2010, President Obama appointed Taylor as the Deputy Commissioner of Foods, despite his campaign promise to insist GMO foods be labeled as such.[22] But don't get your political panties in a bunch. Corruption crosses the aisle when compromise is profitable.

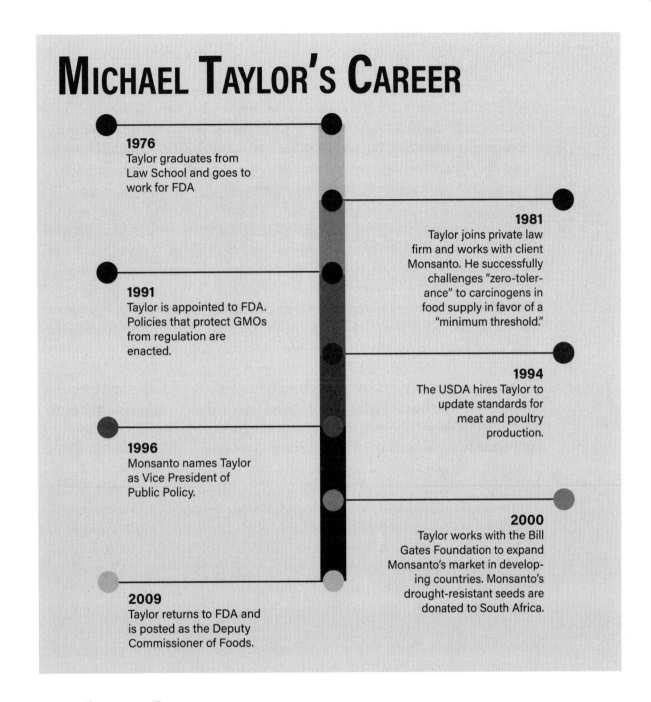

Michael Taylor's Career

1976
Taylor graduates from Law School and goes to work for FDA

1981
Taylor joins private law firm and works with client Monsanto. He successfully challenges "zero-tolerance" to carcinogens in food supply in favor of a "minimum threshold."

1991
Taylor is appointed to FDA. Policies that protect GMOs from regulation are enacted.

1994
The USDA hires Taylor to update standards for meat and poultry production.

1996
Monsanto names Taylor as Vice President of Public Policy.

2000
Taylor works with the Bill Gates Foundation to expand Monsanto's market in developing countries. Monsanto's drought-resistant seeds are donated to South Africa.

2009
Taylor returns to FDA and is posted as the Deputy Commissioner of Foods.

> "The worse *disease* in the world today is *corruption*. And there is a cure. *Transparency*."
>
> Bono, lead singer of Irish rock band U2

DANGEROUS AGVENTURES

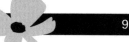

Pay Dirt

Big Pharma, Big Industry, Big Food and the military use behind-the-scene suppliers for ingredients that enhance products and increase consumer demand. Monsanto is one of the "Big Six" (BASF, Bayer, DuPont, Dow Chemical Company, and Syngenta) corporations that design and produce chemicals. Each organization has a specialty and many overlap.

Chemical companies provide the magical ingredients of modern life. I certainly don't want to go back to driving a horse or list my shipping address as Cave #4. I love the workout clothes that wick away the sweat from my skin, and sunglasses with polarized lenses. I am thankful for sunscreen, air conditioning and filtered water. There are many benefits to chemical technology. But every scientific advancement has a trade-off. The freedom to choose which to embrace and which to avoid requires complete and accurate information.

Monsanto was founded in 1901 in St. Louis, Missouri. The first product they took to market was saccharine. The demand was created by the sugar shortages during World War 1. Despite its status as a suspected carcinogen, saccharine is still in use today. History offers many examples of chemical "solutions" that are designed with good intention, only to have time reveal them to be harmful.

Professional integrity calls for high standards of safety and full disclosure of risk. But the FDA has placed the burden of our safety on the same corporations that profit at our expense. The last one hundred years reveal that Monsanto's most valuable product is money. The following examples show the damage Monsanto has inflicted on people and the environment is neither accidental nor minimal.

Remember Agent Orange? Monsanto developed the deadly chemical. Environmentalists describe Agent Orange as "perhaps the most toxic molecule ever synthesized by man."[23,24] Monsanto did inform the government of the dangers. The military ordered it anyway. Over 20 billion gallons were dispensed during the Vietnam War. Millions of Vietnamese and U.S. soldiers were killed and disabled as a direct result. Agent Orange also destroyed the jungles and ecosystems of the Vietnam countryside. The country is still dealing with the effects of contamination today.[25]

PCBs were banned in 1979, but do you know why? PCBs were developed as industrial coolants. But their disastrous effects on the environment were impossible to ignore. (Except by those whose only "green" concern is money.) PCBs are highly carcinogenic and cause disfiguring dermatitis in animals and humans.

Monsanto manufactured them for over 40 years *after* realizing that levels of PCBs in the streams and waterways near their production facility were 7,500 times the legal limit. This resulted in a massive fish kill and numerous health problems for people in nearby communities. Monsanto did nothing to prevent further damage or clean up their mess. Instead, executives suppressed the evidence. They ordered their own scientists to change the conclusions of internal PCB studies from "slightly tumorigenic" to "does not appear to be carcinogenic." Legal battles to protect their monopoly on PCB sales continued long after research confirmed them as global pollutants.[26]

Most recently, Monsanto has shut down about 90 small farms to protect their investment in genetically modified seeds. They monitor their farmers to enforce the contractual obligation to not save seeds. They also survey surrounding farmland for evidence of cross-pollination in neighboring fields. Small farms are sued for patent infringement despite this being an unavoidable natural occurrence.[27] In an ideal world, Monsanto would be held responsible for contamination. In the real world, unlimited cash is required to fight this Not-so-"Jolly"-or-"Green"-Giant. People brave enough to bet the farm in order to stand up for what is right end up losing it.

> **Our lives begin to end the day we become silent *about things that matter.***
>
> Martin Luther King, Jr. (1929-1968) civil rights activist

DEADLY DAIRY

For the past 20 years, much of the nation's milk supply has come from cows injected with a genetically engineered growth hormone known as rBST. The hormone doubles the amount of milk produced by the cow.[28] This is why conventional milk produced on large factory farms is so much cheaper than organic milk.

Yet the price is the only notable difference when consumers read labels and compare brands. The FDA does not require rBST be disclosed as an ingredient. Furthermore, Big Dairy has challenged the right of their competitors to label milk as rBST-free. A judge sided with Big Money and mandated a disclaimer: *"The FDA has determined no significant difference has been shown between milk derived from rBST and non rBST treated cows."* [29]

That statement is the biggest lie since the 1944 declaration by the American Cancer Society that there is no evidence that smoking causes lung cancer. In fact, multiple studies have been done and multiple problems have been found. Milk with rBST increases the naturally occurring, tumor-promoting hormone IGF-1 (Insulin-like Growth Factor) by a factor of twenty.[30] The unnaturally high levels multiply the risk of breast cancer in women under 50 by 7-fold.[31] (A 7-fold increase translates to 700 percent.) Chances of prostate cancer increase 4-fold.[32] In fact, high blood levels of IGF-1 inflate the risk for all cancers more than any other factor discovered thus far.[33]

The U.S. is the only developed nation that allows rBST in their milk supply. The rest of the world is laughing at us. All 27 nations in the European Union have banned the hormone. Canadian scientists released an insulting *Gaps Analysis* Report that highlighted the criminal omissions and contradictions in the FDA's approval process.[34] A summary of their conclusions is on page 95.

The government may have approved rBST for use in milk, however we all have the right to exercise our own authority and ban it from our homes.

"It's dangerous to be right *when the government is wrong.*"

Voltaire (1694-1778) French writer and philospher

LIFE OFF THE LABEL

IT'S COLD IN CANADA

Our northern neighbors are not huge fans of the FDA. Apparently, they missed the memo that America is the "Leader of the Free World." They refuse to acknowledge that our regulatory processes set the bar. Take notes, world wanna-bes. "FDA-Approved" is the ultimate designer label.

WARNING

May contain traces of sarcasm

Canadians are probably mad that the United States blocked the import and sale of their pharmaceuticals to the American people. We the people believe only Lady Liberty can guarantee due diligence when it comes to drugs. Cheap Canadian counterfeits don't make the cut. Sorry, guys.

The Canada Health "Gaps Analysis" is clearly a juvenile retaliation. Their analysis of the FDA's approval process of rBST contains 39 pages of boring empirical data. The take-away message is clear: Canadians do not understand the politics of science.

Their scientists reviewed our scientific justification for using rBST in dairy cows and found it laughable. Accusations made by Health Canada (the FDA's counterpart) include:

- The data package submitted for review is "extremely scant and sketchy."
- "The review procedures that apply to new drug submissions do not appear to have been followed."
- The approval process appears to disregard all concerns for human safety.
- There is no evidence that supports the FDA's conclusion that "rBST poses no hazard to human health."
- Monsanto pursues aggressive marketing tactics, compensates farmers for veterinary bills associated with rBST use and covers up negative trial results.
- The adverse effects to the rBST treated animals are well documented. The drug is deleterious to herd health and used only for economic benefit.

International relationships might improve if the Canucks followed the basic rules of political etiquette. A bogus "our committee will call your committee" would have been sufficient.

> "Truth will *always* be truth, regardless of lack of *understanding, disbelief, or ignorance.*"
>
> W. Clement Stone (1902-2002) American philanthropist and self-help author

CORNFUSED

GM corn produces its own pesticide. Genes from bacteria are inserted into corn DNA that stimulate the production of a toxin called Bt protein. The toxin destroys the gut lining of insects. Spores germinate and cause death within a couple of days.[35]

Genetic modification transforms corn from a plant into a *plant-pesticide* hybrid. You cannot wash the toxins off. Manufacturers (Monsanto) assure the FDA that the human digestive system can safely eliminate the toxin from the body.

There is no research that supports that assurance. To the contrary, a group of Canadian doctors found that 93 percent of pregnant mothers and 80 percent of umbilical cord blood tested positive for the Bt protein.[36] There is also evidence that the Bt protein damages the liver and kidneys,[37] destroys red blood cells, disrupts clotting and causes organ and tissue damage in mice.[38]

The FDA's approval of Bt corn is not justified.

Over 85 percent of the corn in the US is genetically modified to produce the Bt protein. Furthermore, upwards of 75 percent of all processed foods on supermarket shelves contain GM corn.[39]

BUZZ KILL

In 2006, GM corn manufacturers began coating seeds with a *neonicotinoid*. This insecticide affects the central nervous system of insects, causing paralysis and death. Coating the seed prior to planting allows the chemical to penetrate the plant as it grows, eliminating the need for further application. The machines that plant the corn use air pressure to shoot the seed into the ground. The force of the impact consequently blows toxic dust into the surrounding air. The concentration level of the toxin in the air after planting is 700,000 times what a honeybee can survive.[40]

In 2007, one year after the introduction of this new technique, up to 90 percent of the honeybee populations disappeared in areas surrounding its use.[41] This sounded alarm bells amid growing concerns that insecticides pose significant threat to the health of our ecosystem. Essential crops such as berries, nuts, fruits and vegetables rely on honeybees for pollination.[42]

Few scientists are willing to directly attribute what has been termed the *colony collapse disorder* to the use of neonicotinoids. Monsanto (and Bayer CropScience AG)[43] protect their patented products with the ferocity of a mamma bear. But poking the beehive only to find dead bees will have grave consequences. The disturbing findings have prompted the European Commission to ban this class of insecticide for a period of two years. They are calling for conclusive evidence that proves them safe before re-approving the product.[44]

I guess they'll be getting their data from the United States. Our EPA (Environmental Protection Agency) has chosen to re-evaluate the chemicals *without* restricting its use.

Watch and learn, Europe. And Godspeed to the honeybees.

Godspeed to us all, actually. Conventional American agriculture is threatening the health of the entire planet. Albert Einstein warned, "If the bee disappeared off the surface of the globe, then man would have only four years of life left. No more bees, no more pollination, no more plants, no more animals, no more man."

SOYCLONE

We grow and use almost as much soy as we do corn in America. Nearly 94 percent is genetically modified. Either a lot of people are overstocked on soy sauce or it's found in far more foods than we realize. Most GM soybeans are used to make vegetable oils. This includes the partially hydrogenated varieties that are so dangerous. Concerned moms worry that giving soymilk to little boys will lead to man boobs. But the large amount of soy hidden in cookies, crackers and processed foods is a much more dangerous threat.

Studies have shown that GM soy can trigger allergic reactions in children

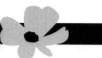

who are *not* allergic to non-GM soy. The immune system of the plant has been altered to produce a protein that is similar to the allergens in shrimp and dust mites. This genetic modification allows the plant to survive large doses of the companion herbicide Roundup. But the mutation may play a key role in many types of human allergic reactions, including peanut allergies and life-threatening anaphylactic shock.[45]

GM soy consumption is linked to more than just allergies. Studies show that it may trigger disorders like irritable bowel syndrome, digestion problems, chronic fatigue, headaches, lethargy, acne and eczema.[46] This may be due to the fact that Roundup-Ready GM soy requires far more herbicide than non-GM soy. These toxins accumulate in plant cells, which makes it impossible to simply wash away the concerns. Farmers wear full-body hazard protection suits when they handle these chemicals. Yet we eat them with nothing more than a napkin to wipe our mouth.

Secret Soy

Store baked goods and baking mixes

- candy
- cereal
- chocolate
- deli meats
- energy and nutrition bars
- imitation dairy foods
- ice cream
- infant formula
- margarine
- mayonnaise
- meat products with fillers
- nutritional supplements and vitamins
- peanut butter
- protein powders
- sauces
- gravies and soups
- smoothies
- vegetarian meat substitutes such as veggie burgers and imitation meats

Many ingredients in processed foods may contain soy:

- bulking agent
- gum arabic
- guar gum
- lecithin
- natural flavoring
- stabilizer
- thickener
- vegetable oil
- shortening
- starch
- vitamin E
- chicken and vegetable broth
- bouillon cubes and MSG

Learn how to identify MSG on food labels on page 65.

ColleenKachmann.com/members

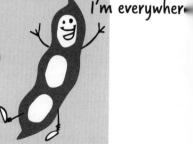

I'm everywhere

The statement that genetically engineered crops reduce the use of pesticides is a lie. Pesticide use has doubled since the introduction of GM crops. And their sales provide the income that sustains their destructive impact.

Consumer Fraud

Genetically engineered crops are not miraculous inventions that will save the world. In fact, they are leading to our demise. GM crops require more pesticides and herbicides, not less. The attempt to manipulate Mother Nature has produced super weeds, super bugs, and highly resistant bacteria and viruses. The destruction of essential biodiversity is impossible to deny.[47] And the introduction of these chemicals to our food supply has coincided with a huge increase in human disease.

And for what? Twenty years' worth of data shows that GM crops offer little to no improvement in yields.[48] Ah, but the yield of profit to Big Agriculture is well documented.

Nearly 80 percent of the processed foods in America contain GM ingredients. Consumers are unaware of the growing evidence that offers more questions than answers and even proof of harm.[49] Many scientists now believe that GMOs trigger the inflammation that is at the root of most modern diseases.[50,51] The correlating data for this legitimate theory cannot be dismissed.

Since the turn of the 21st century the number of Americans suffering from chronic diseases has more than doubled.[52] Asthma, heart disease, autoimmune disorders and diabetes are overwhelming us. Infant mortality is increasing. The health of our nation is in a downward spiral.

Other countries around the world are taking action. In 2015, nineteen countries have banned the cultivation of GM crops.[53] Sixty-five countries have laws that require GM ingredients to be listed on food labels. Yet in America, the majority of consumers don't even know what the GMO acronym means. This is not because our citizens don't care. American food producers spend a lot of money to ensure that their right to profit trumps our right for information.

Even the impoverished people of Haiti are more educated on this issue. After the 2010 earthquake devastated farms, over 10,000 people took to the streets to support the farmers who rejected a donation of $4 million worth of Monsanto's hybrid seeds.[54] The seeds require an application of a highly toxic

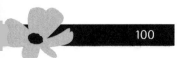

GMO Labeling Around the World

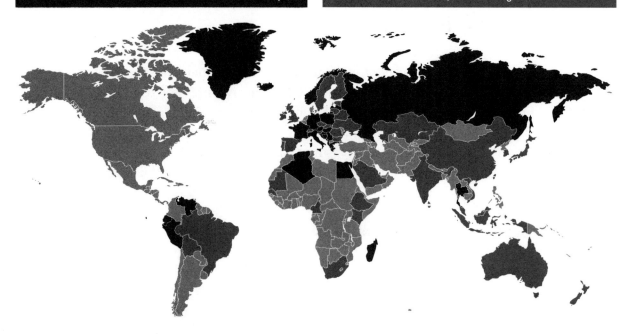

fungicide. Protective clothing must be worn when it's applied. In America the fungicide is sold only for professional use. It is deemed too dangerous for nonprofessionals. Novice gardeners and small farmers may not read the directions or take the necessary precautions.

The Haitians wanted to rebuild their crops with sustainable farming practices. They did not accept the poisonous handout that would ruin what little quality soil they had left.[55] Good for them. Our people and our farms deserve the same choice.

The United States is a country founded on freedom. But the Bill of Rights does not include the freedom to know what's in the food and products that we purchase. Corporate America has revoked our access to this information. We debate an individual's right to access healthcare, yet fail to ask why our nation is so sick. It is apparent that our laws contribute more to corporate profit than individual wellbeing.

Grass root movements are fighting for our freedom. Currently, eight counties in the states of California, Oregon and Washington do not allow GM seeds to be planted. Legislation is being introduced in many states that will require GMOs to be identified on food labels. Activists are working hard to spread the word. What can you do? Vote with your dollars. Boycott deception.

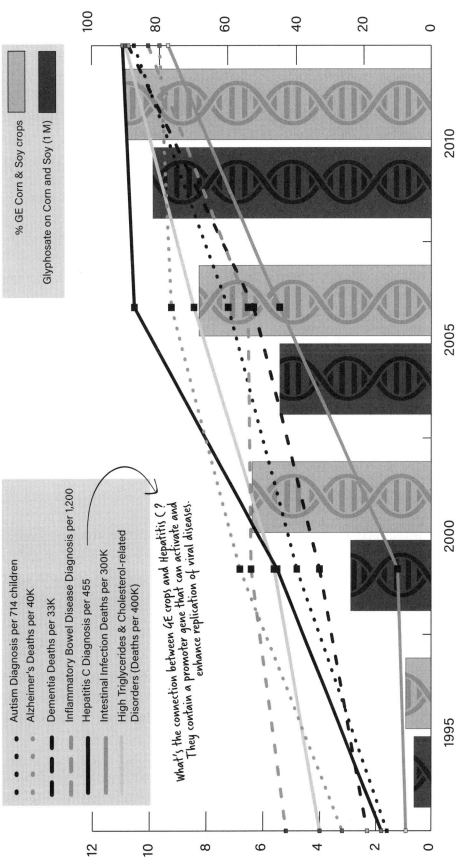

RISING DISEASE RATES AND ROUNDUP READY CROPS

There is no proof of safety for genetically engineered crops or their companion herbicide, glyphosate. Analysis shows a highly significant correlation between the alarming increases of 22 diseases (only 7 shown here) and the increased use of these products. Unfortunately, the burden is on the public to provide proof of harm.[56]

 (ColleenKachmann.com/members)

In 2012, the state of Washington brought Initiative 522 to the voters. The law would have required "clear and conspicuous" disclosure of genetically modified ingredients. Forty-nine percent of people voted in favor of this. But political opposition proved too costly and brutal in this inaugural battle. The opposition spent over $22 million to block the mandate. Monsanto, Dow, Kellogg, Nestle, Pepsico and Coca Cola flooded airwaves and mailboxes with propaganda. Fifty-one percent of voters believed the law would hurt small farmers and make food more expensive for working families.[57]

Are we gullible enough to believe that profitable corporations are spending millions of dollars to protect small farms and working families? No successful corporation spends shareholder's earnings to save their competitors. Where does Big Food get the money for these feigned altruistic endeavors? Go look inside your pantry. Is your own grocery money undermining your freedom?

Food producers proclaim their ingredients are safe. If they are so confident, why do they oppose label laws and the consumers right to know? Label laws were also defeated on California's Proposition 37. The $27.3 million spent on the "vote no" propaganda overwhelmed the mere $2.8 million raised to "vote yes."[58]

These defeats are fueling the passions of consumer activists. Everyday people like you and me are heeding the call to action. In 2015, Vermont took the honor of being the first state to pass a label law. Go Vermont! But one victory does not end the war. Quite the contrary. Monsanto's official response was to express dismay at a law that "creates confusion and uncertainty for consumers."

Monsanto claims to be protecting the consumer by hiding information behind a curtain of patronizing assertions. Evidently, the company has decided that we American Consumers are not qualified to participate in a free market economy.

Excuse me?

Monsanto is taking legal action against the state of Vermont. And label laws are the smallest of their concerns. Their long-term strategy is to lobby for "a friendlier, pre-emptive set of federal rules."[59] They intend to nullify state and individual rights.

In 2013, Congress passed a spending bill to provide temporary funding for government programs. Many lawmakers did not read beyond the "business as usual" language. The fine print is referred to as the "Monsanto Protection Act." The bill restricted federal courts from interfering with the sale or planting of GMO seeds, even if they prove harmful to consumers.[60] The message is clear: Profitable corporations can disable the federal courts by lobbying Congress.

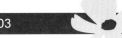

Big Business is holding us hostage. We will only know real freedom when we wake up aware; aware of the evidence, aware of the behind-the-scene players, and aware of the dire consequences of greed.

Monsanto, and the rest of the Big Six, wants to stifle the free flow of information. The only way to stop them is to stifle their free flow of cash. You deserve the right to know what's in your food. No human studies have shown that genetically modified crops are safe. Independent research emerges on a regular basis that says they are not. Yet the FDA continues to allow non-trustworthy corporations to vouch for products that generate billions in revenue. The official FDA policy is, "Ultimately, it is the food producer who is responsible for assuring safety."[61]

That statement is false. Only one person is responsible for assuring the safety of your food. Grab a mirror and introduce yourself.

And please boycott GMO Products - if only on principle.

Proof of Harm

The significant correlations between GE Roundup Ready Crops and rising disease rates are NOT coincidence.

Glyphosate is the active ingredient in Roundup. It is the most widely used herbicide for urban, industrial, forest and farm use in the world. It's in the air, water and food, and accumulates in our bodies.

Glyphosate:

- inhibits the body's ability to remove toxins and enhances their effect. The negative impact manifests slowly over time as inflammation damages cells throughout the body.
- may activate viruses like Hepatitis C and HIV by introducing proteins required for their replication and interfering with the uptake of nutrients that inhibit immunity.
- damages DNA, causing mutations that lead to cancer.
- builds up in the tissues of humans and animals, which means eating meat and dairy increases our exposure. Chronically ill people have high residues of glyphosate in their urine.
- kills the beneficial bacteria in our gut, leading to a steep rise in intestinal diseases.
- blocks and mimics hormones, which disrupts normal functions. As hormones work in very small doses, low-dose exposure over long periods of time leads to very serious illnesses.

The industry has not proven GE crops or the corresponding herbicides to be safe. The burden is on the public to show proof of harm.

FIGHT BACK

Our food supply has been hijacked. Regardless of what you choose to eat, you have the right to know what the ingredients are. Check out these websites, follow them on social media and join your local chapter. Lend your voice.

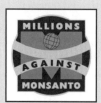

Millions Against Monsanto:
https://www.organicconsumers.org/campaigns/millions-against-monsanto
https://www.facebook.com/millionsagainst

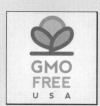

GMO Free
http://gmofreeusa.org
http://www.youtube.com/user/gmofreeusa

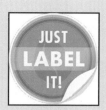

Just Label It
http://justlabelit.org
https://www.facebook.com/justlabelit

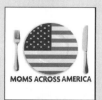

Moms Across America
http://momsacrossamerica.com
https://www.facebook.com/MomsAcrossAmerica

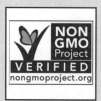

Non-GMO Project
http://www.nongmoproject.org
https://www.facebook.com/nongmoproject

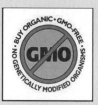

GMO Awareness
http://gmo-awareness.com
https://www.facebook.com/gmoawarenessusa

 ColleenKachmann.com/members

Speak Up

Enter your zip code on the "Just Label It" website to connect with Congress, the FDA and Big Food. Pre-written emails and petitions make expressing your opinion almost effortless.

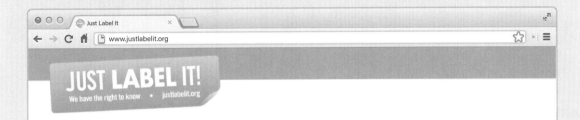

Tell the Senate: Label GMOs on the package!

Stand with Just Label It and tell your senators you want to see a GMO labeling solution without loopholes!

There's a compromise in the Senate that would craft the nation's first mandatory GMO labeling system. As written, this compromise might not even apply to ingredients derived from GMO soybeans and GMO sugar beets.

Tell your senators that you won't stand for Big Food's tricks and you want to see a GMO labeling solution without loopholes.

Use this form to tell your senators to support true mandatory GMO labeling today!

Subject:

Support GMO Labeling without loopholes

Your Letter:

As a Just Label It supporter, I support mandatory GMO labeling on the package, not just high-tech gimmicks.

Americans have a right to know what they're eating — just like consumers in 64 other nations. We shouldn't have to own smartphones to know what's in our food or how it was grown.

The current compromise before the Senate would not only allow food companies to hide GMOs using QR codes, but it would also exclude ingredients derived from GMOs, like soybean oil.

As your constituent, I urge you to support a mandatory GMO labeling solution without loopholes.

Normal vs Healthy

What foods do you eat that contain genetically modified corn, and diary? Think beyond your own kitchen. Include food in restaurants, at work, on-the-go-convenience and in other peoples homes.

How will you reduce consumption of genetically modified foods?

Vegetarian, dairy and gluten-free foods can masquerade as healthy options. If it's not organic, it's likely filled with genetically modified and artificial ingredients. What foods have fooled you?

If you have to ask about the food on your plate, don't eat it. Organic foods are clearly identified. Identify the possible sources of hidden GMOs in your diet and investigate them.

 ColleenKachmann.com/members

PS I left this facing page blank for you.
Fill it with whatever you like. Questions, comments, to-do's, thoughts, etc.
You're welcome . . .

Chapter 6

Prescriptions for Pain

"The doctor of the future will give no medication but instead instruct his patients in the care of the human body, knowing that diet is both the cause and prevention of disease."

THOMAS EDISON (1847-1931)
AMERICAN INVENTOR AND DEDICATED VEGETARIAN

MORE MEDICATION. MORE HEALTHCARE.

The last time I got a flu shot was in 2009. That year, the anticipated swine flu was the lead story on every news channel. The H1N1 virus had the potential to be a modern reenactment of the 1918 pandemic.

The Spanish flu killed 50 million people worldwide. Healthy adults between the ages of 20 and 50 years were most susceptible, perishing within 24 hours of falling ill. Most of the afflicted were WW1 soldiers in the trenches and civilians living with terrible wartime sanitary and nutritional conditions. The virus claimed more lives over a 24-week period than the AIDS virus has in 24 years.[1]

The vaccine for H1N1 was hailed as the promised savior. But expected shortages appeared to be a significant threat to public health.

Prior to the sensationalized pandemic and subsequent national emergency, I held little regard for the flu shot. If I happened upon an opportunity to the get the vaccine, I took it. If I waited too long or forgot, I didn't worry. Each year, I either got the flu or I didn't. From my perspective, the two seemed unrelated.

But it was impossible to remain apathetic to the risks of the impending swine flu. The simmering anxiety was infectious.

Healthcare officials urged everyone to get the shot. Each day, grocery stores, banks and schools hung updated notices in their windows. Television and radio announcers described the symptoms along with reports of confirmed and suspected cases.

Manufacturers could not keep up with the demand. There would not be enough vaccine for everyone.

A media-provoked frenzy gripped the community. Schoolwork was forgotten. Public meetings were canceled. Everything was on hold. The focus was singular and clear: get that flu shot or die trying.

When a clinic announced the arrival of a fresh batch, mobs of people swarmed before the doors even opened. Friends and neighbors bartered inside information in hushed conversations. Several times, I waited for hours with my four children only to hear the last shot had just been given to someone ahead of us.

As I shuffled through the long lines of fellow anxious customers, my sense of impending doom gave way to skepticism. The national emergency seemed surreal. What if this was just another flu season?

I observed. I listened. I began to wonder.

What if I didn't watch the news or read the paper? What if I failed to ask "how high?" when the officials instructed me to "Jump!" Would I perish in ignorance? Or would I either get the flu or not, and live to tell the tale?

I was unaware that a similar scenario had occurred thirty years earlier.

In 1976, it was believed the swine flu caused the influenza pandemic in 1918-19. (We now know it was an avian virus.) When autopsy reports for a single soldier at Fort Dix revealed the H1N1 virus, vaccine makers sprang to action. The government purchased 150 million doses of the vaccine. President Gerald Ford announced the, "Get a Shot of Protection" campaign to inoculate every man woman and child from the swine flu.[2]

The vaccine was problematic. It had the potential to cause neurological problems such as Guillain-Barré syndrome, a disease involving muscle weakness, paralysis and sometimes death. The government knew this, but did not disclose the risks. (Sometimes fear is profitable; sometimes it is not.) Instead, Americans were pressured to help prevent the spread of the virus. Public Service Announcements urged everyone to, "Get the shot. Just roll up your sleeve."[3] Famous people appeared in advertisements to foster an "everyone who's anyone is doing it" mentality.

Some celebrity names were used without permission. When Mary Tyler Moore saw her name listed as one of the vaccinated, she went on record to correct the lie.

Before the program was halted, 46 million doses were distributed. There was no pandemic, epidemic or even outbreak. However, 4000 claims were made for injuries caused by the vaccine.

Unaware of any of this, I joined the herd in 2009 and got the shot. Joining the crowd was easier than standing alone. Nevertheless, three weeks later I was among the casualties of the traditional cold and flu season that tumbles through communities like falling dominoes.

I commiserated with fellow suffers. But I stopped short of giving thanks to vaccine manufacturers for bestowing partial protection via the better-late-than-never flu shot. (Though I was on my knees praying to the toilet god to please make it stop.)

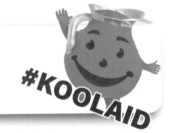

I tried being normal once. Worst two minutes of my life.

#KOOLAID

Something changed for me that year. I stopped believing what I now perceive as total bullshit. I turned off the television. I recycle the newspaper before it gets opened. I've stopped listening to the warnings of illness and risks of disease layered between the reports of natural disasters and horrific crimes. These stories no longer serve any purpose for me. I now view fear-based entertainment as a vehicle that delivers political and financial capital for the powers that be.

My new policy became an old cliché: No news is good news. If something requires attention, I trust it will arouse mine. I operate on a need-to-know basis. Staying "educated" on all of the extraneous threats puts the common consumer at an emotional disadvantage. Mental energy is better invested in efforts that lead to happiness, hope and health.

Ignoring the negative chatter goes against the social norms. It's normal to watch bad news while eating bad food. Once I realized this, my hypothesis was born: being normal is inversely proportional to being happy and healthy.

PRESCRIPTIONS FOR PAIN

The Immunity Challenge: Use It or Lose It

Society's germ-o-phobic culture is weakening the herd. We sanitize our hands, cough into our elbow and stay home for 24 hours after a fever ends. Yet every year, cold and flu season arrives as expected. Most of us get sick at some point despite the vitamins, exercise and immunizations that promise to protect us.

Safety standards dictate that everything we purchase be sterilized, homogenized, pasteurized and disinfected. But our hyper-hygiene efforts do not appear to deliver the desired outcome. These practices indeed reduce our exposure to everyday microbes. The problem is that many of these microbes are necessary and beneficial. In fact, a well-balanced gut flora is essential to the health of our digestive and immune systems. We're killing the good with the bad.

The ability to fight infection improves with exposure to germs. Like the brain and muscles, the immune system gets stronger when challenged. You can't train for a marathon by driving the race route. You don't learn to ride a bike by pedaling a stationary. As with any skill, use it or lose it. Healing is a practice.

It's impossible for modern day medicine to provide protection from the constantly evolving viruses and bacteria that we come into contact with every day. Even quarantine efforts can be contaminated. Traveling to a foreign country where rare pathogens are life-threatening is one thing. I'll roll up my sleeve and stick out a vein for the vaccine before my passport is stamped. Otherwise, I prefer to let my immune system handle the day-to-day operations.

> **HEALING is a matter of *time*. But sometimes, it's a matter of *opportunity*.**
>
> Hippocrates (c. 460-370 BC) considered the Father of Western Medicine

When I feel a case of the sniffles coming on, I embrace the challenge. I don't avoid sick people. I don't need to. I give them a hug, boost my diet with antioxidants and probiotics and tell my body it's "game on."

The first day of school each year is bittersweet. I am not unhappy watching my sweet babes trudge to the bus stop in the warm glow of the dawning sun. Lazy summer days are replaced with football games, bonfires and baked cinnamon apples. I try to hide my excitement as I kiss them goodbye. I embrace the peaceful quiet as the door clicks shut.

But the respite fades when they trample through the door in the bright afternoon, already sniffling from exposure to a plethora of new germs. There is excited chatter of new rules, mean teachers and old friends. Colorful stacks of "Welcome to (X+1) Grade" papers are dumped onto the counter. And hidden amongst the cheery introductions are the god-awful, heinous "supply lists." Mandates for hard-to-find essentials are the epitome of mommy hell.

I grab the lists and pile my four young hooligans into the car. I realize too late that I make the same mistake every year: I allow them to come so they can "help." I peruse the requirements. One kid needs 52 crayons. But they come in packs of 48. Another needs five plain pocket folders, each in a different color. We find only four colors in that style. Next? Four large glue sticks (sold in three-packs).

"Can we just get six small ones?" I ask.

The response is a chorus of, "No!"

One teacher requires 27 colored pencils. They are sold in boxes of 12 or 24.

"Is this a misprint?" There is a pleading tone in my voice. My brain is starting to hurt.

"Not a chance, mom," The middle child's voice is certain. "The teacher said we must follow the directions."

The pressure is intense. If I screw this up, any bad grade will be my fault. (Will I get partial credit for good grades? Nope. I'll get billed for their efforts.)

Each kid is asked to contribute three bottles of hand sanitizer, two boxes of tissues (square only, please) and one roll of paper towels. Additional items include things like hair samples from a squirrel, a 3.1" by 8.6" (exactly) picture of themselves with the mayor, and a family genealogy map that spans 18 generations.

We are at the first store for three hours. We go to other stores for things we couldn't find. I do the best I can to meet the demands. Ok, I might cheat a little. What? The 27 colored pencils had three repeats? Hmm. My bad.

I do refuse one request, however. I will not buy the hand sanitizer. And I tell my kids not to use it. (Yeah, I'm *that* mom.) Why do I take issue with disinfectant? Don't I know that kids touch toilet seats and then pick their nose? Yes. I'm well aware. But I also know that common sanitizers contain the bactericide *triclosan*.

Triclosan is toxic. Yet it's everywhere. It's on the wipes provided to decontaminate grocery carts. It's used in promotional products and passed out with company logo pens. Travel sized bottles are in our handbags, cars and desks. Industrial sized bottles are expected on counters of businesses, public bathrooms and restaurants. It's also found in soap, toothpaste and deodorant.

This powerful chemical doesn't just kill germs. It has been shown to interfere with muscle function and alter hormone regulation.[4] It suppresses thyroid function and accumulates in our fat cells. It also increases the risk of drug-resistance to antibiotics. Research has shown that triclosan is no more effective than simple soap and water for preventing infectious disease.[5] Yet most of us use it every day because we are not aware of the risks.

I send a bar of soap with each kid and attend Back to School Night incognito.

Our commitment for cleanliness and medications is not keeping us healthy. It is making us sick.

Drugs Don't Cure Disease

Consider that many of our ailments are more complicated than they appear. Most disorders and diseases do not have a single cause or culprit. Our genes, environmental irritants, infection and even stress are factors that co-create our susceptibility to illness. Doctors often prescribe pills that control symptoms. But if this approach was effective, why are so many medicated people still suffering? Medications can restore our productivity and allow us to "keep going" for a little or even a long time. But drugs affect the *entire* body and have many off-the-label consequences. Just when one problem seems curtailed, another pops up. It's a life and death game of Whack-a-Mole.

As a culture, we're conditioned to think that illness is something that happens to us. Yeah, we could all eat better and lose a little weight. Yet there is collective acceptance that disease is inevitable. We might prolong our health with due diligence to diet and exercise, but if disease is our fate, the inevitable is only delayed.

TAKE THE IMMUNITY CHALLENGE:
STAY WELL DURING COLD/FLU SEASON

Avoid sugar. Fructose is fertilizer for pathogenic bacteria, yeast and fungi. An unbalanced gut flora disables the immune system. Take a probiotic and eat lots of colorful vegetables to maximize your defense.

Use a Neti Pot. No one likes the sensation of water in the nose. But a two-second sting beats clogged sinuses. Mix about ½ tsp. salt into 8 oz of lukewarm distilled water. Tilt your head and pour into one nostril. It will run out the other and down your throat. Repeat on the other side. Do this preventively or at symptom onset. It works.

Drink more water. Urine should be lightly colored with no smell (unless you just ate asparagus). Water improves liver and kidney function, flushing the system and preventing stagnant germs from breeding.

Gargle with salt water. Or dilute three percent hydrogen peroxide in a one to one blend. Kill those throat germs!

Sweat! Cardiovascular exercise increases white blood cell activity. Heavy breathing clears the lungs of allergens. (Sex counts, if you do it right.)

Take breathing breaks. Exhaling deeply stimulates flushing of the lymph nodes.[6] Breathe into the belly then contract the abdominals to force all the air out of the lungs.

Lemons are a clown car full of vitamins and minerals. Drink lemon water at room temperature or even lukewarm. Lemons boost immunity, reduce inflammation, keep the skin clear and help fight viral infection.

Place a few drops of diluted oregano oil under the tongue. It wards of fungus and viral infections and reduces Candida (yeast) and parasites. It tastes terrible but it works miracles. If you can't handle the intense flavor, add oregano oil to a vaporizer. Inhale as you work or sleep.

Zinc taken within 24 hours of symptom onset reduces the duration of cold symptoms. Zinc lozenges offer maximum absorption (versus tablet or syrup).[7]

Garlic inhibits the growth of many harmful microbials. It counteracts Gram-negative and Gram-positive bacteria, including drug-resistant stains of E. coli. It's particularly effective ainst Candida albicans (yeast overgrowth). It also counteracts human intestinal parasites.[8]

Sleep more. The body restores and repairs itself during uninterrupted rest. Use an old-fashioned alarm (don't take your phone to bed) and sleep for seven to eight hours a night. The benefits of beauty sleep are well documented.

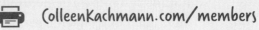

ColleenKachmann.com/members

The belief that illness is inevitable is wrong. Emerging research proves that what we eat and how we live have the most significant influence on our health. Many diseases can be avoided, managed and even reversed with diet and lifestyle changes alone. For example, cholesterol medications effectively lower cholesterol for most people. But so will a diet based on plants (cholesterol free) and whole foods (no refined sugars or grains). Exercise and quality sleep also keep us well.

While statins (the class of drug used to manage cholesterol) may appear to help, they undoubtedly create other problems. Nearly 900 studies show that statins can cause liver damage, kidney failure, Type 2 diabetes, neurological problems, muscle degeneration and erectile dysfunction.[9] Furthermore, statins require a lifetime commitment. They only control cholesterol for as long as you take them. And the risks of negative side effects increase over time.

In contrast, there are never adverse consequences to positive changes in diet and lifestyle.

The bottom line is that our approach to health care is outdated. Medical pioneers in the early 20th century developed antibiotics and vaccines. They were able to eradicate infectious diseases as the leading cause of death in a single generation. This amazing accomplishment saved countless lives. However, modern medicine is out of balance. Our sterile environment eliminates the good germs with the bad. Overkill on inoculations has impaired our innate ability to fight for ourselves.

> "Let *food* by thy medicine.
> Let *medicine* by thy food."
> — Hippocrates

Less than 100 years after the invention of penicillin, 80 percent of ailments qualify as chronic disorders. Unlike strep throat, symptoms do not have a single cause. And the pill-for-the-ill approach does not offer a cure. Anti-inflammatories may reduce the swelling and pain in our joints, but arthritis is not the result of an acetaminophen-deficiency. Drugs are designed to promote, alter or block a specific process in the body. When these same functions are altered in healthy organs, symptoms metamorphose into alternate disorders.

The western approach to health fails to acknowledge that every system in the body connects to the others. For example, it is considered normal for males over 50 to consult a urologist for the awkward issue of erectile dysfunction. But a lack of blood flow to a peripheral organ is often an early symptom of vascular disease (the buildup of cholesterol in the arteries). You may look and feel sexy enough to warrant a daily dose of Viagra, but the problem isn't in your penis.

The disease delusion[10] in America is that illness is mostly an expression of our genetic makeup. Extensive risk forms that document family histories aren't as significant as we've been lead to believe. Genes don't cause most illnesses. Drugs don't cure disease. We must address the environmental and lifestyle factors that co-create disease if we want to heal.

Consider the BRCA gene. In 2013, women who carry this gene have an 85 percent increased risk of a breast cancer diagnosis. That is terrifying. Courageous, high profile women reveal they've undergone double mastectomies to avoid the nearly inevitable.[11] But in 1940, the BRCA mutation indicated only a 24 percent risk increase of cancer.[12] How can this be? It's the same gene. Yes, but our environment is quite different.

Gene expression is turned on and off by the environment. I may have the gene for exquisite beauty but I have yet to be diagnosed as a supermodel. We have the power to create our health (or lack thereof). Our state of wellness is influenced by more than just who sneezed on us or what diseases run in our family. Wellness is the cumulative effect of exponential variables. It is critical to understand what those variables are in order to maximize our potential in life.

Hippocrates reveals the irony of modern medicine. People used to think that suffering was punishment from the gods. Most Americans no longer believe that. But many of us do believe the Creator designs our DNA. The assumption that genes cause illness is a 2000-year setback. Hippocrates was right. Unfortunately, the modern medical oath that bears his name does not honor his convictions. Genetics and the pathogens that cause infection do not have the final say in determining our state of health. Immune function, stress levels and what we put in (and on) our bodies are just as important.

I have eliminated "junk" from my diet. I fight illness with nourishment. The results are clear. I look and feel better in my 40s than I did in my 20s. I agree with Hippocrates. Food is medicine. I take food as serious as I take drugs. I'd rather be hungry than eat chemical ingredients. Processed food is not food. Processed foods are poison.

I am no longer under the impression that health and beauty can be purchased. The industrial age sparked a culture of consumption. The digital revolution rapid-fires us with scientifically enhanced merchandise. Fortified food labels promise complete nutrition. Cosmetic labels promise to reverse the aging process. Medication labels promise to relieve symptoms. Satisfaction is guaranteed (side effects notwithstanding). Yet, we are facing a national health crisis. This reveals the truth. We've been blinded by false hope and poisoned with false assurance. Comfort food, feel-good pills, and smell-good supplies are contaminating the proverbial fountain of youth.

Look beyond the labels. Take off the blinders. Life is filled with chemicals. People are plagued with disorders. Connect the dots.

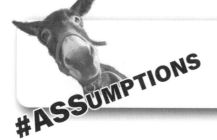

#ASSUMPTIONS Whenever you see the words "fat-free" or "low-fat" think "chemical shitstorm."

Man or Machine?

The body is a biological machine. It functions properly when internal pulleys are oiled and gears turn at the appropriate speed. If screws are corroded, the nuts and bolts won't hold them in place. Henry Ford didn't invent the assembly line; he simply copied the concept from Mother Nature.

In a factory, if the product that comes off the assembly line isn't right, production grinds to a halt. Blaming the flaw on the last guy on the line is futile. The entire process must be examined for flaws. Perhaps a third-party supplier has delivered defective parts. Maybe maintenance failed to fix a machine or someone fell asleep on the job. One problem renders the entire system inadequate.

Our health is also an assembly line product. No organ, tissue or cell is self-sufficient. The whole body is one organism, not a collection of independent systems. Disorder occurs long before illness manifests. The body has remarkable capacity to compensate for shortages, recover from injury and fight infection. But even small deficiencies will eventually have a negative impact on overall health.

If a car comes off the line with a defect that costs lives, the company with its name on the bumper is ultimately held responsible. It is the same with your health. Every choice you make today has influence on tomorrow.

Side Effects Included

For most of my life, I dismissed the potential side effects listed on warning labels. Side effects occur in old, sick and hypochondriac people. I'm young, healthy and have a high tolerance for pain. Also, I'm super smart. Isn't taking acetaminophen before drinking wine standard protocol in hangover prevention?

Physicians are experts of human anatomy and physiology. They work with pharmaceutical reps who sell medications and bioengineering firms that specialize in diagnostic tools. They are trained to evaluate symptoms as signs of disease. They learn how to treat diseases with available products. The medical community is a commercialized system. The reality is that doctors aren't trained to manage health; doctors are trained to manage illness.

Look at the simple problem in Med School 101—Pop Quiz. The answer requires only a dose of common sense, but the alternatives offer insight as to why our expensive healthcare system results in very little actual health.

Med School 101—Pop Quiz

If a patient presents with a blister, what is the correct course of treatment?

1. Prescribe anti-inflammatories for the pain. Begin a course of antibiotics to avoid infection. Schedule a follow up visit in a month.
2. Do an extensive risk-factor assessment. Identify family members who are also prone to blisters. Order genetic testing to determine if they have the "blister gene."
3. Refer the patient to a podiatrist to screen for orthopedic anomalies that may indicate the need for surgical intervention.
4. Ask about recent footwear purchases and apply a bandage. Advise them to wear comfortable shoes until the blister heals.

The answer may seem obvious. But in today's world of chronic ailments, common sense isn't all that common.

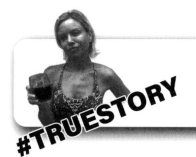

Common Sense is not a gift. It's a punishment because you have to deal with everyone who doesn't have it.

#TRUESTORY

Don't Disable the Fire Alarm

These days, most of us have at least minor health issues. Irritating symptoms are normal. We are not surprised when they seem to get worse each year. It's expected and accepted.

We've all worn the sexy shoes and tried not to wince while we walk. We stop wearing the shoes so the blister can heal. Life goes on. We learn from our mistakes. The next time fashion trumps comfort, we apply a bandage in advance and lose the shoes when it's time to hit the dance floor.

When something bothers you, pain serves as the motivation to remove the irritant. If your sunglasses pinch your nose, take them off. If the music is too loud, turn it down. If small children are ruining the movie, relocate to another part of the theater. (Unless they're your kids, in which case you're probably legally obligated to supervise them. Best to retain licensed counsel or a babysitter before leaving children unattended.)

Ailments are caused by inflammation. Prolonged inflammation generates more inflammation. The cycle self-perpetuates. When this happens, inflammation becomes a disease in and of itself. These diseases usually end in "itis;" arthritis, dermatitis, sinusitis and gingivitis are all caused by inflammation.

When allowed to run its natural course, our body's inflammatory response begins and ends as needed. Drugs may provide temporary relief from the pain of inflammation, but they do not provide healing. Medications for inflammation have side effects that affect everyone. Consequences are the trade-off. The longer such drugs are used, the more problems arise as a result.

Pain and inflammation signal that something is wrong. They are Mother Nature's way of getting your attention. Using drugs to control a symptom is like disabling the fire alarm without investigating the source of the smoke. Only our diet can provide the necessary nutrients to counter inflammation naturally. Failing to see that we are what we eat makes us victims of illness and disease. Do you want to be a victim or a survivor? You can't be both.

Recently, my running partner called to cancel our training session because she was coming down with a nasty head cold. Her voice was raspy and nasal. Phlegm choked her painful cough. She wanted to go to the doctor and get an antibiotic. She wanted me to bring her some DayQuil or NyQuil. She didn't care if she got sleepy or wired. She was desperate for anything that might bring relief.

I wanted to help. She may not be able to run, but I wasn't leaving my wingman. (When we run long distances, we wear Top Gun "Maverick" hats. Neither of us answers to "Goose.") I put on my Wonder Woman costume and filled my invisible jet with super-hero antidotes. I landed on her doorstep and followed a trail of crumpled tissues to her bedroom. Her bed-head hair and bloodshot eyes complimented her foul sense of humor.

She could not hide her agitation when she saw the Wonder Woman get-up. "I told you I'm really sick! I'm can't run. I thought you could be nice for once and bring me some medicine. You're not funny." Exasperated, she pulled the covers back over her head.

Undaunted, I headed to her kitchen and got to work.

I made a steaming hot bowl of miso soup and gave her a few drops of pungent oregano oil to put under her tongue. I juiced bright green spinach with fragrant cilantro and a few sweet oranges. A ripe lemon served as the base for my homemade *Nature's Flu Shot*. (The recipe is on page 64.) She took my "medicine" and fell asleep. An hour later, I told her to put on her shoes, if only to stand on the porch for a few minutes. She complied.

> "Shallow men believe in *luck* or *circumstance*. Strong men believe in *cause* and *effect*."
>
> Ralph Waldo Emerson (1803-1882)

It was an overcast day, but rain had infused the moist air with the scents of pine and lavender. She felt refreshed. We decided to "try" a short walk. After a mile, we picked up the pace to a slow run. An hour of deep breathing and laughter served as the final boost her immune system needed. The bad-guy germs that had violated our shared policy to be awesome every day were defeated.

The fact that fighting a cold is exciting to me is twisted. And true.

The experience reinforced the fact that immunity can be strengthened and drugs can be avoided. It now excites me to realize that I might be coming down with something. I fight back and I win. I'm healthy, not immortal. But every time I support my body with nourishment instead of medication, I get stronger.

Inflammation Versus Anti-Inflammatories

We've all experienced inflammation. From mosquito bites and sore throats to sprained ankles and broken bones, the body's response is standard. Painful, swollen and stiff areas are red and warm to the touch and serve as the bright yellow Caution! tape. The internal crime scene is roped off as the defense system is activated.

Inflammation is the body's natural healing process. It stops the bleeding, removes damaged tissue and initiates new cell growth. Increased blood flow to an injured area delivers white blood cells that attack foreign pathogens. Pain demands that we modify our activities until the process is complete.

We've been conditioned to treat the symptoms of inflammation as though they are the problem and not the solution. But popping a pill so that you can continue the activities that are creating the pain make the problem worse. The side effects of medications often trigger more illness. It may be normal to treat common ailments with drugs, but it is not healthy.

The most popular medications have significant drawbacks. Steroids, anti-inflammatories, pain relievers and antibiotics interfere with the body's natural ability to heal.

Steroids like prednisone are frequently used to treat autoimmune disorders and allergies. They relieve the pain and discomfort associated with inflammation. Steroids reduce the activity of the immune system by blocking production of antibodies and histamines. This can prevent organ and tissue damage caused by acute disease. But interfering with the body's ability to heal and protect itself is a slippery slope. Steroids have significant side effects. The more

5-Minute Miso Soup

You don't have to go to a Japanese restaurant for this immune boosting treat. Keep miso paste on hand and make a bowl whenever you feel a chill. Miso also makes a great base for vegetable soups and Asian salad dressings.

INGREDIENTS
- 1 cup water
- 1 Tbsp. miso paste
- Optional: sliced green onions, diced tofu, grated ginger or whatever suits your taste buds

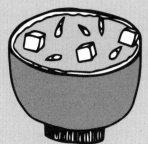

DIRECTIONS
Bring water to a boil. Remove from heat. Cool for about a minute. Boiling temperatures destroy the probiotics. Whisk in the paste and desired additions. Serve immediately.

MISO VARIETIES:
- **White (Shiromiso)** is the least fermented and lowest in salt compared to the other two varieties. The mild, delicate flavor blends well with other ingredients. Great in warm-weather soups, dressings, and light sauces, it can even be used in place of dairy in some recipes (think miso mashed potatoes).
- **Yellow (Shinshumiso)** is fermented slightly longer than white miso, and ranges in color from light yellow to light brown. Flavor is mild, and blends well into soups, glazes and salad dressing.
- **Red (Akamiso)** is fermented longer than other varieties. Red miso is salty and has an assertive, pungent flavor. It's best suited for heartier dishes like rich soups, braises, and marinades or glazes.

6 HEALING PROPERTIES OF MISO:[13]
1. Contains all essential amino acids, similar to an egg minus the 200 mg of cholesterol.
2. Contains probiotics that balance the gut flora, support digestion and enhance immunity.
3. Great source of B_{12}, which is naturally deficient in a plant-based diet.
4. Improves blood quality and lymph fluid. Support detoxification.
5. Captures heavy metals so they can be excreted from the body.
6. High in antioxidants that neutralize free radicals.

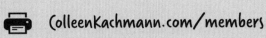

ColleenKachmann.com/members

Side Effects of Steroids[14]

- Weight gain, fluid retention, high blood pressure and the tell-tale rounded "moon face"
- Agitation, irritability and insomnia
- Gastrointestinal bleeding and ulcers, especially when combined with NSAIDS
- Interference in the metabolism of key nutrients, including folic acid, vitamins B_6 and B_{12}, potassium and zinc leaves the body vulnerable to infection.
- Reduced vitamin D and calcium levels interfere with bone development in young people, decrease bone density and lead to osteoporosis.
- Thin skin that bruises easily and a loss of muscle mass
- Elevated blood sugar levels, increased risk of diabetes and heart disease
- Infertility in males and menstrual irregularities in females
- Cataracts and glaucoma

Suppressing Inflammation with NSAIDs:

- inhibits the function of the immune system and increases risk of infection.[15]
- increases frequency and severity of allergic reactions such as rashes, wheezing, throat swelling and gastro-intestinal distress.[16]
- accelerates the breakdown of cartilage in joints, which is especially ironic given that NSAIDs are often used to relieve the pain of osteoarthritis (degeneration of joint cartilage).[17]
- increases hypertension diagnosis by nearly 40 percent.[18]
- triples the incidence of gastro-esophageal reflux disease (GERD) and heartburn symptoms.[19]
- doubles the risk of heart failure. Seniors with a history of heart disease are ten times more likely to experience heart failure.[20]
- reduced blood flow to kidneys, renal dysfunction and failure in those with a history of kidney problems.[21,22]
- may lead to rebound pain after you stop taking them. Headaches and dizziness are symptoms of withdrawal.[23]
- interferes with ovulation. After 10 days of treatment, 93 percent of women taking diclofenac and 75 percent taking naproxen or etoricoxib did not ovulate.[24]

Trying to have a baby? Did you know . . .

ColleenKachmann.com/members

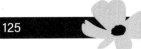

steroids are used, the more detrimental the repercussions.

Non-steroidal anti-inflammatory drugs (NSAIDs) include aspirin, ibuprofen (Advil, Motrin and generics), naproxen sodium (Aleve and others), as well as powerful prescription strength varieties. They relieve pain and control inflammation for as long as they are used. The body's natural cycle of inflammation and anti-inflammation is designed to function without interference. Suppressing the process weakens it. The benefits of short-term symptom relief must be weighed against the long-term consequences.

The most common side effect is stomach upset. When taken with food, and regardless of personal tolerance, regular use leads to the inflammation, ulceration and erosion of the stomach wall and intestines. Aspirin is often used to reduce the long-term risk of coronary artery disease. But the blood-thinning effect increases bleeding and makes it more difficult for wounds to close and heal. Using medication to reduce inflammation can result in serious, prolonged health problems.

Acetaminophen is the most common drug used for pain relief. It is the main ingredient in medications for headache, muscle soreness, cold and flu symptoms and allergies. Free samples are passed out like candy in hospitals and doctors' offices. It's a staple in our first aid kits, medicine cabinets, book bags, briefcases and car consoles. Acetaminophen is the "normal" first line of defense. Yet the drug inhibits the immune system and aggravates the symptoms it's promised to suppress.[25] It may be normal to treat illness with acetaminophen. But it's not healthy.

A single dose of acetaminophen:
- significantly decreases the production of t-cells and b-cell antibodies in the liver. These antibodies destroy foreign invaders, eliminate cells already infected and provide immunity when re-exposure occurs.[26]
- depletes stores of a key liver enzyme (glutathione) that processes toxins, repairs DNA and neutralizes free radicals.[27]
- damages the lining of the lungs and increases the frequency and severity of asthma symptoms.[28]
- stimulates histamine production, which inflames the nose and eyes. Allergic reactions to pollen, dander and ragweed and hay fever are more frequent and severe.[29]

A 2012 European study of acetaminophen use surveyed 20,000 children. The findings indicate the drug is a significant threat to our children. Children ages six to seven years who received the medicine once a year had an increased risk of asthma of 70 percent. Those that were given a dose once a month or more had a 540 percent increase.[30]

Heads up, folks!
When was the last time you gave your child medication that contained acetaminophen? Has your child ever asked for a dose? In light of this information, is it ever justifiable to give this medication to our kids? Think about it.

Aspirin is often combined with NSAIDs or acetaminophen in over-the-counter drug cocktails. Data reveals the combinations of these drugs do more damage to the gut than the sum of their individual effects. Regular use of "cocktail" medications for headaches, arthritis and joint pain and even children's fever medications can lead to ulcers, bleeding ulcers and perforations (holes in the stomach.)[31]

Antibiotics are standard treatment options for many common ailments. They are used to treat colds, ear and sinus infections and stomach bugs. Often, they are prescribed for "just in case" reasons. The problem is that antibiotics destroy good bacteria as well as bad. They cannot discriminate. A balanced microbial flora is essential to the digestive and immune systems. Wiping them out creates a breeding ground for further infection.

Our bodies contain 10 times more microbes (bugs) than human cells.[32] That is a perplexing concept that challenges our core identity. We call ourselves human. In reality, our bodies are predominately microbial. That's a philosophical conundrum better left to the existentialists.

A single course of antibiotics disrupts the delicate balance of the microbe population (gut flora). Negative consequences can linger for years. Essential microorganisms protect us from opportunistic and disease-causing pathogens. Some microbes produce biotin and vitamin K.[33] Others digest food[34] or regulate immunity and inflammation.[35] The destruction of these beneficial bacteria can cause "leaky gut" syndrome. (I'll share my experience with gut disorder in Chapter 10.) When antibiotics wipe out the "good guy" bacteria, foreign invaders multiply without competition. Opportunistic fungus like Candida (yeast) and harmful bacteria then dominate the bowels. This initiates an inflammatory response that can become systemic and impede other systems in the body.

Antibiotics are not inherently bad. Most certainly, they can and do save lives. But if your life is not in danger, it's best to let your body fight infections. A healthy immune system is built over time. A course of antibiotics is a serious setback. If you want a strong immune system, allow it to be challenged. Use it or lose it.

"Good Guy" Microbes Do Good Things[36]

- break down undigested carbohydrates via fermentation
- enhance absorption of fatty acids
- contribute to the synthesis of vitamin K and the B vitamins
- metabolize bile acids, cholesterol and fats
- compete with pathogenic microbes for nutrients
- keep the lining of the gut healthy and intact
- train the immune system to differentiate between pathogens and non-harmful antigens, reducing severity and frequency of allergic reactions

 ColleenKachmann.com/members

Well Baby Visits

The glossy brochures presented to expectant parents gave me the impression that giving birth would commence a luxurious spa-like weekend. A private, state-of-the-art birthing suite touted five-star accommodations, concierge service and valet parking. Pain-free labor and a plethora of caring staff would facilitate the blessed event. Elegant menu options included champagne, caviar and sea-salt truffles. I would enjoy a full night's sleep while my newborn received round-the-clock care in the soothing ambiance of the neo-natal nursery.

The stark contrast with reality was evident the moment my water broke.

Cuffs, belts and clamps strapped to my body monitored blood pressure, contractions and oxygen. A tourniquet was tied around my bicep so that my veins would rise to the surface. Needles were jabbed into my arms and spine and secured to my body with tape. I was afraid to move lest I jar something loose and have to go through it all again. Tiny lights of all colors blinked in cadence with irritating beeps and buzzing vibrations. A revolving door of personnel fanned the antiseptic air that was filled with questions.

"On a scale of one to ten, how is your pain?"

"Can I see your insurance card?"

"Would you like steak or shrimp after baby is born?"

The intrusions intensified after the new little patient took his first breath.

Security bracelets were attached. Safety policies were explained. Medications were administered. Ointments were applied to every orifice on both of our bodies. I peed into a measuring cup; my baby's diapers were weighed. Breast milk and poop were evaluated. I had to watch videos about shaken baby syndrome and proper car seat use. For 48 hours, circadian cycles were negated by rigid procedures and protocols. Numerous tests were done to ensure we'd survive on our own once released into the wild.

For each of my four children, the first year of life was an exercise in endurance. Naps and routines were interrupted by exhausting trips to the germ-infested waiting room of a pediatrician's office. Government mandated vaccination schedules dictated I pack bags filled with toys, snacks, blankets, pacifiers and diapers. I needed extra clothes for the inevitable vomit or poop that we all wore as perfume. I'd strap my little ones into their car seats and head to the doctor because that's what I was expected to do. Height, weight and head circumference were measured. Results were ranked by percentiles and plotted on bell-curve growth charts. Dietary guidelines and development milestones were carefully explained. Shots were administered and duly recorded.

The advice was standardized. Deviation from the norm (however "normal" is defined at any given time) was blatantly frowned upon. Well-baby visits felt like report card days for mommies.

More often than not, my "well-baby" morphed into a "sick-baby." Two of my children were repeatedly diagnosed with ear infections at routine check ups. I thought fussiness and occasional low-grade fevers were part of the teething and tummy aches of toddlerhood. I was told I was wrong. I'd leave the doctor's office with prescriptions for antibiotics, samples of acetaminophen and a screaming child. Antibiotics wreak havoc on little digestive systems. The acidic diarrhea left second-degree burns on their little bottoms. The medications did not result in wellness. Both had surgery to place tubes in their ears at approximately age two.

Ear pain is excruciating. After suffering through countless infections, our doctor offered to prescribe numbing drops. He placed a sample of the gel in my third child's ear canal. The relief was instant. By the time we checked out, squeals of delight had replaced her painful cries. I was grateful, yet confused. I recalled many tedious days and sleepless nights over the years. Why hadn't I been told about these drops before?

After we left, I skipped the trip to the pharmacy for antibiotics. We went to the park instead. She giggled as I pushed her swing in the crisp, sunny fall afternoon. Cheerful energy kept us busy the rest of the day. I reapplied the drops the next morning. No further symptoms appeared. If there had been an infection, it subsided on its own. I used the drops as the first course of action thereafter. I never filled a prescription for antibiotics again.

In 2015, the FDA banned my miracle eardrops amid concerns about inappropriate dosing and contamination. (Well, that's the official reason.) I was dismayed until I discovered that mullein garlic drops offer a safe, all-natural alternative. Studies show mullein (clove) oil is as effective of an anesthetizer as benzocaine (the numbing agent used in the banned drops can trigger allergic reactions.[37]) Garlic has a variety of antimicrobial properties that inhibits a wide range of Gram-negative and Gram-positive bacteria.[38] The drops are available in health food stores and on Amazon. Follow directions carefully.

Ear infections are over-diagnosed and antibiotics are over-prescribed. Symptoms include: fever, pain, rubbing of the ear, and reports of feeling blocked. But the signs are unreliable. Forty percent of children with infections do not have symptoms. Seventy-two percent of children with symptoms do not have an infection. A red and slightly bulging tympanic membrane is not proof of infection.[39] And regardless, most ear infections are viral. Treating them with antibiotics increases the risk of future infection.[40] This explains why many of us find ourselves stuck in the revolving door of the pediatrician's office.

Children's Eustachian tubes are not slanted as they are in adults. Without the assistance of gravity, fluid doesn't drain as well from lymph nodes and ears. This leads to congestion that puts pressure on the eardrum. Eighty to ninety percent of infections clear up without antibiotics.

Furthermore, medications that reduce fever also lower immunity and prolong the illness. Fever is an immune response that has beneficial effects in fighting infection. There is no need to treat a fever under 102 degrees in an otherwise healthy child.[41]

The best way to treat ear infections is to reduce the risk of getting them in the first place. Dairy products contribute to congestion. The mucus provides a breeding ground for infection. Inflammation in the Eustachian tubes traps fluid that harbors bacteria. It is estimated that up to 80 percent of recurrent ear infections are due to allergic sensitivities.[42]

Doctors are not educated on the nuances of nutrition. They are trained to treat illness, not prevent it.

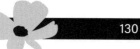

Take-home packets for new moms include samples of dairy formula. (Side effects include a decrease in the length of breastfeeding in lieu of the easier option.[43]) Samples of acetaminophen syrup promise to comfort a crying child. Infants are new customers for big business. Tired moms are easy targets.

MEDICATION MANAGEMENT

Sometimes, using acetaminophen, NSAIDs and antibiotics is warranted. If you must take medication, protect your digestive health and boost your immune system with proactive measures.

1. Take supplemental prebiotics and probiotics.
2. Eat fermented foods such as sauerkraut, kombucha, kefir, and yogurt, which deliver beneficial bacteria to the intestinal tract.
3. Promote detoxification in the liver with ginger, milk thistle and green teas, roasted soy nuts, bone broth, garlic, onions, and cruciferous vegetables like broccoli, kale, cabbage, cauliflower and watercress.
4. Supplements such as 30 g/day of glutamine,[44] 600-1000 mg/day of N-acetylcysteine (NAC),[45] and 400-1600 mg S-adenosyl methionine (SAMe)[46] can counter the negative effects of NSAIDs and acetaminophen on the liver. Consult an integrative physician for advice.

 ColleenKachmann.com/members

The Chickenpox Chit-Chat

The chickenpox vaccination is now standard. The first dose is given at age one. I was unaware of the controversies that surround vaccines when my kids were born. I did not question medical authority. But when I learned that only a natural case of the chickenpox creates a lifetime of immunity,[47] my instincts kicked in. I took the old-fashioned option.

I had chickenpox when I was eight years old. It was summer time. A warm breeze wafted the scent of honey-suckle through the window. I could hear the laughter and shrieks of children playing outside. I longed to climb my favorite tree where I spent hours each day observing life from above. Instead, I was stuck in bed, my body covered with itchy, puss-filled blisters coated in Caladryl. The smell of camphor and mint do not elicit fond memories. It was a miserable week.

My suffering intensified when my mom saw my indisposal as an opportunity to educate me on the "birds and the bees." She gave me a book and left me to read in private. Besides graphic details of human anatomy, there was bad news about puberty. *The Joys of Becoming a Woman* would include a week of heavy bleeding. Mood-swings, fatigue and painful cramps would punctuate the rest of the month. I was disturbed. Nancy Drew mysteries had not prepared me for such horrors.

A week of chickenpox is not fun. But I'll never have to go through it again. That's comforting. I wanted my son to have the same security. When a friend announced that her child had chickenpox, I scheduled a play date and cleared our calendar. His moderate outbreak lasted a week. Caladryl kept him comfortable. I gave him a book on potty training but he wasn't ready to deal with the joys of becoming a man. I did not push the issue. We read *Clifford, The Big Red Dog* until we knew the words by heart.

My son conquered the chickenpox virus the old-fashioned way. He won't need a booster shot. He won't have to read a book called Shingles: Chicken Pox for Senior Citizens (the virus is different and more severe in the elderly). We invested a week and earned a lifetime of immunity.

Prescription for Health

For too many years, I had it backwards. I did not think of food as medicine. I thought what I ate affected only my weight, and that medications were the answer to health problems. The first question I asked when faced with an ailment was, "which drug is right for me?" The promise of relief was far more pleasant than the aches and pain of reality. Why suffer through cramps, tension headaches, head colds and marathon training? My mantra was, "I'm not applying for a spot on *Survivor*. Give me medicine or give me death!"

I wince thinking about the damage medications have inflicted on me, and worse, my kids. Formulations taste like candy and are recommended for everything from low-grade fevers to muscle pain after a vigorous workout. I have even used drugs to induce the placebo effect for hurt feelings and homework headaches. I didn't know any better. My medicine cabinet was always stocked with one of everything from the drugstore. If relief wasn't immediate, I saw my doctor for a prescription. I believed the promises on the labels. Why wouldn't I?

Commercials promote medications directly to the consumer. "See your doctor if you experience the following symptoms." So I did. And sure enough, a drug was prescribed. What an insult this is to doctors! Physicians go through years of medical school and residency. Patients see 30-second advertisements or read something on the internet and feel qualified to make their own diagnosis and suggestions for an appropriate treatment plan.

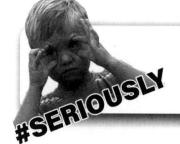

Trust me. I Googled it.

#SERIOUSLY

Frequent use of medications undermined my healthier-than-normal diet and took me to the threshold of disease. Various NSAIDs, acetaminophen, and antibiotics left my internal organs (especially my gut) vulnerable to dysfunction. I mistakenly thought the disclosed side effects carried only the potential for risk (for other people). I assumed I would beat the odds. I was wrong. Eventually, chronic inflammation in my intestines and a host of random and perplexing symptoms overwhelmed me. I did not begin to heal until I swore off the over-the-counter pharmaceuticals.

A bird's-eye look at our current approach to healthcare reveals that disorders are a profitable product. Medications interfere with healing and contribute to the need for more. A vaccine may provide protection from a single disease, but we do not need as many as we are being sold. Side effects of medications and vaccines accumulate. Unrestricted use perpetuates an expensive cycle of illness. Medications can provide a reprieve. But a reduction of symptoms is temporary and should not be mistaken for wellness. Healing (with or without medication) requires nutritional support.

If you consider good health to be something people are either born with or not, you are underestimating your own personal power. True, some of us are more genetically susceptible to certain diseases. But even if our genes contain ticking time bombs, diet has the power to minimize or even prevent the explosion.

Stop using medications when your life is not threatened. Stop giving them to your kids. Explore alternatives. Listen to your body, not the commercials. Figure out what is causing the problem instead of muting the symptoms. The next time you feel a cold coming on, take the *Immunity Challenge* (see page 115). Avoid the syrups and pills—you'll live. Ask *why* your head hurts, not which medication will stop the pain. Headaches are not the result of an acetaminophen deficiency. A pill does not cure the problem causing the symptoms. Only nourishing foods have the power to foster strength. Help your body heal on its own. Avoid the instant gratification of the "quick fix" that throws systems off balance. It may be a few days before you feel better, but when your immune system is trained to fight back, healthy will become normal.

> **The FOOD you *eat* can either be the *safest* and most *powerful* form of medicine or the slowest form of *poison*.**
>
> — Ann Wigmore, founder of the Living Foods Lifestyle program

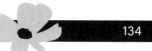

PURCHASING PROBIOTICS

Maintaining the right balance of good microbes (probiotics) in your gut is a challenge. Medications, low quality foods and inflammation disturb the delicate population of micro-flora. Probiotics adhere to the lining of the gut and compete for nutrients with infectious pathogens. They also support immune activity and counteract inflammation.[48]

The best way to sustain digestive health is to eat prebiotic and probiotic foods on a daily basis. Prebiotics foster the growth and activity of beneficial microbes. These can be obtained from fruits and vegetables that contain insoluble fiber. Probiotics-rich foods are sauerkraut, kefir, yogurt, tempeh and miso soup. Consuming pre- and probiotic foods with each meal can eliminate the need for expensive supplements.

Don't be fooled by labels. Processed and pasteurized food imposters are not quality sources of microflora or needed digestive enzymes. Only half of the probiotic products on the market deliver as promised.[49] Worse, many are desserts in disguise, feeding yeast and other pathogens with dangerous amounts of sugar.

Science has yet to clarify the "ideal" populations of beneficial gut flora in individuals. There is no test that can determine if the composition of microbes in your gut is problematic. Eating (or supplementing) large quantities of probiotics does not produce immediate changes. It can take weeks or even months for healthy microbes to flourish, and reduce the food sources and populations of pathogens.

Probiotic supplements are safe for most people. Various clinical studies have noted that doses up to 15 billion CFUs (colony forming units) will maintain digestive health and reverse occasional irregularities.[50] If you have chronic or severe symptoms, discuss high doses with a gastroenterologist or functional and integrative medicine doctor.

Not all probiotics are alike, and not all formulations are effective. Potential side effects pose little threat, however.[51] Seek professional advice if symptoms of bloating, loose stool and itching in the area between the pubic bone and tailbone arise (or intensify).

The expense of a quality probiotic is nullified if the bacteria are not delivered alive and well to the gut. Bacteria must survive the manufacturing process, storage, and journey through stomach acid. Valid strategies include controlled-release (enteric) capsules, "beadlet" technology and refrigeration. Regardless, probiotics need to be protected from exposure to light, heat and moisture.

Buyer Beware: Quality supplements explain how their products work and have clear explanations. LabDoor is an independent research company that checks for label accuracy, product purity, nutritional value, projected efficacy and ingredient safety. Review their findings before you buy.

Medicinal Media

Remind yourself and teach your kids about the impacts that food and medications have on health. Documentaries can help you with important conversations. Add these to your watchlist and invite your spouse and kids to view them with you. It's easier than ever to make wellness the top priority in your home.

Available on Netflix

- Plant Pure Nation
- Forks Over Knives
- Forks Over Knives Presents: The Engine 2 Kitchen Rescue
- Fat Sick & Nearly Dead
- Fat Sick & Nearly Dead 2
- Food Chains (also on Amazon Prime)
- The Healing Effect
- Food Inc.
- Food Matters
- Cowspiracy
- Supersize Me
- Fed Up
- Hungry for Change
- Prescription Thugs

Free stream on original (legit) websites

- The Future of Food
- Heal Yourself Heal the World
- Dying to Have Known
- The Gerson Miracle
- The Beautiful Truth
- The Marketing of Madness
- Bought
- The 11th Hour
- A Chemical Reaction

YouTube

- Big Sugar: Sweet, White and Deadly
- Mask of Deception

Amazon (Prime/Rent/Buy)

- Overfed & Undernourished
- Food Beware
- Food FightChow Down
- Pink Ribbons Inc.
- That Sugar Film
- GMO OMG
- Uprooting the Leading Causes of Death
- Doctored
- Queen of the Sun: What are the Bee's Telling Us?
- Vanishing of the Bees
- Burzynski: Cancer is a Serious Business
- King Corn
- Heal for Free
- Bag It: Is Your Life Too Plastic?
- The Perfect Human Diet
- Food Stamped
- Sicko

Check out Dr. Michael Greger at NutritionFacts.org. He reads every issue of every nutrition journal (so you don't have to). There are thousands of short, informative videos on his website.

 ColleenKachmann.com/members

PRESCRIPTIONS FOR PAIN

Normal vs Healthy

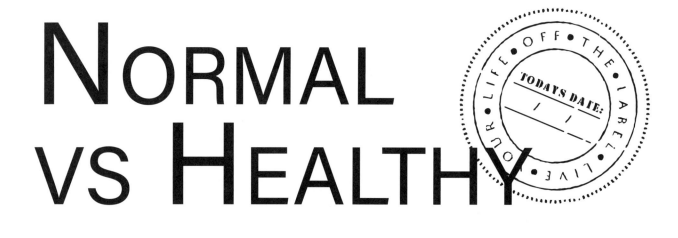

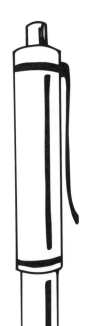

How often do you take antibiotics? Use steroid creams, pills or injections? Rely on acetaminophen and NSAIDs to reduce pain and inflammation? What negative side effects do these medications have on your health?

Take medications only as a last resort. Anticipate and counteract the side effects. For example, take a probiotic with an antibiotic. Supplement with methionine or N-acetyl cysteine if acetaminophen is necessary.[53] Develop a plan to support your immune system before you get sick. What proactive steps will you take each day to reduce your vulnerability to illnesses?

What illnesses are inevitable if you continue to live as "normal?" Do you believe antibacterial soap, antibiotics and vaccines improve or reduce immune function? What habits do you have that are suppressing your immune system?

Is your immune system strong? Develop a plan for the next time acute symptoms present.

 ColleenKachmann.com/members

PS I left this facing page blank for you.
Fill it with whatever you like. Questions, comments, to-do's, thoughts, etc.
You're welcome . . .

PRESCRIPTIONS FOR PAIN

CHAPTER 7

THE GREAT DEBATE: ORGANIC FOOD

> *""People are fed by the Food Industry, which pays no attention to health, and treated by the Health Industry, which pays no attention to food."*
>
> WENDELL BERRY, AMERICAN NOVELIST, ENVIRONMENTAL ADVOCATE, CULTURAL CRITIC AND FARMER

THE INCONSISTENT TRUTH

The inconsistent truth is that organic foods don't always contain higher levels of nutrients. Factors such as growing conditions, storage and harvest times make it impossible to claim they are always the superior choice. The "organic" label doesn't guarantee a vitamin-packed, perfectly flavored fantasy. So why bother breaking the bank for produce that isn't shiny enough to check your teeth?

The benefits of organic foods are best understood by looking at what's not in the food as opposed to what is. Remember that genetically modified corn doubles as a pesticide. Chemical fertilizers settle into plant cells—you can't wash them off. The antibiotics in meat and dairy are causing an evolution of super-immune bacteria and viruses. Furthermore, unless you want to be a cow when you grow up, growth hormones need to be avoided. Why? Consider that the onset of puberty for boys and girls has dropped by an average of one to two years over the last generation.[1,2]

Living with a PMS-ing ten-year-old is super fun," said no one. Ever.

Thanks growth hormones!

THE GREAT DEBATE: ORGANIC FOOD

PMS Comfort Food

Periods are helpful when they punctuate a sentence. They are not as convenient when they punctuate the month. Premenstrual symptoms can affect everyone within earshot, even (and especially) oblivious males. Conquer symptoms and satisfy cravings with this easy recipe.

Ingredients:
- 2-3 frozen bananas (Don't throw away these over-ripe gems. Peel and store in the freezer.)
- 7-10 fresh mint leaves or a dash of peppermint essential oil
- 1 oz. dark chocolate (high in cacao)

Place bananas in a high-speed blender or food processor. After a few minutes, they will be as creamy as ice cream. Add the mint and chocolate and give it another whirl. Feel free to stick a cherry on top.

Bananas contain potassium and melatonin. They help with muscle cramps and sleep issues. Fresh mint is soothing to the digestive tract and helps with tummy troubles. Dark chocolate is low in sugar, full of antioxidants and has plant-based fats such as oleic acid that improve cognitive function. A one-ounce serving delivers 30 mg of iron.

 ColleenKachmann.com/members

The negative effects of conventional agriculture (non-organic farming) on the environment are huge. Harsh chemicals contaminate our waterways and drinking supply. Dead zones kill millions of fish, and those caught alive arrive on your plate filled with toxins. Fertilizers and pesticides injure wildlife and pollute ecosystems. They damage the vitality and productivity of soil and cause erosion.

Everyone concerned about global warming should take note: factory-farmed meat production introduces more greenhouse gases into our atmosphere than all the transportation vehicles on earth. There are 9 billion chickens, 113 million pigs, 33 million cows and 250 million turkeys produced (and consumed) every year. These animals fart, burp and crap into our environment. Livestock generates 130 times more solid and liquid waste than the 7 billion humans on the planet.[3]

I have always considered myself to be a conscientious consumer. Who doesn't? I thought I ate mostly healthy. Don't we all? But our food supply is not what it appears. Catchy jingles and familiar brand logos give us comfort and confidence that what we are buying is healthy. It's not. The foods that fill "normal" pantries have profound negative consequences on our health and the environment. The truth is so obvious it can hide in plain sight.

I wasn't motivated to become vegan by the ethical dilemma of eating animals. I respect the food chain. But when I learned that torture is standard on factory farms, I could no longer support the system.

Inhumane practices are used to raise and harvest the animals that supply our food. Profitable meat and dairy industries hide their atrocious methods from consumers. Special interest protection laws provide a thick cloak of secrecy. Labels with images of happy livestock frolicking on picturesque farms keep us from asking questions. The answers are ugly.

I grew up in a farm state surrounded by cornfields. Yet I shopped in asphalt-covered pastures topped with super-sized big-box stores. These fields have no sunrises or sunsets. Twenty-four hours of fluorescent light bathe acres of aisles stocked with bags, cans and boxes. The first frost in autumn and fragrant blooms of spring do not announce the arrival of a new season. Instead, holidays mark the passage of time with changing colors of candy wrappers. Halloween orange fades to clearance when diesel trucks offload pallets of merry reds and greens.

There is a huge disconnect between the food on our plate and the source of that food. Most of us do not realize this blind spot exists. I was traumatized as a kid to learn hamburger doesn't come from a cow (like milk). It is the cow. A dead cow. I just thought hamburger came from the giant freezers behind the meat counter. As adults, most of us still suffer from a similar form of that naive ignorance. We are unaware that every dollar spent on conventionally raised livestock is a vote for the inhumane practices and toxic chemicals of Big Agribusiness.

As a new and inspired vegan, I read books and watched documentaries that fueled my motivation. I jumped on the organic and locally sourced food bandwagon (for the summer, anyway, when the bandwagons go to farmer's markets filled with fresh produce). I returned to the grocery store when the summer harvest faded. It did not take long to see that organic produce is more expensive than the alternative. And sometimes it went bad before I had a chance to use it.

I was discouraged. My kids were unimpressed.

USDA Certified Organic: What Does that Mean?

The USDA-Certified Organic label ensures:

- crops and livestock are raised without fertilizers and pesticides.
- there are no genetically modified ingredients.
- there are no synthetic additives like MSG, nitrates, food dyes or preservatives.
- there are no chemically altered ingredients like hydrogenated/trans fats or HFCS.
- the food has not been processed with industrial solvents or irradiation.

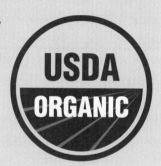

There are 127 non-organic ingredients approved for use in certified organic food.[4] (Compare that to the nearly 10,000 additives allowed in conventional food.) Exceptions are made for chemicals that are deemed necessary to the production or handling of an organic product, not harmful to human health or environment, and have no organic alternative. Substances like yeast, baking soda, certain vitamins and minerals, hydrogen peroxide, and gases like carbon dioxide and oxygen cannot be produced organically. This provides for a wider range of organic products. For example, you can't make bread without yeast and baking soda.

The USDA-Certified Organic label applies only to food products. Beauty products and household supplies can be labeled "organic" for any reason the manufacturer deems fit. No FDA certification process restricts use of the word. The "organic" label on nonfood products guarantees about as much as the words "all natural ingredients" do on food labels. Chapter 14: *Afford the Best on a Budget of Less* reveals how easy it is to eliminate the expense and risks of common home and beauty products.

 ColleenKachmann.com/members

Good Food Goes Bad

Shiny, crisp apples are available regardless of the season. Juicy bright colors tempt you to take a bite, just as the Evil Queen lured Snow White. But did you know that conventional fruit sold in grocery stores might be over a year old when you buy it? A preservative known as SmartFresh™ makes this possible.

SmartFresh inhibits the release of ethylene gas, which ripens and softens fruit. Of course, it is FDA approved. So was DDT. At this point, that provides no guarantee of safety. It's quite clear the FDA values corporate profit more than the health of individuals. Their seal of approval is only valuable to the corporations who spend a lot of money to get it.

Organic food contains nutrients that sustain life. Bugs, slugs and molds need to eat too. Humans find this disgusting. But ponder the reality. If a worm won't eat conventional corn (or dies after doing so), should we be eating it? An organic potato left on an open counter will quickly rot. But McDonalds French fries stay "fresh" for weeks. Bacteria won't touch many of the foods our kids eat regularly. Multiple YouTube videos feature McDonalds hamburgers that look the same after four to six years![5] Sounds delicious, right?

Just kidding.

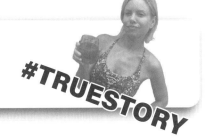

Of all the lies I've ever told, "just kidding" is my favorite. #TRUESTORY

The higher prices on organic food appear to be inflated. That's a fallacy. Introduce me to a rich organic farmer and I'll eat some non-organic crow. Growing sustainable crops (I'll explain that term next) is a farmer's labor of love for both the food and the environment. The process of becoming USDA certified is tedious, time consuming and expensive. Many small farmers don't have the overhead to buy rights to the "organic" label. Our government charges the good guys to prove they are doing it right while paying billions in subsidies to the big guys doing it wrong.[6] Tax dollars support the toxic pesticides and fertilizers that pollute the planet and our health. The price of organic food is not high. The cost of conventionally grown food is artificially low.

When food is labeled "sustainably-grown" (as opposed to organic), it means that a small farm has done everything possible to raise food without chemicals. They save seeds, plant cover crops, rotate fields and nourish the soil with compost. Sometimes a single application of a mild pesticide might be deployed in order to save a crop. That's why "sustainable" is not guaranteed to be completely organic. Also, it's illegal for anyone but the USDA to label food "organic."

The intention of sustainable farming is to work in harmony with the environment. The cost of growing unpolluted food barely covers the cost of doing business. These farmers work sunrise to sunset, seven days a week for the benefit of us all. I support them with my dollars whenever possible. They've earned my trust.

There are times when local, sustainably produced food is superior to certified organic offerings. When organic produce at the grocery is out of season, it's likely to have been shipped from foreign countries. This is where organic food gets a bad rap: good food goes bad. Fast.

The freshness of seasonal offerings will encourage your transition to local and sustainably grown foods. Most citrus fruits are ripe from January through early summer. Asparagus, arugula, cherries and sugar snap peas kick off the spring season. You'll be so sick of zucchini, tomatoes and cucumber by the end of summer, the first frost will be a relief. Root vegetables and squash provide sustenance through the winter. Pomegranates and cranberries are cold-weather holiday traditions because they are in season.

Sustainably produced, local foods are better for the environment than organic options shipped halfway across the globe.

Sustainable versus Organic

Government regulations serve as a trade-off for the safety of civilization. Toxic sludge will be thrown into rivers to save a buck if no authority is watching. Sometimes evil is intentional. Sometimes evil is just ignorant. In theory, checks and balances create accountability.

Demonstrating compliance for the organic certification process takes a lot of time and money. Small producers of high quality food often cannot afford the excess crap required to fertilize their brands with an official stamp of approval. Farmers label their food as "sustainably grown" and quietly go about their business.

I learned the difference between "certified organic" and "sustainably grown" labels when I discovered a scrumptious, vegan and gluten-free "meatball," made by Phoenix Organics. I could not reproduce the flavor and texture in my own kitchen despite my best efforts. So I made a habit of ordering them by the case.

Phoenix Organics was located in Spencer, West Virginia. I travel in that direction a few times a year to play in the New River Gorge. When my sacred supply dwindled to one pack, I decided to take a road trip. I drove my four kids, two large dogs, bikes, kites and gear to West Virginia for some playtime. I paid a visit to Phoenix Organics on the way.

Bill Quick, the owner, agreed to meet with me. He was a burly looking mountain man with a kindred soul. We were instant friends. I accepted his offer to tour the facility. Some of his equipment had been in use for nearly 100 years. Unlike large factories with automated processes that increase efficiency (and profit), Quick believed in old-school integrity. He carefully explained the benefits of his laborious and traditional approach. His recipes contain only non-GMO soybeans and organic ingredients. The man took great pride in doing things right.

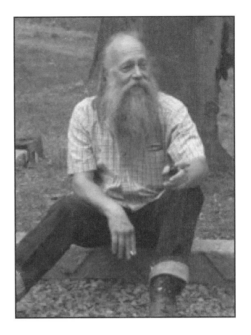

Bill Quick passed away on May 16, 2013. Hopefully, his legacy will continue to grow and be prosperous for his family and community. Rest in peace, Bill!

Prior to 2013, Phoenix Organics was USDA certified organic. The process took four years to complete. Annual fees totaled $793. But a subsidized cost-share program returned $702 in rebates. It took a lot of time, but less than $100, to demonstrate Phoenix Organics was compliant with organic standards.

On inspection day, a USDA agent spent six hours reviewing tedious paperwork. Quick was prepared to give a thorough tour of the facility, similar to those required by the Health Department. A tour was not necessary, however. The busy agent only wanted to ensure Quick's forms were certified organic (and his money was green).

Quick was disillusioned. He framed the experience with another story. When a rabbi came to certify Phoenix Organics as "kosher," the forms were an afterthought. The rabbi wanted to *see* that the operation was kosher. The rabbi explained. "Paperwork is irrelevant. I answer to a higher authority."

In 2013, the updated Farm Bill eliminated cost-sharing and rebate assistance.[7] The price tag for certification increased to $2,400. Phoenix Organics could not afford to prove that they were (still) doing things right.

Quick made the decision to stop playing games with the USDA. But the consequences proved costly. The word "organic" belongs to the USDA. The company could no longer do legal business as Phoenix Organics. Operations were suspended as they waited for a new trademark to be issued. Packaging and labels had to be redesigned. Their former website domain and marketing materials were useless. The company reopened as Spring Creek Tofu using the same organic processes and ingredients. But it was now illegal to "claim" they were organic.

THE GREAT DEBATE: ORGANIC FOOD

The nonsense of this story is that tax dollars subsidize conventional commodities (responsible for much of the planet's pollution) to the tune of $20 billion per year. Yet organic farmers are charged high fees to show they *aren't* using fertilizers, pesticides and unnatural processes. The irony is absurd. Organic farming should be rewarded. Conventional agriculture should be held responsible for damages.

Big Food is quickly responding to consumer demand for certified organic products. Production facilities are being industrialized. They have the money to lobby lawmakers, and to challenge rules that are costly and inconvenient. Farm Bill updates are modifying guidelines that reduce profits for large manufacturers.

The message that Bill Quick wants people to know is: The USDA's "certified organic" is only a set of political parameters. It's business as usual in Corporate America. Buyer, beware.

PRIORITIZE YOUR ORGANIC BUDGET

Finding the money for organic food can be a challenge. But, as you will see, it can be done. Start by switching to organic snacks and frozen foods. These do not contain MSG, HFCS, preservatives, artificial colors or GMOs. This important step will lead to weight loss, fewer allergy symptoms, improved digestion and a reduction in cravings for foods that aren't good for you. There are many affordable options, especially online. I find the best deals on prepared organic foods at Costco and Vitacost.com.

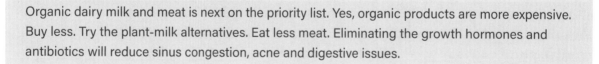

Organic dairy milk and meat is next on the priority list. Yes, organic products are more expensive. Buy less. Try the plant-milk alternatives. Eat less meat. Eliminating the growth hormones and antibiotics will reduce sinus congestion, acne and digestive issues.

Little Organic Brands[8] Sell Big Food

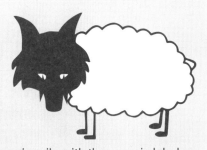

Organic consumers tend to be less brand conscious, identifying primarily with the organic label itself. This creates a halo effect around organic brands, and a gold mine for large corporations who want a share of the growing market. (Organic food sales have tripled in the last ten years.) Once acquired by Big Business, organic recipes are prepped for large scale production in factories. Labels and websites lead with the previous "Our Story" to conceal the stealth new ownership.

Coca-Cola
- Green Mountain Coffee
- Odwalla
- Honest Tea
- Suja Juice

JAB Holding
- Kurig Green Mountain
- Peet's Coffee 7 Tea
- Caribou
- Einstein Bros./Noah
- Stumptown
- Intelligesta

Pepsi
- Naked Juice
- Stacy's Pita Chips

Campbell's
- Bolthouse Farms
- Plum Organics
- Wolfgang Puck
- Garden Fresh Gourmet

Mondelēz
- Boca Foods
- Back to Nature
- Green & Black's

Nestle
- Sweet Leaf Tea
- Tribe Mediterranean Foods

Hain Celestial
- Rudi's Organic Bakery
- Ella's Kitchen
- Blue Print
- Earth's best
- Nile Spice
- Spectrum Organics
- Garden of Eatin'
- Arrowhead Mills
- Debole's
- Imagine
- Rice Dream/Soy dream
- Health Valley
- Casbah
- Celestial Seasonings
- Westoy
- Little Bear
- Bearitos
- Westbrae
- TofuTown
- Maranatha
- FreeBird
- Mountain Sun
- Walnut Acres

General Mills
- Annie's Homegrown
- Immaculate Baking
- Muir Glen
- Cascadian Farm
- Food Should Taste Good
- LaraBar
- Rythem Superfoods
- EPIC Provisions

ConAgra
- Blake's
- Lightlife
- Alexia Foods

Dannon
- Stonyfield
- Brown Cow
- Happy Family
- Helios
- Lifeway
- First Juice
- Fresh Made Dairy

Kellogg
- Bare naked
- Wholesome & hearty
- Kashi
- Morningstar Farms
- Natural Touch

M&M Mars
- Seeds of Change

Snyder's - Lance
- Late July
- Kettle

Pinnacle Foods
- Earth Balance
- Evol
- Udi's

 ColleenKachmann.com/members

The Great Debate: Organic Food

Pick Your Poisons

Our environment is filled with chemicals. Medical breakthroughs, agricultural enhancements, and new methods of food preservation are part of normal, everyday life. That's why it's easy to get irritated with organic activists demonizing everything from palm oil to plastic containers.

I once rolled my eyes at any reference to "all natural." After all, who wastes money on DEET-free bug spray? And why would any modern woman choose to have a baby without drugs? Seriously. Ouch. Isn't the whole point of science to live better through chemistry? Chill pills, diet soda and Miracle Grow transform people into happy, skinny, successful gardeners. If vaccines and antibiotics can prevent death, why shouldn't we embrace technologies that promise to enhance life?"

Because they don't.

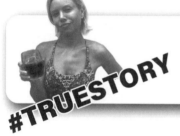

#TRUESTORY When you are dead, you don't know you are dead. It is only difficult for those around you. It is the same when you are stupid.

As I conduct my own life experiments and eliminate more and more chemicals from my diet and home, I feel the truth. Correction, I see, taste and feel the truth. Make no mistake; I'm not chemical free. I just understand that minimal toxic intake maximizes my body's ability to process exceptions that I deem worthy of risk.

I eat a plant-based, organic diet. My food is packed with antioxidants, vitamins, minerals and fiber. This keeps my detox abilities running on all cylinders. I avoid processed foods, dairy and antibacterial soaps. Not that any one of these is worse than anything else, but because collectively it all adds up. I fill my health account with as many points as I can. I spend them wisely and enjoy life. I don't need "World's Oldest Woman" carved on my gravestone. I'll settle for "Lived Well. Died Happy. Looked Tan."

But being tan has its drawbacks. Weathered skin only looks good on burly sailors. And skin cancer is often deadly. However, avoiding a tan is also problematic. A new warning has been issued: sunscreen is toxic. The ingredients penetrate the skin, disrupt hormone, reproduction and thyroid systems and aggravate allergies.[8] This presents a traumatic conundrum to dermatologists, moms and light-skinned people. What's the alternative? Sunburn? Stay inside and watch television?

Skin is our largest organ. Slathering it with chemicals to prevent cancer is logically counter-productive. I see that.

When I failed to tighten the lid on a small tube of sunscreen in my purse, I really saw that. The cream seeped into my wallet and corroded all of the coins. The money was rendered useless. And I rub that onto my face?

Sometimes. I use sunscreen when necessary because I'm more concerned about age spots, wrinkles and skin cancer. Sun damage is not my poison of choice. I have banned the graphic images of those faceless quarters and pennies from my consciousness. I have blond hair, fair skin and the freedom to choose. I wear hats and sit in the shade whenever possible. But when I can't hide from the sun, I close my eyes, hold my breath and spray myself from head to toe.

This leads to yet another dilemma. Sunscreen prevents a healthy glow. Sporting ghostly translucent skin in the middle of the summer doesn't boost my self-confidence. I want to feel cute in that sexy little sundress. So when I'm headed to a special event, I strategically create the illusion of tan. I paint my body with either a sun-kissed sepia or brushed-bronze brown. Thankfully, it's a new millennium. The obvious-orange of the '80s is a relic of the past. The spray even contours my abdominals, making it look like I have a dedicated workout routine. That's quite a bonus.

Ah, but what exactly is in the magical potion that turns this ice princess into a Caribbean Queen? I don't know. Please don't tell me. In this situation, I'm filing for protection under the "ignorance is bliss" cliché.

> "People who do not find time for *healthy* living will need to make time for *illness*."
>
> Edward Stanley (1826-1893), British Statesman

Life is a marathon. I've run a few of those so I have earned 26.2 analogies. The last few miles are grueling. A kickass playlist and a gear belt filled with energy gels provide my mind and body with the fuel to finish. I train for months. This includes 20-mile practice "jogs." I maximize my potential with extra rest, hydration and healthy food. I minimize exposure to chemicals that age prematurely and diminish the body's ability to keep going. If we want to stay healthy and finish strong in the marathon of life, we must protect ourselves from things that slow us down.

Notice I said to *minimize* exposure to chemicals. I did not say eliminate. I want to finish the race at a comfortable pace. I am not looking to take first place.

Buy organic foods and products as often as possible. Yes, they are more expensive. So is medication. American's spend 7-10 percent of their income on food, and 20 percent on healthcare. The reverse is true for European countries that follow a Mediterranean diet. If we allocated more time and resources to quality food, we'd spend less on healthcare.

Consider what your money is buying. It is possible to eat well if you are motivated to do so, regardless of income. Stay tuned for Chapter 14. *You can Afford the Best on a Budget of Less* and reclaim the funds wasted on "normal" products that are not healthy.

Step #1: Don't Panic

This chapter put my editor into a panic. "Colleen, the reader is only halfway through the book. The information is overwhelming. Busy people will think, 'I can't afford to know more!' They will put the book down, disheartened, and miss the helpful solutions you explore in later chapters.

"The politics of American agriculture, pharmaceuticals and government are ugly. The reader now sees that everything 'normal' is a lie. They will want to pull the covers over their head and go back to sleep. Please lighten the mood. Add some realistic 'how-to' and 'hands-on' sections. Give us some good news."

Her sentiment reminded me of the (first) time I dropped my phone into the lake. I rescued it before is sank, but the effort seemed futile. The screen was as black as the wet mascara running down my face. Insurance does not cover water-damage. I Googled, "Help! My cell phone got wet!" There were many step-by-step instructions for salvage. But they all had one directive in common: Step #1. Don't panic.

GOOD FISH, BAD FISH

Fish can be a lean and healthy source of protein, with heart and brain healthy omega-3 fats that reduce inflammation in the body. But with all the fresh-caught versus farm-raised options, it's difficult to know which offer more benefits than toxic risk. When in doubt, look for the blue Marine Stewardship Counsel (MSC) ecolabel.[9]

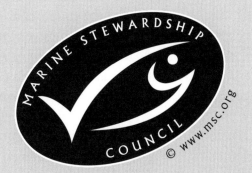

Five healthy fish to include in your diet are:

- salmon: Wild-caught Alaskan or freshwater-farmed Coho.
- albacore tuna: Troll- or poll-caught from U.S. or Canada. Canned is good.
- oysters (farmed): Best to avoid raw unless you are certain they are fresh.
- rainbow trout (farmed): Lake trout are high in contaminates. Freshwater "raceways" are protected from contaminates.
- sardines: These pack more omega-3s than nearly any other food on the planet. Also, sardines are one of the few foods that are naturally high in vitamin D. Look for wild-caught Pacific.

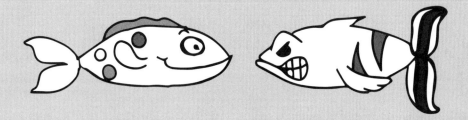

Five fish to avoid:

- bluefin tuna: High levels of mercury and PCBs.
- Chilean sea bass: Methods used to catch them are very damaging to the environment. They also have high levels of mercury.
- grouper: High levels of mercury.
- salmon (farmed): Atlantic salmon farms are rife with parasites and diseases. They are fed antibiotics and contain high levels of PCBs.
- orange roughy: Toxins (especially mercury) accumulate in these fish, which have a lifespan of nearly 100 years.

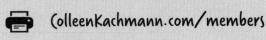

ColleenKachmann.com/members

THE GREAT DEBATE: ORGANIC FOOD

Let me offer some encouragement. This book is the culmination of my own years of experience and extensive research. Skip around when you are tempted to give up. See how you can save money living this way. The last few chapters suggest small, simple changes. Make one and see for yourself. Try a recipe. Observe "normal" life through the filter of "healthy."

This book is a resource. It can guide the creation of your own brand of health and happiness. Digest the information at your own pace.

PS: Place a water-logged phone into a bag or rice. Seal. The rice will absorb the water. Wait 24 hours. Regardless of the outcome, don't panic.

INDEPENDANT ORGANIC COMPANIES[10]

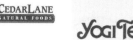
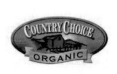

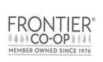
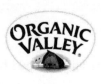

Dominant corporations seek to control our food supply from seed to supermarket. Organic brands are fetching 2-3 times their annual sales in corporate buyouts. These companies have remained independent despite the tempting financial payoff.[11]

 ColleenKachmann.com/members

The Good News in Fast Food

The collective demand for healthier options is increasing the supply of high quality offerings in chain restaurants. Companies that use real food to compete with fast food deserve kudos. Support them when you can.

Panera Bread: Most of their chicken and dairy is antibiotic and hormone free. (This varies by region.) Organic ingredients are used whenever possible. Most importantly, they are the first major chain to stop using GMO ingredients. They have delicious soups, salads and breads, with vegan and gluten-free options.
Chipotle: Served buffet style, customers build burritos, tacos and salads with fresh and local ingredients. Chipotle's corporate commitment to organic, hormone- and antibiotic-free meats and produce is raising the bar for industry standards.
Jason's Deli: With such creative salads, you might miss their wide selection of mouth-watering sandwiches.
Au Bon Pain: These pioneers in healthy fast food offer yummy low-cal soups, hormone-free chicken and nutritious, creative salads and entrées.
Noodles and Company: Lean, hormone and antibiotic free options like chicken, beef, shrimp and even organic tofu are available. They specialize in three fares: Asian, Mediterranean and American. High quality, healthy oils are used for sautéing. This is a go-to favorite for me and my kids.
EVOS: Air-bakes French fries and burgers are made with naturally raised beef and organic milk. They use Fair Trade products. Bags and cups are biodegradable. Renewable wind energy supplies one-third of their energy.
Lemonade: I ran across this gem in the Los Angeles airport. Best layover ever! Fresh salads and soups include many organic, gluten-free and vegan ingredients. And carnivores are welcome. Delicious, high quality meat and dairy items delight carnivores as well. Currently, they are located only in California. Hopefully, demand will expand their base.
Lyfe Kitchen: This growing chain of healthy restaurants is committed to serving local and sustainably sourced food. Founded by the former president of McDonalds, the brand stands for "Love Your Food Everyday."

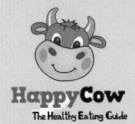

There is great news to compliment the good news. There's an app for all of this information. Check out The Happy Cow whenever and wherever you are searching for a home-style meal you don't have to make at home. It will guide you to the restaurants that have what you want.

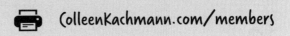

Normal vs Healthy

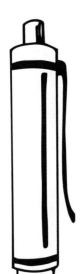

Do you know where your food comes from? Okay. Where? Trace it all the way back to the farm that it came from.

How will professional and social situations affect your new priorities?

How much money do you spend on food each month? How much do you spend on over-the-counter and prescription medications?

What challenges will you face as you reduce your dependence on medication and increase the quality of your food?

 ColleenKachmann.com/members

PS I left this facing page blank for you.
Fill it with whatever you like. Questions, comments, to-do's, thoughts, etc.
You're welcome . . .

THE GREAT DEBATE: ORGANIC FOOD

CHAPTER 8

THE
DAIRY
DILEMMA

"He who has the gold makes the rules."

BRANT PARKER AND JOHNNY HART,
CREATORS OF WIZARD OF ID NEWSPAPER CARTOONS (1971)

NO MAN CAN SERVE TWO MASTERS

The gold standard for "official" nutritional information comes from the United States Department of Agriculture (USDA). This agency issues the dietary guidelines that shape menus for hospitals, cafeterias and health clubs. Dairy is promoted as an essential food group, with 2-3 servings recommended per day. Physicians, dietitians and schools are required to follow the criteria (if they operate on tax dollars). Unfortunately, the standards pay more homage to corporate politics than nutritional science.

We have blind faith in the USDA's Food Pyramid® and Choose My Plate® guidelines. It's ironic that we protest government "intrusion" in businesses, religions, and bedrooms, but we don't blink at being told what to eat and drink. The same outspoken individuals who argue, "Guns don't kill people, people kill people," accept that milk is part of a nutritious breakfast without question. Oh, and please pass the donuts.

Close examination of the staff at the USDA (Remember Michael Taylor in Chapter 5?) reveals many experts wearing lab coats over expensive executive suits. It is a mistake to accept their self-serving information as infallible science.

Handshakes, back slaps and money-making deals turn the political cogs in all governmental agencies. Sadly, the USDA is not above this behavior. A fundamental conflict of interest in the agency's two-fold mission presents a significant dilemma. Tasked with educating the American public on what to eat, the USDA is also responsible for promoting American commodities (dairy, meat and food crops). Therefore, all recommendations must support domestic agricultural products. In essence, the USDA is an advertising agency for the farming, meat and dairy industries.

Corporate agribusinesses receive $20 billion a year in tax-funded subsidies to produce (or not produce). The marketing (disguised as USDA-approved nutritional advice) is worth far more. Big Food is getting quite a deal. This is why processed foods are so cheap, and why vegetables and organic foods are so expensive in comparison.

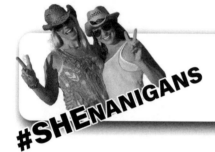
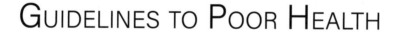

I declare shenanigans!

GUIDELINES TO POOR HEALTH

The Milk Mustache and Got Milk? campaigns are the most successful in marketing history.[1] Drinking milk is synonymous with strong teeth and healthy bones. There is big money being made. But it's not the little dairy farmers that are getting rich. These licensed trademarks can be found in a range of corporate consumer goods. Big Business wins again.

Milk is as American as apple pie. Toddlers and seniors alike are bombarded with infomercials that promote dairy products as wholesome, necessary and nutritious. Doctors and dietitians tell us dairy is essential for adequate intake of calcium, protein and vitamin D. Just try mentioning to your pediatrician that you don't give your child milk. I recommend you wear a helmet, kneepads and shin guards when you do.

The FDA-approved USDA's dietary guidelines seem to be based on the science of nutrition. They are not. The millions of dollars spent on education and health awareness initiatives generate a lot of profit for the dairy industry. Doctors, teachers and policy makers are trained to serve as mouthpieces to the public. Millions more are spent on commercials and PSAs (public service announcements) that appear in every medium to every age group. Corporate individuals clothed in TEAM CONSUMER uniforms write policies that make it all possible. The system is a political sham.

The government-promoted belief that "Milk Does a Body Good" is cemented into our culture. We are cautioned that a lack of dairy causes broken bones, rotten teeth and osteoporosis. But over 34 million Americans have low bone mass.[2] In fact, the United States has one of the highest osteoporosis rates in the world. That's not because our obese population doesn't eat enough cheese. It's time to free ourselves from the dogma of the "official" guidelines and see them for what they are: successful marketing plans.

Got Osteoporosis?

Commercials, dietitians and doctors reiterate the idea that calcium in milk is necessary for strong bones and healthy teeth. But low calcium intake is not responsible for osteoporosis and bone fractures.[3] Most of us get adequate amounts of calcium. It's getting it into our bones and keeping it there that is problematic.

The amount of calcium we consume is only relevant to the amount we excrete. It's the net balance that matters. High protein meats, dairy, soda pop and processed foods increase the acidity of our body. Viruses and pathogenic bacteria flourish in acidic environments. This leads to frequent illness, a lack of energy, pain and more. The body attempts to restore the pH balance by leeching potassium, calcium and magnesium from organs and bones and teeth.[4] These minerals neutralize acid. The resulting salts get flushed down the toilet.

You are what you ~~eat~~ pee.

FUN FACT

A woman loses 28 mg of calcium after eating a burger.[5] Substances that deplete calcium include:
- animal proteins (excess amino acids are neutralized with salts like calcium)
- salt, refined sugars and grains
- alcohol, nicotine, caffeine
- antacids and acid-reflux medications
- antibiotics
- steroids (cortisone and prednisone)
- thyroid medication

ColleenKachmann.com/members

Osteoporosis accounts for more days in the hospital than diabetes, heart disease and cancer.[6] The average American preschooler has 6-10 cavities.[7] We consume more dairy than most other people in the world, and our bones and teeth are not stronger or healthier because of it.

An Irish dentist named Tomas Murray noted a striking comparison in dental health when he served on a relief mission to a remote area of South Sudan. The country has the lowest level of milk consumption of any civilized country. They consume 0.0 kg/person.[8] That's right. They don't drink milk. Many of the people Murray examined had never seen a dentist in their life. Regardless, there was little dental decay and gum disease. He attributed this to good brushing habits using chewed sticks and more importantly, to the lack of sugar in their diet.[9]

In fact, eliminating dairy (and sugar) from the diet would significantly improve the health of Americans. In 2011, Harvard published the Healthy Eating Plate[10] in response to the USDA's Choose My Plate.° Harvard created guidelines using unbiased scientific research. Harvard encourages *limiting* dairy to 1-2 servings a day. Their report went on to criticize the USDA for making recommendations in support of sales goals of dairy producers. Harvard noted that high dairy consumption is directly linked to cancer rates, and that calcium is best obtained through greens and legumes.[11]

That's not information you'll hear on the news. Corporate advertisers fund television. Research that conflicts with the USDA's endorsement of 2-3 servings of dairy a day will not make the airwaves. The media cannot publicize ideas that demonize their sponsors. How would they sell the ads that pay for their programming? The next time you watch a news program, pay attention to the commercials. How can anything funded by pharmaceutical and fast food dollars be objective? It can't be. And it isn't. Critique the quality of information by the benefactors who make it available. Discriminate between what they want you to think and what you need to know.

"They call it the *American Dream* because you have to be *asleep* to *believe* it."

George Carlin (1937-2008) comedian

Dairy in Disguise

For those of us who live, work and play in the real world, eliminating dairy from our diet is harder than giving up meat. Giving up dairy isn't difficult—that's the easy part. Avoiding dairy is the challenge, especially if you want your children to be dairy-free as well (and believe me, you do!). It's simple to manage at home, where you can shop and cook for yourself. But it takes a Herculean effort to evade dairy when you are out and about. It's everywhere and in everything. Even the moon is apparently made of cheese.

The first time I gave a presentation on the vegan diet was at a potluck for a support group called Healthy Beginnings. The people in the audience were recovering diabetics and heart attack survivors who had adopted a strict plant-based diet. They were celebrating undeniable transformations from sickness to health, thanks to the changes they'd made in their diet.

I prepared an informative speech filled with strategies for surviving in a world of carnivores. I contributed a mouth-watering, sweet-yet-spicy "sloppy Joe." I even included copies of the recipe. (Okay, so it's just finely chopped mushrooms combined with some cooked quinoa, crushed garlic and a bit of BBQ sauce. No biggie.) I set a package of whole-wheat buns next to my homemade creation. The setting sun decorated the cheerful room with bright colors. The aromas of delicious food mingled with pleasant conversation as everyone filled their plates. Ah, bliss.

An awkward silence descended and the food line ground to a sudden halt. The director was looking at the label on my package of buns. I heard her say my name with a polite undertone of distress. "Um ... Colleen? These buns have *whey* in them."

One of my greatest skills in life is being wrong. My contribution contained contraband and my cover as the "vegan specialist" was blown. I had no idea what whey is or why it was a problem.

Before I could educate them on the joys of being vegan, they taught me that dairy contains more than just lactose. Cow's milk also has two other potential allergens: casein and whey. Dairy is obviously in milk, cheese, and ice cream. But lesser-known milk proteins are used as flavors and thickeners in a lot of processed foods such as breads, condiments, soups, and snacks.

Whole-wheat buns contain diary. Who knew? I didn't. But I do now ... and so do you.

I was duly humbled. The group responded in kind. A bit of self-effacing humor on my part had everyone was laughing. In the end, they graciously forgave my *faux pas*. Still, I learned a valuable lesson and added the information to my list of "Things Every Vegan Should Know."

The group was an inspiring example of how diet can make a remarkable difference. They had skirted death thanks to invasive medical procedures. But giving up animal products had brought them back to life. Many of them discussed how they are now labeled as "radical" because they refuse to compromise their diet. But as one man said, "How radical is it to have open heart surgery because you refuse to stop eating cheese?"

> GUNS *may* or *may not* kill people, but BAD food *certainly* does.
>
> Colleen Kachmann, founder of Life off the Label

Undigested Dairy

Removing dairy will rejuvenate everything from your mood to your skin. It is the most significant dietary step you can take for your health (after you quit drinking soda pop).

Why? Despite widespread consumption, dairy is one of the most common sources of allergies, second only to peanuts.[12] Evolution explains the common intolerance. All mammals require milk at birth, preferably the milk of their own species. Humans can tolerate the milk of other species such as cow and goat. But our bodies gradually reduce and even stop the production of the necessary digestive enzymes needed to process that milk around the age of five.[13]

The natural decline of these digestive enzymes makes sense. If someone offered you a glass of human breast milk with a cookie, you'd gag. We instinctively shun it because it's not a substance that is meant for us. With good reason. Simply put, milk is a hormone delivery system designed to promote the rapid growth and development of an infant. Dairy milk is the hormone delivery system for an infant cow. The purpose of cow's milk is to turn a calf into a 1,500-pound heifer or bull. Humans neither need nor want to resemble cattle.

GOT SYMPTOMS?

Signs of dairy sensitivities include:[14]

- congestion of the nose, sinuses and throat. Infections often accompany chronic congestion.
- coughing, sneezing, wheezing, asthmatic symptoms or tightness in the chest.
- gastro-intestinal problems, including bloating, gas, heartburn, burping, ulcers, diarrhea, constipation, nausea, vomiting and general discomfort.
- allergies and asthma; watery, puffy eyes with dark circles.
- ear infections; dizziness, vertigo or poor balance.
- headaches and migraines.
- acne, eczema, skin rashes and canker sores.
- swelling of the hands, feet, face, or other areas.
- muscle aches, leg cramps or twitchy legs (restless leg syndrome).
- cognitive problems, including lack of focus, poor memory and brain fog.
- emotional issues, including depression, anxiety, and anger.
- lethargy, low stamina; insomnia or restless sleep.
- excess salivation, spitting while speaking.

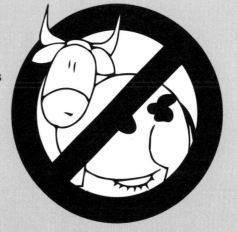

 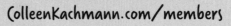

The practice of drinking cow's milk began in central and northern Europe about 7,000 years ago. Back then, the protein and calcium helped people survive in northern latitudes. Individuals capable of digesting milk beyond infancy lived longer and reproduced successfully. At some point, a creative cavewoman discovered that moldy milk has a pungent aroma that pairs nicely with a bison fillet. *Viola!* The first cheeseburger was born.

But that was 7,000 years ago. Life expectancy has doubled. The human body and digestive system have evolved since then. So has our accessibility to fresh vegetables, beans and legumes. The question remains: why is dairy considered an essential part of our modern diet?

Let's examine the claim that low fat milk is an excellent source of protein and calcium.

THE DAIRY DILEMMA

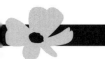

A serving of 2% milk contains (on average) 20 and 30 percent of the daily requirements for protein and calcium, respectively. Sounds healthy. But these numbers are misleading. A serving of two-percent milk also contains five grams of fat. This translates to 37 percent fat. How can such high fat content be labeled as "two percent"?

Ever heard of the bait and switch?

Misleading manufacturers use the *weight* of milk fat instead of the *calories* from milk fat to describe their product. Nutrition labels do the opposite. Two percent milk does not qualify as "low fat" by any standard. But the uninformed consumer only knows that milk does a body good, and two percent seems a happy medium between whole and skim milk.

Adding to the confusion, values for nutrients such as calcium are calculated per *serving* as opposed to *per calorie*. As serving sizes vary widely, it is difficult to compare apples to cheese.

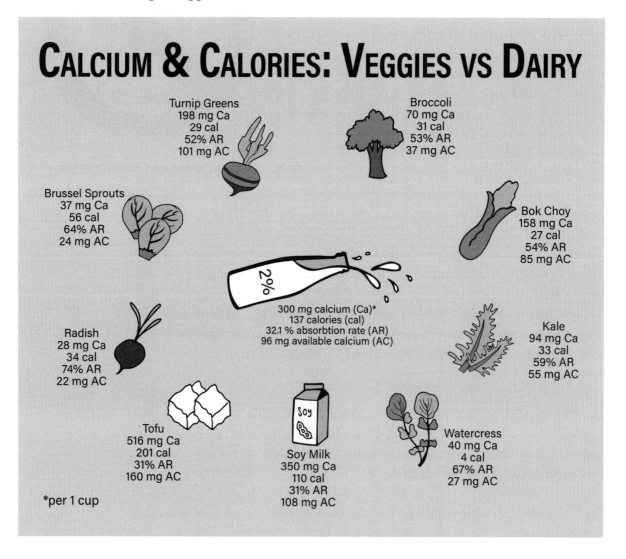

Of further significance, the body doesn't absorb all of the nutrients listed. Less than one-third of the calcium in milk is actually absorbed.[15] The nutrient absorption rate for vegetables tends to be higher than dairy—sometimes double. For example, a cup of milk has double the calcium of a cup of bok choy (but five-times the calories). Yet the body absorbs about the same amount of calcium. Also, an equal serving size of bok choy (Chinese cabbage) offers the same amount of protein, and much higher levels of vitamins A, C, K, B-complex, as well as iron, fiber and minerals. In contrast, 2% milk has cholesterol, saturated fat, three teaspoons of sugar and 120 mg of sodium.

Dairy is promoted as a good source of protein. But "protein" is a generic term. There are thousands of proteins. They are not created equal. Some are far more useful (or problematic) to the body than others.

Casein accounts for 80 percent of the protein found in dairy. It coagulates easily, making it an ideal thickener. It is used as a coagulant in processed foods, adhesives, paints, and other industrial products. We often think that milk allergies are due to lactose intolerance. Lactose is a sugar that makes up seven percent of cow's milk.[16] People use lactase digestive enzymes and lactose-free milk and continue to consume dairy. But casein allergies are more serious, and often overlooked and undiagnosed. The concentration of casein in dairy is two to four times greater than human milk, specifically designed for rapidly growing baby cows.[17]

To get a visual for how casein affects the body, think about the slime that glazes the freshly boiled pasta as you drain and rinse. This gelatinous goo is wheat gluten. Casein is very similar to gluten in structure. It is a sticky film that coats the digestive tract and airways, and causes irritation. Subsequent inflammation produces excess mucus. Stagnant gunk blocks the absorption of essential nutrients and is a breeding ground for infections. Casein is implicated in many respiratory problems.[18]

The remaining 20 percent of protein in dairy is whey. Whey protein is easier to digest than casein. The body absorbs whey within an hour or two, versus the seven or eight hours necessary to break down casein.

This is why whey protein is found in many protein supplements. However, the current trend to "get more protein" is unnecessary and potentially unhealthy. A typical 30-gram scoop contains 27 grams of protein, more than half the recommended daily requirement. Unless you are training for the Olympics, excess protein increases the risk of dehydration, kidney stones and disease, osteoporosis and cancer.

Furthermore, a 2010 Consumer Report found traces of heavy metals in

15 samples of popular commercial whey isolates.[19] Toxic levels of arsenic, cadmium, lead and mercury accumulate in organs and cause long-term neurological damage. Symptoms of low-level heavy metal poisoning include muscle and joint pain, fatigue, headaches and constipation.

Plants have smaller amounts of high-quality proteins and fewer contaminants. Plant proteins are the best source of nutrients for building and repairing muscle.

Many of us, including our doctors and dietitians, never make the connection that dairy consumption contributes to the symptoms we suffer. This is because the two do not appear directly related. Most of us can recognize an allergic response. But symptoms of intolerance can be intermittent and inconsistent. Many symptoms we normally treat with medication can be alleviated when problematic irritants (especially dairy) are avoided.

TIPS FOR TRANSITIONING OFF DAIRY

- **Use less.** We often use dairy without thinking. Explore the alternatives. Try adding humus or mashed avocado to create rich textures. Enhance flavors with dried spices. Learn to make cream sauces from cashews, squash or tofu. If you do cook with cheese, use half of what you normally would. Replace breakfast cereal and milk with fresh fruit and scrambled eggs. Drink water!
- **Buy organic.** Conventional dairy products have growth hormones and antibiotics. Removing them from your diet is one of the easiest ways to improve your health. Organic dairy is more expensive. Buy and consume less. Your body will thank you.
- **Discover plant milks.** There are a wide variety of plant milks. Each has a unique flavor and texture. Many are fortified with as many (or more) vitamins as dairy milk. Almond milk has half the calories of other varieties. Soymilk is high in protein. (Buy organic to avoid GMO soybeans.) Coconut milk is great for baking and cooking. It's creamy and filled with heart-healthy fats. (Fats are necessary for the absorption of vitamins A, D, E and K.) There are blends that taste delicious. Experiment to discover your preferences. Mix and match until you find a suitable alternative.
- **Split the difference.** Continue to buy whatever milk you prefer. Purchase a plant-based milk (my family prefers regular almond milk). Pour them together at whatever ratio you can tolerate. Increase as taste buds adjust. A healthier flavor of normal is just ahead!
- **Choose wisely.** Cultured yogurts and sour cream contain many microorganisms that are beneficial to the gut. Butter, ghee, feta, whole milk ricotta, Neufchatel and cream cheese are higher in fat and lower in dairy proteins, thus easier to digest.

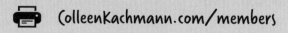 ColleenKachmann.com/members

THE DIRTY DETAILS ON NON-ORGANIC DAIRY

Growth hormones and antibiotics are used to increase milk production in cows. Conventionally raised cows produce more than double the milk of untreated cows.[20] The increased output results in a significant decrease in bovine health. Cows develop infections, cancers and reproductive disorders. The resulting puss ends up in your glass.

The large doses of antibiotics used in conventional dairy farming foster drug-resistant superbugs. Crowded conditions on concentrated animal feeding operations (CAFOs) mingled with the side effects of growth hormones are breeding grounds for illness. The media reports that family practice doctors are over-prescribing antibiotics. That may be true. But 80 percent of the antibiotics in this country go to farm animals.[21] We're getting drugs from our food, not just the pharmacy.

If you look behind the milk mustache smiles, you'll see Big Tobacco's devious methods alive and well. The two largest dairy lobby groups, the National Milk Producers Federation and the National Dairy Council, are pushing the FDA for exclusive rights to the term "milk." This is because plant milk alternatives compromise their profits. Trivializing healthier options as "imitation" milks and plant "beverages" implies they are inferior.[22]

Like their predecessors (the Tobacco Industry Research Committee), cash-rich non-profit groups generate "research" that vilifies non-dairy alternatives.[23] They are succeeding. The USDA's 2015 Dietary Guidelines continue to claim, "Consuming dairy products provides health benefits—especially improved bone health."[24]

Remember Hitler's strategy: "Make the lie simple. Keep repeating it and eventually, everyone will believe it." Oh, and smile. Got milk?

The myth that dairy is an essential part of a healthy diet is perpetrated by Big Business and supported by our government. Best-case scenario: milk is not necessary. Most-likely scenario: our love affair with dairy is making us sick.

It is normal to trust the government's nutritional suggestions. It is not healthy. The USDA's dual mission compromises the integrity of the system. Their recommendations keep the agricultural industry profitable. As a result, health class curriculums double as massive marketing campaigns. From preschool through medical school, Americans are taught that milk is "nature's perfect beverage."

It's not. Drink water.

The effects of dairy intolerance vary from person to person. Lactose and casein intolerances lead to inflammation. Some individuals experience profound relief when dairy is eliminated. Other people find the effect negligible. If you don't eliminate dairy, limit consumption to organic products. Drugs given to non-organic dairy cows are destructive to our health.

Eliminating dairy will improve your health. There is no doubt about it. At first, it's not easy—creating a new normal never is. You have the right to sustainable wellness; but you must accept responsibility for your day-to-day actions. The question is, how bad do you want to feel good?

> "The distance between what you want and what you get *is what you do.*"
>
> Author unknown

Dairy and Gluten-free Mac & Cheese

This easy comfort-food recipe is the perfect blend of classic and clean. Dark orange squash or sweet potato add depth to the flavor and a deep cheddar color to the sauce. Who knew macaroni and cheese could be both delicious and healthy?

INGREDIENTS:

- ½ lb. raw cashews
- 2 cups squash or sweet potato
- ½ cup yeast flakes (more to increase pungency)
- 2 Tbsp. apple cider vinegar
- 1 Tbsp. + 1 tsp. yellow mustard
- ½ organic ranch seasoning packet
- ¼ tsp. cayenne, red pepper, black or white pepper (optional)
- gluten-free pasta of choice (or baked spaghetti squash)
- gluten-free croutons (optional)

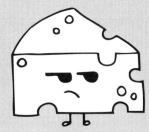
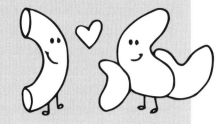

DIRECTIONS:

Soak cashews in water at least one hour. Soaking four to eight hours is ideal. Color fades as the nuts plump, similar to soaked beans. Drain and rinse cashews in a colander.

Bake whole squash or sweet potatoes for about 45 minutes (less if small) at 375°. No need to cut and seed before you bake. It's easy when it's soft and cool! Use a cookie sheet to keep drips contained. After it cools, cut in half and remove skin and seeds.

Add ingredients (except pasta and croutons) to a blender. Puree until creamy and smooth. If sauce is too thick, add ¼ to ½ cup of water. Do a taste-test before adding extra or optional seasonings.

Prepare pasta according to directions. Add 1-2 tsp. salt to the water once reaches a boil; pasta will absorb and pop with flavor.

Pour sauce over pasta, top with crumbled croutons and serve.

 ColleenKachmann.com/members

HOW TO FOLLOW A PLANT-BASED DIET

A plant-based diet can prevent, treat or reverse every single one of the fifteen leading causes of death in this country.[25] Time and money are our favorite excuses for why we can't eat better. Yet illness reduces our quality and quantity of life. Disorders and disease are far more expensive than wellness in many ways.

Following a plant-based diet is not a religion. Terms like vegan, vegetarian and paleo are defined by what you *don't* eat. Too often, all-or-nothing mindsets serve as an excuse for those hesitant to make changes. If there are foods you can't give up, don't! One serving of macaroni and cheese won't kill you. Focus on the day-to-day meals that matter most.

Studies of people who adopt plant-based diets have found that participants feel so much better within a few weeks, they refuse to go back to their baseline diet.[26] Adopt these healthy habits and you won't want to go back to normal either!

- Don't keep junk food in the house. Conquer the temptation by removing the choice.
- Only allow processed foods if they increase your consumption of whole foods. For example, if adding bacon bits to your salad is the only way you'll eat it, then bacon bits are the sugar that makes the medicine go down.
- Most families rotate through the same eight or nine meals. Transition in three steps:
  1. Tweak three plant-based meals you already enjoy (like spaghetti) with whole grains and added veggies.
  2. Adapt three meals you already eat (like switching from beef to bean chili).
  3. Learn to prepare three new meals. Google "whole-food, plant-based recipes."
- Focus on what you need to eat, not what you should avoid. Strive to eat the minimum servings of essential plant-based foods each day.[27] (See checklist on the next page.)

 ColleenKachmann.com/members

> ## "Plant-based diets are the nutritional equivalent of quitting smoking."
>
> Dr. Neal Barnard, President of Physicians Committee for Responsible Medicine

Plant Based Foods:
Minimum Serving Cheatsheet

Use this check list developed by Dr. Michael Greger (and check out nutritionfacts.org) to make sure you meet the minimum servings of your plant based foods each day. FYI: If you print and laminate this list, you can reuse it daily as a write-on/wipe-off list.

☐☐☐ Beans and Legumes

☐ Berries

☐☐☐ Other Fruits

☐ Cruciferous Vegetables

☐☐ Greens

☐☐ Other Vegetables

☐ Ground Flaxseed

☐ Nuts and Seeds

☐ Spices (turmeric, dried herbs)

☐☐☐ Whole Grains (oats, rice, quinoa, corn)

☐☐☐☐☐ Beverages (water, tea, coffee)

☐ Exercise (90 min moderate or 40 min vigorous activity)

Focus on fiber: The original "Paleo" diet included 70-120 mg of fiber. Compare that to the average American's intake of 15 mg. Increase your fiber intake (via plant foods) and transform your health.

ColleenKachmann.com/members

Normal vs Healthy

What symptoms of dairy intolerance do you have?

The dual mission to promote dairy, meat and agricultural products taints the USDA's recommendations. How does this affect your faith in their guidelines?

How many servings of dairy do you consume in a day? In a week?
How many servings of vegetables? What changes in these numbers are necessary to improve your health?

How much (and what kind) of dairy will you continue to consume? What factors lead you to this decision?

ColleenKachmann.com/members

PS I left this facing page blank for you.
Fill it with whatever you like. Questions, comments, to-do's, thoughts, etc.
You're welcome . . .

THE DAIRY DILEMMA

CHAPTER 9

THE ALLEGORY OF ASTHMA AND ALLERGIES

"A great deal of intelligence can be invested in ignorance when the need for illusion is deep."

SAUL BELLOW (1915-2005) NOBEL PRIZE WINNING AUTHOR AND SOCIAL COMMENTATOR

Illusions of Illness

Our culture has been conditioned to head to the pharmacy for every mild irritation. Hundreds of over-the-counter (OTC) medications promise relief for all combinations of complaints. Even grocery stores and gas stations have aisles of options. Chronic allergies and asthma are now expected and accepted as a normal part of life. When your stock of medication runs low, chances are good that a friend or coworker has extra. You don't even need a prescription for Claritin anymore. Samples fall free from the sky with the last snowflakes of winter.

Plato's parable, *The Allegory of the Cave*, can lend thoughtful perspective to our modern malaise. The story contrasts illusion with reality.

A group of men are chained in a dark cave, unable to turn their heads or see anything that goes on around them. Imprisoned since birth, the prisoners have no concept of freedom or life beyond the cave. They spend their days mesmerized by shadows that flicker across the cave wall. Their captors create the shadows using firelight and puppets, distracting the prisoners with entertaining dramas. The men hear echoes of words, but do not know that fire or other people exist. To the prisoners, the shadows are independent entities that live in the cave with them.

One of the prisoners escapes to the outside world. He returns with the truth. He tries to convey the news to the prisoners, but they don't want to hear anything that challenges what they "know." The cave is their home. The shadows are real. This life is normal.

The allegory reveals the power of perception. The men are held captive by the shadows, not the shackles. The shadow-makers are masters of deception. Their intentions parallel the industrial masters who profit from disease. The prisoners are distracted by the shadows; they study their movements. We are distracted by diseases; we study their symptoms.

We're conditioned to see allergies and asthma as diseases of chance. Symptoms are unavoidable. Medications are necessary. What if this is wrong? What if, like the prisoners, we're analyzing the data of illusion? Meanwhile, we're overlooking the inflammation (fire) creating the symptoms (shadows). We know that Big Business sells products filled with irritating chemicals and medications that alter functions in our body. Yet we don't see that the more we buy, the more we need.

Chronic disorders limit our lives and wear us down. The good news is that awareness is freedom. But we have to be open to it. Evidence must be examined without assumption. Medications do not cure these diseases; they perpetuate the disorder. The only way to prevent the symptoms is to identify and eliminate the source of the inflammation.

> No question is more *difficult* to answer than the one where the answer is *obvious.*

George Bernard Shaw (1856 - 1950) playwright, author and ardent vegetarian

Mysterious Manifestations

There are hundreds of foods and environmental substances that trigger allergies and asthma. For many of us, the frequency and intensity of these ailments increase each year.

Chronic allergy symptoms include wheezing, watery eyes, sinusitis, skin disorders, gastrointestinal distress and, in extreme cases, mental impairment. The immune system releases an overload of histamines when it doesn't recognize an otherwise harmless substance. This leads to swelling in various parts of the body.

Asthma symptoms are due to bronchial-spasms, sudden constrictions of the tubes that bring air to the lungs. Breathing treatments dilate the tubes and stop the spasms.

But what provokes bronchial-spasms? What causes immune malfunction? Why have asthma rates doubled since 2001? Why do more than half of us have allergies? Our health has not been improved by the endless array of treatment options. The reason for this is simple: we're treating the effects, not the cause.

Millions of dollars are spent to develop drugs that suppress symptoms, they do not make or keep you well. Medications support human productivity; they do not prevent reoccurrence. As scientists shift their focus from subduing reactions to treating the source of the reactions, a common denominator has been identified. Allergies and asthma (in fact *all* diseases and disorders) share one common characteristic: inflammation.[1]

The logical approach to reducing inflammation is to counter it with anti-inflammatories. Inflamed tissues are overly sensitive and produce too much mucous. Excess fluid causes pain and limits range of motion. But inflammation is evidence that the immune system is working. How does disabling this process return the body to a state of health? Obviously, it doesn't. But it takes time and effort to identify the underlying source(s) of the inflammation. It is easy (and expensive) to confuse the *causes* of inflammation with the triggers.

Cigarette smoke and smog can trigger asthmatic attacks. They do not cause asthma. Pollen and ragweed keep many people indoors. But the airborne spores of spring and fall do not cause hay fever. Domestic animals can trigger allergic reactions. Some people wheeze at the sight of a cat or sneeze at the sound of a barking dog. Yet others sleep with their furry friends. The number of people not bothered by common triggers exceeds those who are. Thus, the triggers are not the source of the problem.

Classic allergies are known as Type 1. Predictable and immediate reactions occur with every exposure. People allergic to strawberries break out in hives. Shellfish allergies cause swelling of the lips, tongue and throat; breathing becomes difficult. Hay fever produces dark circles under red, itchy eyes; fatigue and asthma symptoms are common. A blood test confirms Type 1 allergies.

Other allergic reactions change with age, season and stress. They can move from one organ to another. Dairy sensitivity may induce asthma in a small child, skin disruptions in an adolescent and irritable bowel symptoms in an adult. A blood test may identify a specific food or environmental substance as the culprit, but multiple factors are often in play.

Normal people are exposed to thousands of foreign substances every day. The onslaught eventually overwhelms the immune system. Food allergies and chemical sensitivities can develop unexpectedly. Symptoms are often misdiagnosed or mistaken for acute infection. Health is further compromised when a lack of essential micronutrients impairs immunity, and medications interrupt natural cycles of inflammation.

Chronic inflammation in the digestive tract and an imbalance of gut flora leave us vulnerable to asthma and allergies. Allergy medications do not heal the digestive tract, support a healthy gut flora or strengthen the immune system. In fact, they do just the opposite, increasing the dysfunction and subsequent "need" for additional medications.

Internal inflammation and poor digestive health affect everyone differently. Various allergens produce an array of symptoms at different times. Multiple symptoms may not appear to be related and rarely point to the underlying cause. But consider that oceans appear in unique colors all over the world. Infinite factors create brilliant Mediterranean blues and turbid Atlantic grays. Yet water itself has no color. Just so, allergies and asthma can manifest in many ways. Yet they are all caused by inflammation.

Determining the cause of inflammation is an arduous task. There are many possibilities and none exist in a vacuum. Eliminating irritants requires trial and error. This seems archaic in the age of instant gratification. Healing takes time. Because immediate results are in high demand, it is easier to surrender to a disease diagnosis and swallow our medicine like good little patients. This is the fastest way to get back to "normal." It is normal to anticipate the arrival of ragweed season by anticipating a month of misery and stocking up on allergy medications. It is healthy to maximize the intake of veggies and fruit and cut dairy and processed foods. But most people don't do that. Consequently, it's not normal to be healthy.

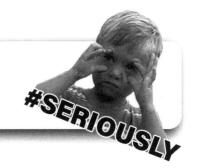

> List of things ain't nobody got time for:
> 1. That.

INFLAMMATION INSTIGATORS

Asthmatic attacks and allergy symptoms occur when snowballing issues overwhelm an already-compromised immune system. Multiple factors co-create inflammation. Individual susceptibility is unpredictable.

Inflammation is caused by:

- injuries and infection.
- medications.
- stress, dehydration, nutritional deficiencies and inadequate sleep.
- exposure to carcinogens, smoking and irritating foods.
- obesity, diabetes and existing inflammation caused by other diseases.

Common foods that provoke inflammation include:

- dairy products; lactose and casein free diets offer profound relief.
- wheat; gluten-free diets can eliminate many symptoms.
- artificial ingredients in processed food; MSG, HFCS, refined and/or fake sugars and fats, trans fat, nitrates and GMOs irritate the gut.
- excess sodium; use fresh herbs to season food.
- excess alcohol consumption.

ColleenKachmann.com/members

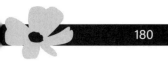

ALLEGORY OF THE TELEVISION SET

I arrived on the planet in 1973. Our home had one of those wooden 4' x 4' box televisions that sat on the floor. As a little girl, I wanted to be an actress. After careful observation, however, I decided against pursuing the career. I assumed I would need to be shrunk. As much as I enjoyed singing and dancing, I didn't want to live inside the little box, waiting for my character's next line. It was mind-blowing to discover that movie stars have red carpet lives in Hollywood. I later penned the *The Allegory of the Television Set*.

I sit on my couch, staring in a trance, I'm living my life, observing the dance.
The room is dark, yet filled with light. Friendship, love and beauty in sight.
My body is still but my mind is filled—Charmed and fixated by those in my guild.

I know the day by the programs that air. Theme songs tell time, their melodies—a prayer.
The jingles make me tingle. Promises are guaranteed.
If only I can buy that, I'll be happy. Yes, indeed.

I will eat that and be thin. I'll apply that to my skin.
My hair will have new luster—If only I can muster
The $19.95 plus shipping, handling and tax. I can pay COD, order by phone, mail or fax.

I dream of these characters, so tiny and small. How can I join them, once and for all?
If only . . . I must find my way into that box! I, too, will dance in the rainfall, sharing my locks . . .
Of love, laughter, beauty and pain. My adventures of singing and dancing in rain.
Without getting wet or making a sound. I will live as I dream: free and unbound.

My world contracts to a small dot of light. Connection severed, I'm lost in the night.
Frantic, I squint at the traces of static. "Turn it on!" I plead. "No. Don't be dramatic."
"Go play." But I was. "Make friends." But I did! Tears swell, then fall. I hate being a kid.

From my seat I untwist, I want—I *need* more. Disappointment tastes sour. Fear grips my core.
Cut off from the source, I cease to exist. I'm just a shadow. I will not be missed.
Their life is my life, so tiny and small. The truth? I live in that box after all.

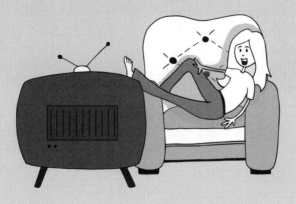

Childhood Memories

My childhood memories include trampolines without nets and bikes without helmets. There were no seatbelts in my great grandmother's car. Neighbors gave out homemade treats on Halloween and scolded each other's children. We hung upside down from rusty monkey bars and cherry dropped onto steaming black asphalt in bare feet.

In the summer, I walked alone to the library and checked out more books than I could fit in my backpack. There was no summer reading program. I just loved to read.

A fictional heroine inspired me to jump off the high dive at the pool. I did not need a permission slip to climb the towering test of bravery. I walked to the edge of the 10-foot plank, shivering with hesitation. Children waiting on the ladder cackled with impatience. The lifeguard winked. He signaled clearance with two thumbs up. The chaos of the free-fall met with silent fluidity; for a moment, I was suspended in light. I surfaced, gasping with chlorine-infused confidence and beaming bright as the sun.

At home, play dates were outside. There was no supervision or schedule of activities. Bushes were forts; climbing-trees were escape. Invariably, there were chiggers, ticks and spider bites.

I stepped on a bee once. That hurt. My mother removed the stinger with a kiss, applied a salve, and offered me a Popsicle. The slam of the screen door as I raced back outside overruled her advice: "Put on some shoes!"

At school, field trip notices instructed parents to send a brown bag lunch and play clothes. The informal permission slips did not serve as legal documents and living wills as they do today. The answer to the question, "Do you have any allergies?" was predictable. Girls replied, "boys." Boys wrote, "girls." The answers were of no consequence. We were forced to ride the same co-ed bus anyway. Stupid grown-ups.

It was normal to be healthy when I was a child. School absences were few and far between. (I tried the "rub the thermometer on your sheet" in middle school. My first attempt registered 110 degrees. I pled guilty and high-tailed my butt to school.) My parents only took us to the doctor when a bone appeared broken. We did not ask for medicine; we avoided it like the plague. It tasted disgusting. I could not swallow a pill to save my life. (No one had to teach me how to hide it under my tongue. That was natural instinct.) The only reason I missed school was because I was literally too sick to get out of bed.

Playing Pretend

Today, one in thirteen kids has food allergies and one in nine has asthma.[2] As a result, medical inquiries preempt every activity. Health conditions, medications, emergency contacts and insurance information are carefully documented, kept on file and reviewed annually. Safety protocols in elementary classrooms rival those in hospitals. My kids cannot even finish their breakfast on the bus. The driver is responsible if someone eats something they shouldn't. Schools clearly identify "Peanut-free zones." Homemade foods are not allowed in classrooms. Offerings to the general population must be store-bought so the ingredient list can be cleared for nuts.

This means Skittles and soda pop are approved snacks. Homemade popcorn and granola bars are to be left at home. How's that for crazy?

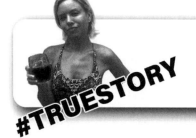

Crazy people don't know they are crazy. I know I am crazy, therefore I am not crazy. Isn't that crazy?

As a child, no one in my family had allergies. I did not anticipate that my own children might be susceptible. My boys were young when I noticed little red blotches on their cheeks. Bumps covered the backs of their arms. It was obvious that something was irritating their skin. I switched to an expensive, hypoallergenic brand of laundry detergent. But the issue persisted. Several mommy friends suspected allergies. They recommended the new allergy and asthma center where most of them *and* their children were patients.

There were colorful advertisements for this state-of-the-art facility plastered on billboards all over town. Commercials sponsoring my children's Nickelodeon programs caught my attention. Highly specialized doctors and well-trained nurses were caring and ready to help. I heard "life-changing" testimonials on the radio during the daily carpool routine. When I saw the waiting room had a jungle gym and free fountain drinks, I made an appointment.

The doctor described a benign-sounding "skin prick" procedure. It would test the boys for 40 different allergies. A grid was drawn on each of their backs with permanent purple marker. I wondered how this would look at swim practice the next day. However, vanity faded to horror when the "pizza cutter" was revealed.

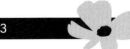

A round, metal wheel with tiny spikes and prickly needles was rolled up and down the columns on my oldest son's back. My younger son bolted for the door. I was so busy comforting his traumatized brother that I made no effort to prevent his escape. Alas, a nurse captured my terrified little guy. I winced. He cried. The pizza cutter was wielded a second time.

Within minutes, welts began to appear on the bloodied checkerboards. (Meanwhile, I broke out in hives.) The doctor diagnosed allergies to grass, strawberries, centipedes and dust mites. He also told me both of them had asthma. To this day I do not understand how he came to that conclusion. Both cases were mild (as in asymptomatic) but inhalers were prescribed as a precaution.

Dazed, I left the appointment with a bag full of sample medications and two whimpering, traumatized boys. I passed my neighbor and her kids waiting for their standing weekly injections of allergy shots. I couldn't even smile.

I joined the ranks of Parents of Children with Allergies despite my skepticism.

Inhalers are standard equipment at baseball fields these days. I had no intention of keeping the boys out of the grass (or dusting every day), so I kept the medication on hand as instructed. The inhalers were rarely used. One of the boys might ask for a "hit" on occasion, but I never heard any wheezing. The "before" was no different than the "after." I also noticed that the haphazard requests were prompted when they noticed another kid taking a puff. It seemed we are participating in a surreal game of monkey see, monkey do.

We eventually grew bored with the novelty. I stopped disclosing the asthma diagnosis on health forms. Doing so required me to provide unopened inhalers to school nurses and athletic coaches. That got old fast.

The blotchy skin issues that initiated the foolish charade disappeared several years later when I removed dairy from our diets. The bumpy cheeks, armpit rashes and back-of-the-arm redness that we'd concluded to be a genetic malfunction (family members had similar issues) vanished without a trace. Coincidence? I think not. Unfortunately, doctors rarely prescribe dietary changes.

Chasing Shadows

Allergic reactions are immediate and obvious. But food intolerances can have subtle effects. Sensitivities exist on a spectrum. Irritations are inconsistent. Multiple factors influence digestion: the amount of food eaten; when and how it's eaten; what other foods are eaten (or not); as well as stress, infection and medication. Some foods (high fiber vegetables) move through the intestinal tract in as little as 12 hours. Others (meat and dairy) linger up to three or four days. Making connections between the foods we eat and how we feel can be a daunting challenge.

We have all eaten a food that we know might make us feel bad. Spicy salsa can cause heartburn. Cheese can leave us constipated. We'll probably regret that oh-so-good-going-down piece of cake. But Free-for-All Fridays come with a price. We buy into the "Eat now, pay later" mantra. Hey, maybe it won't be so bad this time. Sometimes we get lucky . . . or so we think.

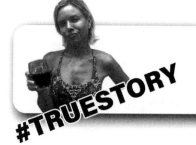

#TRUESTORY

I'm going to pretend that what you just said did not bother me. I will flip out on you later for something minor and irrelevant.

But just as the shrieks of a fussy two-year-old poke holes in our patience, stress, infection, medications and undigested foods poke holes in the intestinal tract. Microscopic lesions allow toxins and bacteria to escape into the bloodstream. Antibodies then form to attack the foreign invaders. These antibodies stay in the system. They serve as protection against future exposures, enabling the body to respond quickly to the foreign substances it recognizes. This is problematic when food particles make their way into the bloodstream. When antibodies form for foods we eat regularly, intolerances develop.

There is hope. The cycle of chronic inflammation can be broken. Just as our patience gradually returns after the two-year-old goes "nighty-night," the digestive tract heals when left unprovoked.

Once intestinal irritations heal, foods can't escape into the bloodstream. Desired foods can be reintroduced on a trial basis. Observing the effects of food on the body is a life-long process. Nutritional needs change throughout life; circumstances must be taken into account. Dairy may be tolerable during winter months; allergy symptoms may require you to eliminate it completely in the spring. Your system may tolerate gluten if you get rid of the dog. Or vice versa. A piece of celebratory cake may have little consequence on a relaxing vacation, whereas a piece of fruit might serve as dessert during times of stress. It's your health and your choice.

SELF-DIAGNOSING ALLERGIES

Food and chemical allergies are often the underlying cause of random and unrelated symptoms. Even mild irritations cause dysfunction over time.

Symptoms of common allergic reactions affect all systems of the body.[3]

Adrenals: low energy and chronic fatigue
Central Nervous System: poor focus, anxiety, headaches, insomnia, and antisocial behavior (It is estimated that food and chemical intolerances contribute to over 90 percent of schizophrenic conditions. Many psychological problems are compounded by allergies.)
Skin: rashes, redness, roughness and swelling
Respiratory: wheezing, shortness of breath, asthma and bronchitis
Cardiovascular: heart pounding, rapid pulse, faintness, flushing, pallor and redness or blueness of the hands
Digestive: Dry mouth, burping, flatulence, heartburn, bloating, canker sores, stinging tongue, diarrhea, constipation, frequent urination, nausea, abdominal pain and rectal itching
Other: muscle aches and joint pain, ringing in the ears

Careful observation of symptoms is critical to healing. Identify and eliminate irritants with trial and error. There are several approaches that can work.

1. Pulse rate can increase 20-40 beats above normal in response to foods that produce an allergic response. Take your pulse before eating and every 30 minutes for the next two hours.
2. Conduct a sensitivity test. At bedtime, take a drop of the food in question (if the food is solid, mash it with water) and place it on the inside of your wrist. Let the drop dry on the skin and leave it overnight. If it is red or itchy, avoid the food. Test the food in the same state that you consume it. For example, don't test with a raw egg if you eat them cooked.
3. Avoid all suspect foods for four days. Every fifth day, try eating one of the foods and observe. Avoid processed foods when establishing a baseline. For example, eat a bowl of cracked wheat as opposed to bread, which contains yeast, sugar and other additives. If you can tolerate the wheat but not the bread, wheat is not the culprit.

ColleenKachmann.com/members

Wellness Wisdom

The structure of the immune system is similar to the design of a spider's web. When an insect is trapped, the sticky strands of silk vibrate in all directions. This alerts the spider to spring into action. Likewise, the presence of a foreign invader triggers a cascade of chemical alerts. The immune system launches an inflammatory response to disable and remove the threat.

Inflammation is a complex response. It allows blood to clot, triggers the heat that destroys pathogens and collects debris in pockets of fluid. Pain, swelling and pus are evidence of inflammation, which is destructive by nature. Extended periods of inflammation deplete enzyme reserves, damage communication receptors and nutrient portals. Prolonged inflammation does more harm than good. Inflammation does not heal the body. It removes obstacles so that healing can occur. Inflammation must be countered with anti-inflammatory processes.

This is not to be confused with anti-inflammatory medications.

Nutrient dense foods support the mechanisms that stop inflammation after it has served its purpose. Antioxidants, living enzymes, vitamins and minerals provide the necessary tools for cells to rebuild and restore function. Colorful, whole and unprocessed foods (especially those high in omega-3, vitamins C, D and E) counter inflammation and reduce the frequency, intensity and duration of allergy and asthma symptoms.[4]

The body's ability to absorb nutrients requires your cooperation. Irritating foods, stress and medications interfere with digestive and immune health. If you won't commit to a diet of unprocessed foods, at least cut out the processed crap when you aren't feeling well. Medications that reduce inflammation camouflage the source. It is better to be uncomfortable for a few days and allow your body to heal on its own.

It is difficult to avoid airborne allergens. It is much easier to avoid foods that inflame the digestive tract. If the sound of a lawnmower makes you sneeze, cut out dairy, wheat and processed foods. This will provide the additional resources your body needs to reduce inflammation. Your immune system will be better able to handle irritants like pollen, ragweed and cat dander if it's not already stressed.

It takes time for consequences of both normal (bad) and healthy (good) habits to manifest. One cigarette doesn't kill but the habit is deadly. Foods that aggravate your body on a regular basis are no different. In *The Allegory of the Cave,* the shadows were distractions created by people and fire the prisoners did not know existed. In *The Allegory of the Television*, the onscreen lives of the little people were illusions of light. Just the same, allergies and asthma symptoms are external expressions of unknown internal dysfunction. It is this underlying dysfunction that causes the immune system to malfunction.

Illuminate the cave of misperception by casting light into the shadows. Freedom awaits.

Grab your sunglasses. Sunlight is blinding when you've been living in darkness.

> "It's not what you *are* today that matters, *it's what you do.*"
>
> — Colleen Kachmann

How to Heal Allergies

Allergies and sensitivities to natural substances are caused or magnified by: 1) impaired digestion and 2) synthetic chemicals. Restoring gut health and removing irritations can reduce and even eliminate symptoms. A high intake of micronutrients restores function to the immune system.

Taking a natural approach to healing feels quite different from taking drugs. Nutrients are not drugs. Drugs have an immediate and noticeable impact. Drugs also have side effects that create additional problems. Nutrient-dense food and vitamins work with the body; positive effects accumulate over time (there are no negative side effects). Drugs counteract functions in the body; they do not belong in the body and must be metabolized and excreted.

Illness doesn't manifest over night; wellness doesn't either. Unique genetics and lifestyles make healing an individual endeavor. Observation and consistency are rewarded in time.

- Bentonite clay pulls toxins from the body. It can be taken internally or applied to the skin.
- Eliminate sugar, wheat, dairy, beef, potatoes, shellfish, eggs, tomatoes, coffee, peanuts, soy, corn, yeast and citrus fruit. Reintroduce a single food every four days. Evaluate all systems of the body.
- A rotation diet is the best menu for preventing allergic reactions. Eat different foods each day. Do not repeat suspect foods for four to seven days. This keeps the body from overreacting to problematic foods (though not all). It also ensures that you are consuming a wide variety of nutrients.
- Maximize micronutrients by eating lots of colorful vegetables, seeds and sprouts.
- Vitamins, minerals and herbal supplements offer additional support during times of stress. Effective dosages are highly individualized. Evaluate your needs, lifestyle and desired outcome. Most health stores have certified specialists. Get several opinions and do your homework.
- Use homemade personal care products. The artificial ingredients in fragrant soaps, sudsy shampoos and creamy shave gels provoke inflammation.
- Use natural cleaning products. Toxic fumes are not a mandatory exchange for cleanliness.
- Clean up your indoor air supply. Use high quality filters in your furnace. Dust and vacuum air vents. Surround yourself with plants, the most effective (and cheapest) air filters on the planet. Change or add new soil periodically as indoor plants can harbor mold if soil becomes stagnant.
- Drink (lots of) filtered water. There are many impurities in drinking water. Plastic containers leech chemicals on hot days. Use metal, glass or BPA-free containers.

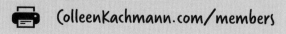

Drugitis: Which Comes First, the Pill or the Ill?

	lower immunity/increased infection	increase allergy and asthma symptoms	indigestion, nausea, diarrhea and/or constipation	unable to absorb nutrients, leaky gut	fatigue, low energy and libido	pain (joint, muscle or bone)	reduced cognition, brain fog	increased blood pressure	increased cholesterol	weight gain/obesity	prediabetes/metabolic disease	depression/anxiety	headaches	neurological disorders/dementia	thyroid disorders/dementia	kidney damage	liver damage
NSAIDs	✓	✓	✓					✓					✓		✓		
Acetaminophen	✓	✓														✓	✓
Antibiotics	✓	✓	✓												✓	✓	✓
Antihistamines	✓		✓														
Stimulants		✓	✓			✓	✓	✓									
Decongestants			✓			✓	✓	✓									
Antacids			✓	✓		✓											
Acid Blockers		✓	✓								✓			✓			
Blood pressure meds		✓	✓		✓					✓	✓	✓	✓	✓	✓		
Antidepressants		✓	✓				✓			✓	✓	✓	✓				
Thyroid meds		✓						✓		✓		✓					
Statins						✓	✓	✓	✓	✓		✓			✓		

Medications are designed to promote, alter or block specific functions in the body. They affect healthy organs as well, throwing the immune system off balance. Side effects manifest as symptoms and demand more medications. It's a vicious cycle of sickness. The only medicine that strengthens and heals the body is nutrient-dense food.

 ColleenKachmann.com/members

Normal vs Healthy

What triggers your allergies or asthma? What illusions of "health" do you buy at the pharmacy and grocery store?

Do you play defense with medications or offense with nutrient-dense foods?

Everyone thinks they are healthy, except for a few problems. But how often does the way you feel prevent you from doing what you want to do?

List the pros and cons of exchanging short-term relief for long-term wellness. What challenges will you need to overcome to allow yourself the time, space and nutrients necessary to heal?

ColleenKachmann.com/members

Life off the Label

PS I left this facing page blank for you.
Fill it with whatever you like. Questions, comments, to-do's, thoughts, etc.
You're welcome . . .

CHAPTER 10

THE GUT-BRAIN CONNECTION

"The mind tells lies. The gut knows the truth. Don't believe what you think. Trust what you feel."

COLLEEN KACHMANN, LIFE OFF THE LABEL

BUGS AND BUTTERFLIES

We all know what a "gut-wrenching" experience feels like. Many of us get "belly butterflies" before a high-pressure moment. The brain and digestive system are intimately connected. Each has a direct effect on the other. Emotions trigger reactions in the gut. In turn, tummy troubles can induce anxiety, stress and depression.[1] If you are struggling with either, both must be addressed.

When food is properly digested, nutrients are absorbed through the intestinal tract into our blood stream. Every cell in our body requires specific molecular tools. When diet is inadequate or digestion is incomplete (as it is during times of stress) bodily processes begin to malfunction.

The body reacts to stressful conditions with "fight or flight," also known as acute stress response. This sharpens our senses and focus. A rise in anxiety levels cues Survivor's *Eye of the Tiger* as the nervous system prepares for a fight. Adrenaline, cortisol and norepinephrine increase our breath and heart rate. Blood is directed to our muscles. Our speech takes on a thick New York accent and we are ready to kick some ass, Rocky Balboa style.

It's easy to understand why some of us thrive on stress. That inner surge of energy is the edge we prefer for the day-to-day boxing matches. But there is a trade-off.

Stress slows and even stops non-essential body processes. The body stops digesting food, repairing muscles, resisting disease and managing emotions when we're in survival mode. Maintenance activities require a state of calm.

When high stress begins to feel normal, we may forget that peacefulness isn't just pleasant—it's necessary. Never-ending delays in getting back to normal develop into dysfunction over time.

The lining of the gut acts as both a barrier and a portal. It keeps problematic substances like allergens, pathogens and undigested food particles from entering the bloodstream. Tiny gateways capture nutrients. Nutrients fit into these doorways like little puzzle pieces. This allows them to be transported to the cells where they are needed. When the intestines are inflamed, nutrients can't get to the doorways.

Poor digestion will render even the best nutritional habits useless. If the gut has been irritated by medications or food intolerances, stress will be the proverbial straw that breaks the camel's back. Intestinal inflammation can lead to new intolerances to foods not formerly problematic. When undigested food gets into the bloodstream, antibodies form. These defenders attack the food each time it's encountered. Frequent consumption leads to chronic inflammation. The gut cannot heal when it is inflamed. Large, unwanted food particles get into the blood; small, essential nutrients don't. This is known as "leaky gut" syndrome.

A leaky gut devastates health. Symptoms are random and vague. The first step to restoring health is to recognize that something is wrong. Stress aggravates gut inflammation which, in turn, increases stress. When either food or emotions aren't properly digested, both physical and mental health decline.

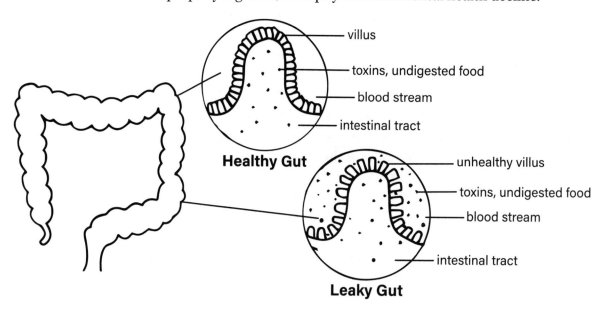

Are You Dealing with Leaky Gut?

Small holes in the intestines lead to a vicious cycle of inflammation. Enzymes needed for digestion are lost in the chaos. The body becomes overfed and undernourished. Food particles penetrate the blood stream and trigger an immune reaction. Drugs that suppress symptoms perpetuate the problem. Gut dysfunction deteriorates both physical and mental health.

The following are symptoms of intestinal dysfunction:[2]

- low energy and bouts of fatigue
- brain fog, chronic headaches, depression, anxiety, ADHD
- food intolerances, sensitivities or allergies
- seasonal, environmental or pet allergies
- joint and/or muscle pain or arthritis
- regular bouts of irritable bowel syndrome (IBS), gastro-esophageal reflux disease (GERD), heartburn, gas, bloating, diarrhea and/or constipation
- skin Issues such as acne, rosacea, eczema, rashes, hives and psoriasis
- autoimmune disorders such as Hashimoto, rheumatoid arthritis, lupus, celiac disease, multiple sclerosis, Type 1 diabetes
- uncontrollable weight gain or loss

The first step in healing is to identify the illness. Don't resign yourself to disease. Accept the symptoms as an opportunity to become well. There are answers. There is hope.

 ColleenKachmann.com/members

Dubious Diseases

Conventional doctors are not trained to recognize leaky gut syndrome. There is no protocol for treatment because it's not recognized as an official disease. Nonetheless, many people are afflicted, myself included. When suffering cannot be explained, anxiety (stress) amplifies the symptoms. I stumbled upon the leaky gut diagnosis via my homeopathic chiropractor. Once I understood the dysfunction, I was comforted with hope that I could heal. But the process has been slow and imprecise.

Leaky gut is a condition that affects the lining of the intestines. Initial symptoms include bloating and cramping, similar to irritable bowel syndrome (IBS). Indeed, leaky gut presents a lot like IBS. The disorders may overlap in theory and real life, but they are not the same. IBS is attributed to irregular contractions of the muscles that move food through the intestines. This leads to constipation and/or diarrhea. Leaky gut is characterized by small openings in the intestinal wall that allow food particles to penetrate the blood stream.

Food particles are not supposed to enter the blood stream. The immune system sees them as foreign invaders and launches an attack. Inflammation is the result. Swelling and excess mucous reduce the intestines' ability to absorb nutrients. Subsequent nutritional deficiencies cascade into a snowball of unpredictable health issues.[3]

Mainstream physicians dismiss leaky gut syndrome with the same contempt once held for fibromyalgia. Fibromyalgia is characterized by widespread pain that has no identifiable cause. Treating subjective pain is controversial. Sufferers are compelled to prove the pain is real and not a product of their imagination (or a desire for narcotics). Validation for fibromyalgia sufferers came in 2010. A diagnosis code was issued; the disease is official.[4] Treatment and medications are now covered by insurance.

I may or may not have fibromyalgia. I definitely have symptoms that qualify. For 15 years, pain greets me daily. Bad days are unpredictable. Good days offer reprieve. I make the best of both. If nothing else, the symptoms upgrade my understanding of autoimmune disorders from theoretical to practical. My experiences provide empathy and lots of great anecdotes. Wisdom comes when adversity challenges our beliefs. I have been blessed with a multitude of obstacles that offer the opportunity to practice what I preach.

Thanks fibromyalgia.

The intestinal inflammation characteristic of leaky gut appeared several years into my vegan journey, and coincided with the end of my 20-year marriage.

I was familiar with the stinky backfires (farts) that can occur when large amounts of vegetables are consumed. But this persistent, painful bloating was new and seemed to be independent of what I ate (or did not eat). No amount of toilet time relieved the pressure. I tried doing deep yoga twists (similar to wringing out a rag) to expel the gas. I called upon the force of gravity, doing headstands in hopes the bubbles would rise to the surface. I swallowed Gas-X, antacids, fiber laxatives and digestive enzymes. Nothing worked. My stubborn, distended abdomen became part of everyday life.

Brain fog is another symptom of leaky gut. As if on cue, I developed a raging case of what appeared to be adult-onset attention deficit hyperactivity disorder (ADHD). I spent days floundering through zero-visibility fog. To this day, I find myself in closets wondering what I am looking for. I head to the kitchen for a cup of coffee and end up cleaning out the refrigerator in the garage. If something interrupts what I am doing or saying, my original intentions are forgotten.

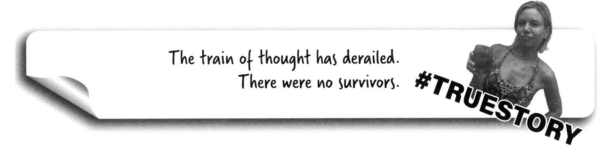

The train of thought has derailed. There were no survivors. #TRUESTORY

Intense pain in my hips and joints accompanied the bloating and brain fog. None of the symptoms could be explained by one known disease or ailment. I consulted various specialists over several years. My gynecologist cleared me of ovarian cancer (bloating can be a symptom). An internist found no evidence of a perforated bowel. Orthopedic doctors ordered X-rays, CT scans and MRIs of the affected areas. My diet and lifestyle were as healthy as could be. In theory, I should have felt like a superhero. Instead, I felt awful.

I tried various anti-inflammatories and pain medications. A steroid injection granted reprieve for about a year but the pain returned with a vengeance. I opted out of a second dose when I learned that steroids cause joint degeneration. Temporary relief wasn't worth the trade-off. I wanted to fix the problem without doing further damage.

My family doctor diagnosed me with stress and prescribed an anti-anxiety medication. I declined. When a gastroenterologist agreed that my symptoms were probably a reflection of mental agitation, I got angry (and more bloated). Stress explained the tension in my neck and back. It probably lowered my tolerance for pain too. But my belly was bloated! Why did everyone keep insisting that the problem was in my head? Something was wrong with my body, not my brain.

I did not yet know the gut and the brain are two sides of the same coin.

I sought alternative therapies and worked hard to self-heal. Details on the supplements I've tried qualify for another full-length book. I got acupuncture and acupressure. I consulted shamans, energy healers and Reiki practitioners. I scheduled regular therapeutic massages. But the pain in my hips and the bloating did not diminish.

A friend recommended a chiropractor. I'd heard about these "wacky" docs, but I was willing to try. The first appointment alleviated my skepticism.

THE GUT-BRAIN CONNECTION

The philosophy of chiropractic medicine is to restore balance to both body and mind. Doctors of chiropractic medicine do not see the body as a collection of systems. They do not believe disease is a list of symptoms. They don't prescribe drugs or perform surgeries (though they refer when appropriate). This natural approach is shunned by mainstream medicine. They aren't feeding Big Pharma. When a patient heals without drugs, expensive tests and procedures, profit margins of other specialties are threatened.

The doctor's evaluation took over an hour. She noted all of my physical symptoms and mental stressors. She asked about my diet. It was clear to her that my health did not reflect my lifestyle. She diagnosed me with leaky gut. Her explanation of the disorder matched my symptoms to a tee.

> **When the student is *ready*, the teacher appears.**
>
> Tao proverb

Taoism is a philosophy that explores the connections between divinity, humanity and nature.

I was eating all the right things, yet I was malnourished. Stress leads to incomplete digestion and medications irritate the gut. Little blisters form and become inflamed. The resulting mucous prevents nutrients from being absorbed. If the blisters are continually irritated, they become holes. Undigested food enters the bloodstream. The immune system attacks unrecognized particles. Inflammation becomes systemic and moves to other vulnerable parts of the body. In my case, gut inflammation was aggravating the pain in my hips.

This felt right. Finally, something made sense! She recommended a two-pronged approach. First, eliminate all foods that can irritate the gut. This would allow the blisters in my intestines to heal. The healing process takes time and is directly affected by stress. The second step was to address the stress load that was overwhelming my body.

That's easier said than done. I can drink smoothies for as long as it takes. But I was going through a divorce. I have four children. I needed to move. I was looking to re-enter the work force after 15 years at home. What size U-Haul could possibly carry these burdens on my behalf?

Digesting Divorce

When life kicks into survival mode it's hard to prioritize creative meals and leisure time. Such luxuries simply aren't available. Instinct leads us to eat "whatever," skip the workout and just keep going.

This compulsion is misguided. Ignoring our needs sets us back further. Sugar and processed foods keep insulin levels high. A lack of exercise and relaxation keep endorphin levels low. You may not be able to change your circumstances right away. But counteracting stress with healthy habits is essential. Protecting yourself in times of weakness is an act of strength.

When my first husband and I got married, we were not old enough to order champagne. We had 4 children and spent 20 years together. We share many happy memories. Our relationship fell apart just when it appeared we'd finally "arrived." We fought aggressively to save our family. The last few years were a blur of battles and confrontations. We learned the painful lesson that you can't fight for peace and expect to win.

The division of our home, finances, parenting time and responsibilities was devastating. Managing my own emotions as well as the feelings of my children, family and friends was overwhelming.

The death of a marriage is indeed a death. Too often, the burden of the loss during divorce is placed on the individuals suffering through it. When a partner dies, loved ones rally to support the survivor. When a marriage dies, blame and accusations come from all directions. Guilt, fear and rejection challenge the sanity and self-worth of splitting couples like nothing else.

Mental suffering has injurious physical affects. Stress hormones rage as the primitive mind prepares for battle. High levels of cortisol and adrenaline are the elements of survival. It does not matter if the threat is the result of social and emotional pain or an actual emergency. Prolonged stress is destructive. Mental anguish leads to physical disorder.

> I've learned to use meditation and relaxation to handle stress. Just kidding, I'm on my 3rd glass of wine.

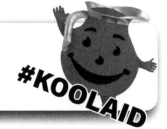
#koolaid

My brain understood and accepted the divorce. But that did not keep my body from reacting to the trauma. Life was filled with chaos and uncertainty. I internalized my fear in an attempt to provide a sense of security for my kids. The chemicals my body produced in response to stress were, quite literally, eating my insides. I wasn't digesting my emotions or my food.

My struggles with stress, pain, multiple medications, and leaky gut offer a case study on the cumulative effects of chronic indigestion. Anti-inflammatories inflame the stomach lining. Acid blockers and neutralizers decrease stomach acid and inhibit digestion. Undigested food irritates the intestines. The resulting inflammation denies nutrients access to the blood stream. A weakened immune system is vulnerable to infection. I did my best to maintain a facade of emotional normalcy but my body was falling apart.

Processed, low-quality foods and many medications create an environment in the gut conducive to bacterial and yeast overgrowth. An imbalance of microflora triggers unhealthy cravings for sugar, carbs and alcohol. These cravings perpetuate the downward spiral of health. Calling unhealthy food "comfort food" is a misnomer. Poor eating habits magnify gut dysfunction and inflammation. There is nothing comforting about that.

The age-old adage "trust your gut" is good advice. Life-interrupting symptoms that are holding you back are a signal to re-evaluate your habits. Taking drugs to suppress the warning signs is the same as telling the body to "shut up." Don't tell your body to shut up; listen! Gut health can be restored when conditions are right.[5] Take action. Give it time. Wellness is worth it.

CYCLE OF CHRONIC INFLAMMATION

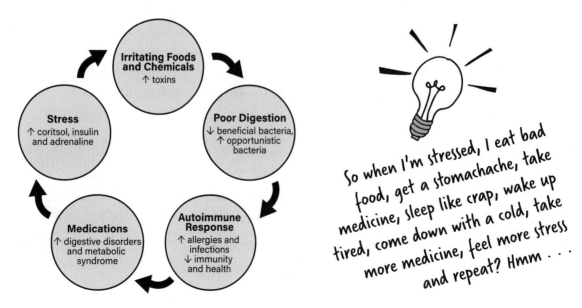

So when I'm stressed, I eat bad food, get a stomachache, take medicine, sleep like crap, wake up tired, come down with a cold, take more medicine, feel more stress and repeat? Hmm . . .

Seal the Gut: Heal the Deal

If you are wondering if leaky gut is affecting you, it probably is. Regardless of the factors that create the dysfunction, healing requires action. Food intolerances will diminish as inflammation subsides and gut flora is restored.

- Eliminating dairy and wheat can bring quick relief. Don't worry. If symptoms don't improve, you'll know it. Try it for a few weeks. If you reintroduce either, choose organic and gluten-free options. Keep a food log and connect symptoms (or lack thereof) with diet.
- Supplement with a probiotic and L-Glutamine (an amino acid that is fundamental to the well-being of the gut). Eat fermented foods (natural probiotics) such as organic Greek, soy and almond yogurts (plain or low sugar), sauerkraut, miso soup and Kombucha tea.
- Avoid packaged and processed foods. For salty or sweet cravings, eat whole foods like nuts, seeds and fruit whenever possible.
- Drink lots of water. Add lemon. Lemons reduce inflammation and blood acidity.
- Avoid over-the-counter medications that irritate the stomach and intestines.
- Eat foods rich in omega-3 fatty acids, which have powerful anti-inflammatory properties (sustainable seafood, walnuts, flax, kidney beans, wild rice, edamame and eggs). Reduce intake of foods high in omega-6 fatty acids, which are pro-inflammatory (refined vegetable oils, turkey, mayonnaise, chicken and pork).
- Check your diet for zinc. Quality sources include raw oysters, crab, lentils and nuts. Studies show zinc supplementation can drastically improve the integrity of intestinal lining.[6]

Substances that Destroy Gut Flora and Facilitate "Leaky Gut"[7]

Medications:
  Antibiotics: This includes the remnants found in non-organic meat and dairy.
  Antacids: When stomach acid is neutralized, the acid-thriving probiotics die. This gives pathogens an opportunity to thrive.
  Birth Control Pills: Increased estrogen levels lead to yeast overgrowth in the vagina and gut.
  Steroids: Intestinal bacteria that metabolize steroids are dominant. Their proliferation reduces resources necessary for other beneficial microbes. Subsequent imbalance inhibits digestion and immunity.
  NSAIDS: Anti-inflammatories damage the mucosa lining of the intestines and increase its permeability. Toxins and food particles gain entrance into the bloodstream.
Foods:
  Industrial fats, processed grains and artificial sugars lack the fiber and nutrients necessary to maintain a healthy microbial population in the gut. Preservatives that prevent foods from spoiling also prevent the "good guy" microbes from thriving.

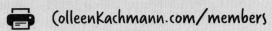

THE STRESS FACTOR

Most problems are products of our own actions and reactions. It's easy to see the self-defeating habits of other people. It is far more difficult to analyze our own words and behaviors for circular patterns. Familiar predicaments disguised as new dilemmas reveal that our worst enemy is usually our self.

Modern day stress exists in the mind. We assess a situation and label it as good or bad. Problems that must be explained in order to be seen and understood exist only in theory. For example, when it rains, things get wet. The farmer sees the rain as a gift; the bride feels the rain is a curse. It could be either. In reality, it's neither. It's just rain.

Natural disaster, war, famine and physical injury are real problems. You don't have to understand them to experience them. Hungry tigers and tsunami waves rarely threaten our survival. The trauma-dramas of our imagination fuel chronic states of fight or flight. We scramble to (and from) intangible illusions like the "suicide runs" in middle school gym class.

Could it be that the insanity that limits our lives is exactly that? *Insanity*!

> *Knowing yourself* is the beginning of ALL wisdom.
>
> Aristotle (384-322 BC), Greek philosopher and scientist

Looking around in this present moment, I see a beautiful, safe and temperature-controlled home. There is plenty of food; my challenge is to not eat too much. I have unlimited information via Google and free shipping on Amazon. My four kids are healthy. We have cats, dogs, cars and bikes. There are plenty of tissues to wipe our tears. I don't see anything wrong. My laundry-list of complaints changes with my mood. Problems are a matter of perspective.

Physical pain is often temporary. It's the fear of impending pain or the memory of former pain that leads to suffering. For example, when a five-year-old knows he's going to get a shot at the doctor's office, he cries and resists. The fear of the shot is far worse than the pain of the shot. But when it's over, it's over. The

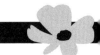

pinch lasts a second. It might ache for a few hours but life goes on, no therapy session required.

(This example is admittedly flawed. If the shot is a vaccine that compromises immunity, it could lead to infection. The resulting course of antibiotics will lead to an imbalance in the gut flora. Allergies, yeast overgrowth and further infections will be a problem . . . But I digress.)

In contrast, if you tell the dog he's going to the vet for a shot, he wags his tail and hops in the car. He greets the other animals in the waiting room with the enthusiasm of a rock star. When his name is called, he prances into the exam room. He is super excited to see the doctor and embraces the hug. He might notice the fleeting sting in his hind end, but the treat offered as reward puts the wag back in his tail. He is grateful when you let him stick his head out the window for the ride home. Overall, it's a dog-gone good day!

Emotions such as the hurt of rejection or the excitement of reward frame our experiences. Perception defines reality. You can't gain advantage when you perceive yourself at a disadvantage. Reasons that explain why you "can't," prevent you from seeing (and then doing) what you can. The only way to interrupt a cycle of negativity is to put space between what you think and how you act. Negative energy does not produce positive results.

Learn more about identifying (and conquering) the thoughts that lead to suffering in Chapter 15.

> Never hold in your farts. They travel up your spine and into your brain. That's where shitty ideas come from. #ASSUMPTIONS

10 Ways to Fix a Bad Day

1. Breathe deep into your belly. Fully exhale to rid the lungs of lingering allergens and toxins. Deep inhalations stimulate the parasympathetic nervous system and reduce cortisol and adrenaline levels.
2. Put on your shoes and get dressed, even if you have no desire to leave. Getting ready to go somewhere increases the chances you'll get there.
3. Turn on music that makes you want to sing or at least hum. Positive verbal expression raises energy levels and increases endorphins.
4. Make a "Things I Am Grateful For" List. Read it out loud. Share it with others.
5. Organize a closet, junk drawer or space that's cluttered. Plant flowers. Try a new recipe. Work on a puzzle. Do something that shifts your focus in a productive and creative direction.
6. Perform a random act of kindness. Turning around someone else's bad day has significant impact on your own.
7. Move. Get out of bed if you are not sleeping. Get out of your chair if you're not being productive. Get off the couch if you aren't smiling.
8. Turn off the computer, phone, and TV. Pulsating lights and constant notifications irritate the nervous system.
9. Get in touch with Nature. Go outside. Breathe deeply. Notice the clouds, the sun, the moon and the stars. Embrace the fragrance of the air. Watch the trees wave in the wind or feel the rain on your face. There is no bad weather, only inadequate clothing.
10. Give away free compliments. Make eye contact. Smile at everyone. Start "the wave" of happiness.

ColleenKachmann.com/members

Love the Skin Within

The mucous membrane that lines the digestive system is called the body's "second skin". Our health depends on it's ability to:

- act as the protective barrier, keeping pathogens out of our blood stream.
- secrete antibodies that provide immunity from infection.
- absorb nutrients and secrete waste.
- buffer acids and maintain the pH of the digestive tract, supporting beneficial bacteria and inhibiting opportunistic microbial populations.

When skin is inflamed, infected and blistered, healing can't begin until we stop irritating it.

No One But You Can Reduce Stress

Don't put the key to your health and happiness in someone else's pocket.

Take control of your attention.

In the first hour of the day do not check email, social media or watch television. When you allow yourself to be distracted before you have a chance to focus, you are allowing the agendas of others to circumvent your own. Directing your attention reduces frustration and improves productivity.

Set your intentions.

Make a to-do list every day, either before bed or first thing in the morning. Make your agenda your top priority. Write down what must be done and activities you'd like to participate in. As you complete needed and desired tasks, cross them off your list. If you don't have time to do everything you want to do, redesign your plan for the next day. Most importantly, celebrate your accomplishments. This creates a sense of purpose and self-esteem.

Identify the top stressors in your life.

What changes would eliminate these issues? Stop complaining about problems for which you have no action plan to change. If you don't have enough money to make ends meet, you have two choices: increase your income or decrease your spending. And if you think your problem is someone else's fault, you're wasting time that would be better spent in search of a solution.* You are either a victim or a survivor. You can't be both. Make a plan, work the plan, and adjust the plan when necessary. Reap the rewards of being proactive.

*Unless you have kids, then good luck.

Stop communication or making decisions in times of emotional distress.

Attempting to resolve conflict when you are upset is equivalent to driving drunk. Negative emotions reduce your intelligence, judgment and problem solving skills. Learn to recognize the early physical sensations of anger, frustration and anxiety (hot flush, hyper-focus on the situation, repetitive thoughts with increasing agitation, an overpowering need for validation that you are "right" and others are on your side). Know your triggers. When you realize you are upset, stop talking and put yourself in a safe place. Calm down by focusing on something that returns your sense of peace and power Get your mind under control before additional words and actions increase the chaos. Your ability to influence others depends on positive and effective communication.

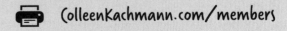 ColleenKachmann.com/members

Normal vs Healthy

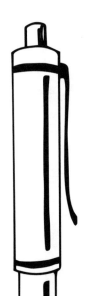

What over-the-counter medications do you take to treat digestive disorders? What medications do you take to treat stress, anxiety and emotional instability?

Look for connections between your physical and mental wellbeing. What thoughts create disorder in your gut? How do digestive problems influence your stress levels?

It's easy to see the self-defeating habits of other people. Can you recognize your own?

Problems that cannot be seen must be perceived. What fresh perspectives can you apply to reduce your stress?

 ColleenKachmann.com/members

PS I left this facing page blank for you.
Fill it with whatever you like. Questions, comments, to-do's, thoughts, etc.
You're welcome . . .

CHAPTER 11

WESTERN DIET FEEDS WESTERN MEDICINE

"Eat food. Not too much. Mostly plants."

MICHAEL POLLAN, AMERICAN AUTHOR, ACTIVIST AND PROFESSOR OF JOURNALISM

IN SICKNESS AND IN HEALTHCARE

Western diseases (cancer, heart disease, diabetes, asthma and allergies, even some autoimmune and neurological disorders) can be reversed or eliminated with a plant-based diet. Food choices have a direct impact on illness and quality of life. You can't wiggle your nose or wave a magic wand and expect your health to improve. But it's a proven fact that you can chew your way to wellness.

Following a plant-based diet doesn't require that you give up meat and dairy. It doesn't require you to give up anything! It's really very simple. Eat more vegetables.

Consider:

- Plant foods do not contain cholesterol. Humans do not need to consume cholesterol. The body can synthesize what it needs from the nutrients in plants.[1]
- Multiple studies demonstrate that high blood pressure and diabetes can be reversed with a plant-based diet. The need for medications can be reduced and even eliminated.[2]
- Heart disease and cancer rank as the number one and two causes of death in affluent countries. Wealthy countries have the highest intake of meat

and dairy. Ironically, they have the highest rates of osteoporosis, far surpassing third-world, poverty-stricken countries.[3]
- Only one percent of U.S. children eat the recommended levels of fruits and vegetables.[4]
- Patients with advanced asthma adopting a vegan diet report "life changing improvements" over a one-year period. In almost all cases, medication was drastically reduced or no longer necessary.[5]
- Allergy medications have serious side effects, including kidney disease and cancer. A plant-based diet has only positive side effects and has been shown to cut allergy symptoms in half. Sometimes symptoms are eliminated completely.[6]

Drugs can save lives, there's no doubt about that. But nutritional deficiencies will devastate them. There are times when pharmaceutical intervention is necessary. But it's critical to ensure that the body is well nourished. Drugs should be the last resort, not the first. Diet is just as relevant as drugs, therapy or any other treatment. Yet most doctors receive less than 25 hours of nutrition education in medical school.[7] Drugs can suppress illness. Nutrient-dense foods facilitate wellness.

Food is not a drug; it's medicine.

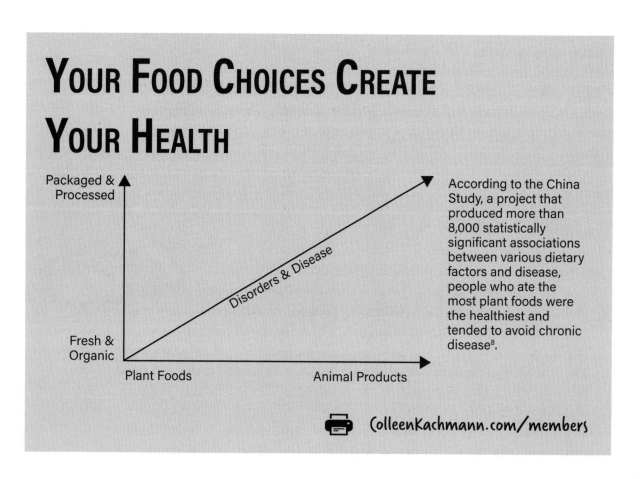

Plants for Patients

Plants have co-evolved with humans. We breathe in; they breathe out. They inhale; we exhale. The human species has been, and always will be, dependent on plants. Nature is an elaborate orchestra of delicate, interwoven systems. Fruits, vegetables, nuts and seeds contain over 12,000 vitamins, phytochemicals, minerals and enzymes.[9] In contrast, fortified foods might contain 10 isolated substitutes. Store-bought supplements can enhance Mother Nature's complex offerings, but they cannot replace them.

Plants live where they take root. They can't just move when their home is invaded or threatened. They cope with challenges or die trying. They synthesize protein, metabolize toxins and ward off pests and disease. Survivors reproduce via fruit, flowers and seeds. The successful adaptations of plants benefit the humans who eat them.

Plants provide the living micronutrients essential to the functions of every cell in our body. As our food supply (and that of livestock) becomes more and more processed, vital elements are diminished if not eliminated. Nutrient deficiencies are on the rise and our health is on a steady decline.

Plants are also the only source of fiber. Americans do not get enough fiber. Fiber is essential for digestion, lowers cholesterol, stabilizes blood sugar and keeps the intestines and colon free of stagnant pockets of undigested food. Plants don't contain cholesterol, unhealthy saturated fats, growth hormones or high amounts of amino acids that increase the pH levels of blood and urine. Plants foster wellness, not disease.

Skip the Statins

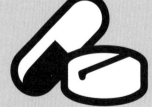

If you have high cholesterol, stop eating cholesterol. This eliminates the need for problematic drugs. Statins are prescribed to reduce onset of heart disease. Ironically, they often accelerate it. Statins increase blood pressure, chronic fatigue and belly fat. They induce insulin resistance and "drug-induced" diabetes, which is often mistaken for Type 2 diabetes and managed with additional medications. Statin users also experience muscle pain, weakness, chronic inflammation and kidney damage.[10]

Only animal products have cholesterol. Lower your cholesterol intake and reduce cholesterol without drugs.

Acidic Aging

We associate hormone dysfunction, weight gain, poor eyesight, memory loss, brittle bones and weak muscles with the aging process. But a shortage of micronutrients impairs the body's ability to detoxify and heal. Inflammatory foods interfere with cellular functions and promote our decline. Over time, toxins accumulate in fat cells and cause premature aging.

Kidney stones, osteopenia, arterial plaque and urinary tract infections are exacerbated by acid-producing foods. The kidneys must neutralize excess acid with calcium and magnesium from the bones. This disrupts electrolyte balance and leads to mineral deposits in our organs.[11]

Fight the aging process by reducing consumption of acid-forming foods.

Acid-forming foods include processed cheeses; red and processed meat; sugary dairy products; processed wheat, corn and rice; alcohol; soda pop; artificial sweeteners (aspartame, saccharine); corn syrup; and some fish (especially lobster and shrimp).

Low-Acid and Alkaline-forming foods include most vegetables, legumes and many fruits (though not all). Whole and unprocessed foods are the fountain of youth.

ColleenKachmann.com/members

Meet Your Meat

I've always had compassion for living animals, so I ignored the fact that meat is produced via death. I grew up believing meat was an essential source of protein. I doubted I could ring the neck of a chicken unless post-Apocalyptic conditions threatened survival. But the neat, sanitary packages of meat at the store removed me from the process.

When I stumbled upon the sobering secrets of CAFOs (concentrated animal feeding operations) my apathy turned to outrage. Images of grass fed cows grazing in sunlit pastures and happy fat pigs rolling in mud are fake. They conceal the horrors endured by livestock raised for food.[12]

Did you know?

- Cows stand in cages with feces up to their knees their entire lives. They can't move or turn around. They are fed unnatural diets (cheap GMO corn) that cause bloating and pain. Many never see the light of day or the calves they birth.

- Chicken beaks are sadistically removed at birth so they can't peck each other to death in an environment that fosters insanity. They are born into darkness and confined in football-field sized coops with tens of thousands of other chickens. Conditions are so cramped there isn't room to spread their wings. Growth hormones are injected or added to food to facilitate rapid growth for earlier slaughter. Their legs often break under their own weight.
- Pigs live in darkness and crowded squalor. They hang by one leg on the conveyor line to slaughter via electrocution. Many are not lucky enough to die. These animals are more intelligent than dogs. They hear the groans and squeal in terror as those ahead bleed out or get tossed alive into the grinder.

The barbarity of meat and dairy production is sickening. Seeing the truth compelled me to commit to a lifelong boycott. I stopped participating in the demand for the unlimited and cheap supply of brutally mistreated "commodities." Independent of my concern for the animals, I did not want to consume the hormones of stress and fear that linger in tissue after death.

I fully accept that well-fed animals, raised with sunlight and space, have a place in our ancestry and culture. But *less than one percent* of our meat supply comes from such farms.[13]

The planet does not have the capacity to support the humane production of sustainable livestock at current demands. According to the United Nations Food and Agricultural Organization (FAO), "Meat production is the second or third largest contributor to environmental problems at every level and on every scale, from global to local. It is the primary culprit in land degradation, air pollution, water shortage, water pollution, species extinction, loss of biodiversity and climate change."[14]

We treasure some animals as pets and classify other animals as meat. There is no logic in our approach. We don't eat cats. But cows and bison are on the menu. It is a crime to eat a dog or a horse. But everyone cheers when Babe is served as bacon. These flagrant discrepancies defy explanation. Are we a culture of hypocrites?

It is not only possible to live on a plant-based diet, it's healthy and delicious. The cliché is true: We are what we eat. Being vibrant and alive versus artificially large and dead is a matter of choice.

Challenging Carnivores

Labels simplify life. Ingredients, directions and descriptions frame the expectations we have for both packages and people. But assumptions about what we are eating (or who we are dealing with) limit our ability to make independent decisions.

The way I promote my diet is to just live and eat. Others can judge for themselves. I don't care to argue. There is no secret vegan club where points are awarded for recruiting new members. Of course I care about people. I hate to see suffering that I know could be eliminated with a change in diet. But unless someone asks my opinion with genuine interest, I chew with my mouth closed (most of the time).

Declining normal foods in social situations can lead to conflict. A polite "no thanks"—and even silent avoidance—can have audible repercussions. Unregistered carnivore customer service representatives mistake the vegan diet for a personal challenge. Try to be polite. You have the right to choose what you eat. And everyone has the right to be wrong.

The dispute often begins with, "You *need* to eat meat for protein and iron. You need milk for calcium!"

I usually respond with, "No, doctor, I don't." (I call nutritional know-it-all's "Doctor" even if they aren't... though many of them are.)

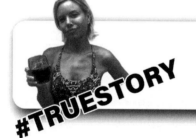

People say I'm condescending.
(That means talking down to someone.)

A plant-based diet provides plenty of protein and superior nourishment. The high levels of micronutrients in plants aren't a McFib. Accurate information should be issued to novice vegans on a laminated, wallet-size card. The fallacy that a plant-based diet lacks protein because it doesn't include meat needs to be corrected.

Within a year of adopting a vegan diet, I had answers for every carnivore concern. I read books, watched documentaries and practiced what I preached. But, as life reveals time after time, theoretical knowledge does not always translate into practical application. Whenever we declare allegiance to a particular ideology, we surrender some of our individual freedom. We exchange autonomy for the acceptance of like-minded people. Let's face it: life is easier when membership has its privileges.

Labels (vegan included) provide standardized answers to complicated questions. Once I was up and running as an official vegan representative, I noticed that elevator-speech explanations for complicated issues were not always accurate.

Nutrition Facts[15]

Amount per 500 calories	Plant Based Foods*	Animal Based Foods**
Cholesterol (mg)		137
Fat (g)	4	36
Protein (g)	33	34
Beta-Carotene (mg)	29,919	17
Dietary Fiber (g)	31	
Vitamin C (mg)	293	4
Folate (mcg)	1168	19
Vitamin E (mg)	11	0.5
Iron (mg)	20	2
Magnesium (mg)	548	51
Calcium (mg)	545	252

*Equal parts of tomatoes, spinach, lima beans, peas, potatoes
**Equal parts of beef, pork, chicken and whole milk.

Meat Geeks vs. Veg Heads Challenge accepted!

RULES VERSUS REALITY

I had been a strict vegan for two years when I began to have trouble with my hair. It was frizzy and fried. The only difference between the fuzz on my head and that of a troll-head pencil-topper was the color (blonde versus bright pink or purple). I assumed my hair stylist was over-processing the highlights. I switched salons. I cut it short. My hair looked bouncy and full. It will grow back, right? I was still cute. Worse things have happened to nicer people.

It didn't grow back, though. The ends continued to split, break, and crumble. My hair was getting shorter, not longer. I suffered unusual bloating and joint pain. I was losing weight. My skin had an ashen pallor. I was tired all the time. I wasn't getting much exercise, yet my muscles were often sore. And, though I'd gone cold tofu on the nicotine mints, my dentist found more cavities.

I did not consider that the problem might be diet related. Duh. I was vegan. How much healthier can you eat? Ah, but I had forgotten that adequate intake of several essential nutrients requires attention and strategy for the plant-based diet.

I took my laundry list of random symptoms to my family doctor. She took one look at my thin frame and anxious demeanor and proclaimed "stress" to be the official diagnosis. (Thanks, Sherlock. But I need to know what's *wrong*.) She knew I was vegan, but seemed to respect the issue as though it's a religion. Indeed, vegans may be motivated by a set of beliefs. But nutritional deficiencies aren't a moral penance. She prescribed an anti-depressant. I declined, requesting a blood panel instead.

The results showed my thyroid was healthy. Immune indicators, iron levels, cholesterol and triglycerides were textbook perfect. But the hallmark signs of the vegan dilemma were there. I had no detectable levels of vitamin B or vitamin D in my body.

This explained a lot. Vitamin B can be stored in the body for 2-3 years. I'd been a vegan for the same time frame. Symptoms of deficiency include stomach problems, depression and thinning skin. A lack of vitamin D results in fatigue, muscle pain and tooth decay. Hello, Ms. Obvious! Deficiencies also impair concentration and memory. Self-diagnosis and healing are impossible when you can't remember that they are options.

I wanted to stick with my plant-based diet. Weekly injections of vitamin B12 and 50,000 IUs of vitamin D were prescribed. Within weeks, I was feeling much better. My doctor had wanted to balance my brain chemistry with an anti-depressant. But my diet was not balanced enough to support healing. Anti-depressants aren't fortified with vitamins. (And why the heck not?) I wanted to be well, not just feel better about being sick.

I am grateful for supplements that allow me to remain true to my vegan ideals. My hair didn't grow for a long time (due to leaky gut), but a cute cut made it look bouncy and full. I received a lot of compliments on the style, so I thanked Mother Nature for the fashion intervention. (I guess ponytails aren't as cute in middle age.)

There was no escaping the turmoil in my life at that time. I was in the thick of a divorce, managing four children and looking for an income after being a stay-at-home mom for 15 years. But the odds of conquering these challenges improved dramatically once I was properly nourished.

My goal was to earn a living without actually getting a job. (Dream big or leave home!) Becoming vegan had launched my journey to wellness. I've fallen into almost every pitfall on the path. My experiences offer valuable insight (mostly in what not to do). Busy people searching for hope need solutions. I developed a strategy to use my problems (both real and perceived) as a guide to help others.

The more I dug in, the more I found legitimate concerns that strict vegans must address. Research shows that a plant-based diet can prevent and reverse illness and disease. That's a fact. But can it keep us healthy in times of stress? I dared to read the labels from opposing camps. I discovered there are no one-size-fits-all-all-the-time answers. Reality doesn't have to play by the rules.

> Rules are for the *obedience* of fools and the *guidance* of wise men.
>
> Sir Douglas Badar (1910-1987) WWII Royal Air Force flying ace

Vegan Propaganda

There is picture of a huge, furry, awe-inspiring ape, with a big wad of grass hanging from his mouth. The caption reads: "If this guy can get all of his protein from plants, why can't you?"

The answer is supposed to be rhetorical. A light bulb moment should follow. Touchdown! Team Vegan.

Carnivores are quick to cry foul. Grass-eating gorillas don't negate cow-eating cavemen.

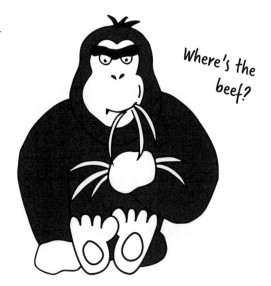

Upon closer inspection, the analogy falls apart. There are fundamental differences between the human digestive system and range-roaming herbivores. Yes, a well-rounded plant-based diet does provide all of the nutrients that human beings need. But accessing and *absorbing* essential amino acids in fibrous foods requires more than swallowing.

Fiber is essential to a clean and functional digestive system. As it moves through the intestines, it absorbs toxins and eliminates waste. This benefits our kidneys and strengthens the immune system. Fiber blunts sugar absorption. This is why fruit is healthy and jellied pastries are not. Fiber keeps cholesterol levels low and maintains bowel health. Fiber also aids in weight loss and lowers the risk of heart disease, diabetes and cancers of the intestines, colon and rectum.

High fiber foods are bulky. They pass through the digestive system faster than animal products. The body has less time to break down and absorb nutrients. Vegetable roughage is eliminated in about 12 hours. In contrast, it takes two to four days to digest a steak.

This contradicts an over-simplified vegan-ism that "meat rots in the gut." Ironically, the opposite is true (though it's a mere issue of semantics). Our bodies produce the enzymes necessary to digest meat proteins. The proteins in vegetables, grains and legumes (beans) are encased in fiber. Humans don't produce the enzymes that break down fiber. Fiber digestion is outsourced to the bacteria (gut flora) that live in the intestines. As the technical definition of "rotting" is decomposition by bacterial or fungal action, vegan speechwriters lose that round.

The secondary concern in fiber digestion is that fermentation of plant material produces methane and carbon dioxide gas. This is why farts are stinky and beans and cruciferous vegetables can make us bloat. It is critical to include probiotics and fermented foods (such as unpasteurized sauerkraut) in a whole-foods diet. The "good guy" microbes digest the tough stuff for us.

The reason that cows, goats and deer thrive as herbivores is because grazing is a full time job. An adult cow produces 100-150 liters of saliva a day and chews for hours. They even regurgitate to keep the process going. (This is called "chewing your cud" not "throwing up in your mouth.") The digestion process of a ruminator (an animal with four stomachs) takes up to three days. In contrast, humans produce 1.5 liters and chew less than 10 times before swallowing. We need the bacteria and yeast in our intestines to ferment (break down) the plant material.

Eating whole plant foods takes effort. I've adjusted my habits to allow for the time and energy to prepare them. Many people have seen me carry around a tub of salad that takes me all day to eat. I don't chew my cud so, technically, I'm not a grazer. But I've adjusted my habits because eating a plant-based diet makes me feel good. It's my "normal."

My approach isn't suitable for everyone. And in chaotic times, I do make concessions. There are days that I don't have the time (or the energy) to chop and chew all day. Stress has poked some holes in my gut, which interferes with my ability to digest high fiber foods. Sometimes for the sake of survival, I eat a "happy" chicken egg or a few bites of organic meat. Starving myself for the sake of claiming strict vegan status only reinforces the nay-sayers objections. I promote compromise and independent thinking as opposed to rigid rules that can be self-defeating.

Health is not just genetic destiny. In turn, diet alone does not guarantee wellness. Knowledge, awareness and the ability to adapt are essential to vitality. There is more to the cliché, "you are what you eat." If life was that simple, I'd be a sophisticated salad and not the fruity cocktail I am.

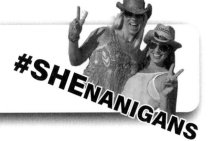

They say you are what you eat.
I don't remember eating a hot mess.

#SHENANIGANS

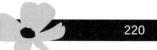

MONEY MANUFACTURERS

Government funding is dwindling. The baby boomers are retiring. Social security is maxed-out. The cost of healthcare is taxing the system. Reduced government aid cripples medical research, and funds for health initiatives are hard to find.

WARNING: May contain traces of sarcasm

Who has money these days? The industries that manufacture money, of course. Unfortunately, the Organic Farmers Association produces vegetables, not money. Grant requests are placed in cheap frames and provide comic relief to the volunteer staff.

Pharmaceutical Companies, on the other hand, make a *lot* of money. (To be fair, they make drugs too.) In turn, self-interest disguised as altruism subsidizes the medical community. Over 98 percent of revenue for medical journals is generated by ad sales to drug makers.[16] They finance college courses, seminars, literature and research; and sponsor community health initiatives. Drug reps even cater lunches for busy physicians all over the country. Their "Happy-to-Help!" efforts cover all the bases.

Will Big Pharma go broke helping all the doctors, future doctors (medical students) and the institutions that train them? Nah. In fact, they'd go broke if they didn't make magnanimous efforts to properly educate the medical community. You see, only doctors can prescribe their drugs. To do that, doctors must be informed about those drugs. The gift is in the giving.

THE SOY CONTROVERSY

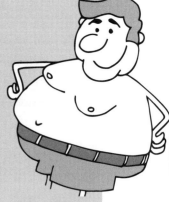

Soymilk and tofu get a bad rap in the media with concerns of breast cancer and man-boobs.[17] Rest assured, whole soy foods are good for you. It's all the hydrogenated vegetable oils, fillers and thickeners American's consume in processed foods that are problematic. And the majority of GM soy is used to feed chickens, pigs and cattle; soy compounds are present in the meat we eat as well.

Soy contains protective phytoestrogens called isoflavones. It's also high in protein and fiber. Soy has been shown to lower the risk of breast cancer, improve survival rates and help reduce menopausal hot-flash symptoms. Isoflavones are protective. They serve as antioxidants, improve immune function and regulate estrogen levels.[18]

 ColleenKachmann.com/members

LIFE OFF THE LABEL

Essential Foods and Supplements for the Vegan Diet

No diet is perfect in all seasons, stages of life or geographical locations. Choosing a plant-based approach for ethical or physical reasons (or both) has amazing health benefits. Understanding the limitations allows you to rise above them.

Probiotics and Fermented Foods: Our bodies don't produce cellulase, the enzyme that breaks down cellulose (fiber). Plants have small amounts, but can't provide enough to sustain digestion. Having the right balance of microbes in the gut is essential to high fiber diets. Quality probiotic supplements and unpasteurized (and homemade) yogurts, sauerkraut, miso and kombucha tea boost nutrient absorption.

Vitamin B_{12}: You cannot get enough B_{12} from plants to sustain healthy reserves in your body. Plants do not store the nutrient in their tissues as animals do. Thus, only minuscule amounts are present. It is present in soil, but eating a few dirty organic vegetables doesn't bridge the gap. Animals can store B_{12} for up to two years. Deficiencies develop slowly and are hard to identify. See your doctor for a blood test to determine your level of need.

When analyzing supplements, look for B_{12} in the form of methylcobalamin. It is the most easily absorbed. Daily requirements are 1,000 to 2,000 micrograms. The synthetic version, cyanocobalamin is cheaper. But it contains traces of cyanide and is not stored in the body for long.

Iron: Iron supplements can be necessary on a plant-based diet. Foods high in vitamin C boost the absorption of plant-food iron. Cooking in a cast-iron skillet is a great way to reduce or eliminate the need for supplementation. This is my approach and regular blood tests confirm my iron levels to be healthy.

Iodine: Using iodized salt can provide adequate supply. Regular consumption of sea vegetables is an even healthier option.

Vitamin D: If you live in a place where winter is dark, it's essential to consume at least 1,000 IUs of vitamin D per day during the winter. You can get this from fortified foods. If you eat mostly unprocessed foods, look for a D_3 supplement or ask your doctor for a prescription.

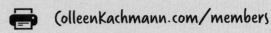 ColleenKachmann.com/members

Normal vs Healthy

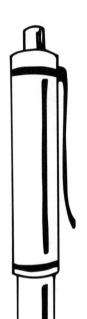

Many people are malnourished, even if they are overweight. Are you one of them? What evidence supports your opinion?

Redesign your plate. The bulk of every meal should be vegetables. One to two ounces of meat per day is optional and adequate. What changes can you make?

What labels define you? Name as many as you can, positive, negative and neutral.

Create an image of yourself from scratch. Compare and contrast the normal and the healthy versions of yourself.

 ColleenKachmann.com/members

PS I left this facing page blank for you.
Fill it with whatever you like. Questions, comments, to-do's, thoughts, etc.
You're welcome . . .

CHAPTER 12

SEEDS OF HEALTH

"If it came from a plant, eat it. If it was made in a plant, don't."

MICHAEL POLLAN, AMERICAN AUTHOR, JOURNALIST AND ACTIVIST

YUMMY VERSUS YUCKY

Fruits and vegetables are the staples of "healthy" food. But why? Most of us out-grow the need to ponder this question. Philosophical musings are the lost luxuries of childhood. We default to cliché answers when our own kids demand redundant explanations. Adult responsibilities eclipse youthful curiosity. Most of us just accept that we need to eat fruits and vegetables because "they are good for you," and move on with life.

The struggle between delicious and nutritious begins with the first taste of strained peas. The drama plays out on dinner tables every evening. We recite our lines from memory:

Parent: Eat your vegetables.
Child: (face scrunched in disgust) But they are yucky!
Parent: (exasperated) Eat them or no dessert!
Child: (near tears, whines) But why?
Parent: (eyebrows raised) Because they are good for you.
Child: (surprised) Why?
Parent: (with clenched teeth) Because I said so.

Vegetables are often served as a mushy, obligatory side dish (unless they are deep fried or smothered in cheese). Good-for-you food is not usually good. We follow complicated recipes for meat dishes and desserts, and heat up corn, carrots or green beans as an afterthought. If any food is left on the plate, it's likely the bland vegetables.

Fruits and vegetables should be the centerpiece of every meal. They are the most critical component of our diet. Why? The worn-out cliché, "an apple a day keeps the doctor away," is best explained with basic biology.

Breathing 101 (Don't Hold Your Breath)

Every cell in the body needs oxygen to function. We can't go more than a few minutes without breathing and live to tell the tale. The oxygen we inhale transforms glucose (sugar) into energy. A lack of oxygen prevents the heart from beating. Carbon dioxide is produced in the reaction. A buildup of carbon dioxide is toxic to our cells. We must exhale to release it.

The exchange of oxygen and carbon dioxide between plants and animals sustains life. Humans breathe in what plants breathe out, and vice versa. This is why having plants in our home keeps the air fresh. That's also why slashing the rainforests is equivalent to removing the lungs of the planet.

Oxygen converts fuel to energy. Substances disintegrate in the process. Oxygen's ability to generate heat, light and movement is known by many terms. Respiration occurs when oxygen produces energy in our body. Oxidation turns an apple brown and decomposes organic matter. Rust is the result of metal decay. Burning a candle produces light. The combustion of oil, gas and coal provide us with power.

When there is not enough oxygen to entirely break down a substance, the reaction is incomplete. Dangerous and unstable intermediates form. For example, using a generator or a gas fireplace in an enclosed room leads to incomplete combustion. Carbon monoxide is the result. Carbon monoxide has only one atom of oxygen, unlike its inert counterpart, carbon dioxide, which has two oxygen atoms. The missing oxygen atom leaves the molecule unstable. Carbon monoxide binds easily to the hemoglobin in our blood, but is ineffective at delivering oxygen to our cells. Thus it is known as the silent killer.

A shortage of oxygen in the body leads to incomplete respiration. Just as incomplete combustion produces deadly carbon monoxide, incomplete respiration leaves dangerous byproducts in our cells. The byproducts, known as *free radicals,* are highly reactive and electrically unstable.

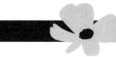

Like an out-of-control, flaming bouncy rubber ball, free radicals ricochet though the body, burning holes in cell structures. Free radicals damage DNA, and destroy essential nutrients, portals and binding mechanisms. They interfere with metabolism, hormone and brain functions. They mutate proteins and prevent the formation of key enzymes.

When the body has the right tools to keep free radicals under control, their powerful energy can be put to good use. Free radicals assist our immune system by zapping invading microbes. They kick our muscles into high gear during intense exercise (anaerobic respiration), and are destructive to cancer cells. Damage won't occur as long as the body can neutralize the free radicals when they are not needed.

Pollution, cigarette smoke, toxic food ingredients and existing disease increase the formation of free radicals. An overload of free radicals causes oxidative stress. Like any stress, the harmful effects accumulate over time and reduce our ability to function.

Free radicals must be neutralized to eliminate oxidative stress. There's only one way to do that: eat fruits and vegetables.

Why fruits and vegetables? Keep reading.

THE BEST VEGETABLE DRESSING EVER

This recipe will transform salads, stir-frys and grilled vegetables into a masterpiece of "More Please!" Vegetable-haters and kids alike will devour everything it coats. The recipe can be tweaked for more sweetness or less. It takes less than one minute to make.

Ingredients:
- Garlic Expressions Classic Vinaigrette Salad Dressing
- nutritional yeast flakes
- maple syrup (the real deal)

Place about ⅓ bottle of Garlic Expressions, ½ cup yeast flakes and 1-2 Tbsp. of maple syrup in a measuring cup. Whisk. Adjust flavor as needed. Done. Enjoy your vegetables!

 ColleenKachmann.com/members

The Physiology of Food

Plants face the same challenges that humans do. Environmental contaminates, pathogens and predators threaten their ability to survive. When plants are in danger, oxidative stress leads to the formation of free radicals. Failure to thrive, disease and death are inevitable as cell functions deteriorate. Humans have the ability to avoid and/or treat stressful irritations. Plants must thrive where they are, with what they have, or die trying.

Plants have evolved a powerful defense against unstable chemicals. Their vibrant colors reveal the presence of protective shielding molecules known as *antioxidants*. Antioxidants serve as sunscreen, insulating the plant from the penetrating rays of the sun. They encapsulate heavy metals. They neutralize industrial pollution, acidic soil and even nuclear radiation.

Antioxidants are Mother Nature's antidote to free radicals. This applies beyond the plant kingdom. Antioxidants also counteract free radicals in humans (who eat plants). They disable the fiery activity of dangerous chemicals and safeguard cellular processes in all living organisms.

That's why fruits and vegetables are good for you. They contain antioxidants which are the only protection we have against free radicals.

PS: Carnivores can relax. Meat does contain some antioxidants. But that's only because the animal ate the plant. Thanks, Babe.

From the movie? Get it? oink oink!

Beef versus Bean Burger

Many restaurants now offer bean burger substitutes. Try them! When prepared and served the same as hamburgers, your taste buds won't know the difference.

The body appreciates the alternative, however. Calorie for calorie, beans and legumes have the same amount of protein as ground beef, a ton of fiber, and there's no fat or cholesterol. The opposite is true for beef. And as beans take up a lot more room in the stomach, you'll feel full and satisfied.

Easy Bean Burger Recipe

- 2 (15-ounce) cans black beans
- ½ cup bread crumbs (gluten-free works too)
- 1 Tbsp. chopped garlic
- 1 egg (or egg substitute)
- ½ medium chopped onion
- 1½ Tbsp. Italian seasoning (fresh is best)
- 2 tsp. each parsley and cilantro
- ½ tsp. red pepper flakes (optional)
- salt and pepper (to taste)

Set aside one can of beans and the breadcrumbs. Blend rest of ingredients in a food processor or blender. Transfer to a mixing bowl and stir in remaining ingredients. Form patties. Using a baking sheet, grill on medium-low heat for about 6 minutes per side. Garnish as desired.

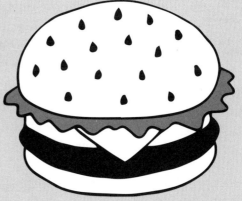

Get creative. Smother small patties with barbeque sauce and top with cabbage and red onion to make sliders. Or substitute romaine lettuce for bread and top with pico de gallo, avocado and cilantro.

 ColleenKachmann.com/members

SUPPLEMENT SUPPORT

Wellness is based on good nutrition. Yet sugar-free gelatin, saltine crackers and Sprite are issued to hospital patients in recovery. The standards of healthcare do not include nutrition. Few doctors argue the importance of a healthy diet. The problem is that doctors believe most people are adequately nourished (including themselves). If this belief were true, wellness would be normal.

Recently, I have come across the field of orthomolecular medicine. It's a field of wellness that is, like many other holistic disciplines, shrouded in vague misinformation. The mainstream medical community is quick to dismiss anything that isn't patentable and thus profitable.

Simply put, orthomolecular medicine considers nutritional deficiencies as (at least in part) both the cause and effect of illness. Orthomolecular physicians have been using nutrition to treat and cure disease for over 80 years.[1] Larger than normal doses of vitamins—used alone and in support of conventional therapies—have proven to be successful for the treatments (and recoveries) of depression, schizophrenia, alcoholism, heart disease and cancer.[2]

The government's recommendations for vitamins and minerals are set just above the minimum doses that prevent deficiency diseases. The vast range between individual deficiency and sufficiency is unknown and ignored. The Recommended Dietary Allowances (RDA) are defined as "the average daily intake sufficient to meet the requirements of most healthy individuals."[3] Sufficient consumption is not a prescription for optimal health. (A car can idle for a long time with little fuel. Going full speed on the highway requires a lot more gas.) Regardless, the majority of us are not healthy. Undiagnosed illness and pre-disease conditions are not the foundations of wellness.

Do you strive for adequate or abundant health (life)?

It's impossible to get all the nutrients we need from a "balanced diet" when the diet is heavy in processed foods. Packaged foods do not contain the same nutrition as whole foods. Produce grown in nutrient-deficient, pesticide-rich soil, picked early for long-distance transport, does not compare with ripened, seasonal offerings from local farms. And fortified foods are not bridging the gap. If they did, you wouldn't be reading this book.

Also, it's impossible to know exactly what nutrients a person needs during various times in life. Multiple factors deplete our nutritional reserves: stress, surgery, trauma, illness, lack of exercise, pollution, aging, medications—life! What's more, individual metabolism varies widely. Biochemical imbalances

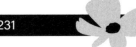

are genetic. The prescribed "adequate intake" may be optimal for some people. In others, it may be so inadequate that debilitation occurs.

Poor nutrition has created a chronically diseased, undernourished and overweight population. The ideal treatment for any illness should begin with, or at least include, substances that are naturally present and necessary in the body, as vitamins are. Vitamins are remarkable for their low toxicity and beneficial effects (versus the side effects of powerful pharmaceutical chemicals). They are inexpensive (compared to illness) and very effective at reducing disease.

When I began the vegan diet, I learned the hard way that nutritional deficiencies disable health. I take my vitamin B and D supplements religiously. When I discovered time-tested research on mega doses of vitamin C, niacin and zinc, I decided to experiment. I am finding relief from chronic issues—anxiety and insomnia to name a few. It will take time to evaluate my long-term outcome, but so far, I'm pleasantly surprised.

And to the extent my children are willing to try, I'm seeing that vitamins can help overcome junk food and sugar cravings, and many other common (normal) ailments. As I share the possibilities with friends and family, I am bearing witness to consistent results.

It is too early in my own research and experimentation to claim understanding of orthomolecular medicine. I do, however, claim hope. If you are looking for additional support in your wellness journey, look for more information about potential vitamin therapies.

Be very careful where you look, however. The largest and most frequented health websites have incomplete, biased and government-generated opinions about vitamins. Information on the Internet (as well as television and print) is heavily influenced by the pharmaceutical industry. Many commercial websites use pseudo-science to pitch pricey supplements. Simple vitamins are not expensive. It's best to look at independent research written by professionals who aren't trying to sell you something.

The Journal of Orthomolecular Medicine (JOM) has been publishing high-dose vitamin studies for almost 50 years. It is read and contributed to by physicians and scientists in over 35 countries. It is not indexed on the United States National Library of Medicine's electronic database, Medline. Questions regarding the omission of this journal go unanswered by government officials. Their responses are illogical. Medline says they only publish journals that are peer-reviewed. Yet JOM is peer-reviewed. The censorship by the political powers-that-be is evidence of corruption.

Use my bibliography to jumpstart your research. I have purchased every book referenced. Each was worth the price. Don't be dissuaded by the fact that many have been in print for thirty and forty years. Therapies that stand the test of time are more credible, not less. The websites I've cited are filled with research and links to additional information. Go to *orthomolecular.org* for the full archive of papers published in *JOM*. The ideal blend of theoretical and practical knowledge comes from physicians experienced in the field. But they are few and far between.

There's a reason for that. Regardless of the vague controversies, you don't need a prescription for vitamins. Examine the myths and decide for yourself.

Myth #1: Vitamins and supplements have not been proven to be beneficial. Actually, they have. Vitamins and supplements safely prevent, reduce and reverse disease.[4] According to the Poison Control Center, multivitamins kill no one.[5] Studies concluding that low-dose vitamin supplements are ineffective are correct. And irrelevant. A cup of water is no match for a raging bonfire. Does that prove water can't put out fires? Of course not! Low-dose vitamin studies simply prove that low doses do not reverse the impact of a nutrient deficient diet. There are many studies, however, that prove higher doses can.

In 2006, the NIH (The United States National Institute of Health) published a report concluding that vitamins are of no benefit to the general population. The report cited limitations in the quantity and quality of research and cast doubt on safety. As a result, vitamins are not included in the medical standards of care. Doctors who prescribe nutritional supplements are vulnerable to malpractice lawsuits (regardless of patient outcome). They are restricted by the politics of healthcare.

The NIH report said the research on vitamins was limited. Indeed, their research was feigned. The panel did not include any medical professionals that use nutritional supplements in combination with conventional therapy. No review was done of the 600-plus studies published by specialists in orthomolecular medicine. They considered only research published in their own database (and none of it included any evidence of harm).[6] The NIH did not find the well-documented truth that vitamins reduce disease because they weren't looking for it.

Myth #2: Vitamins make expensive urine. Vitamin critics use urine spillover to dismiss nutritional supplements as, at the very least, ineffective and wasteful. This argument is hypocritical. The body does not metabolize 100 percent of anything—food, vitamins, supplements or medications. Prescriptive dosages for medications are not based on what the body needs, but

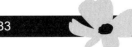

what the body will absorb. The presence of most drugs is easily detected in urine. In fact, 85 percent of a one-gram dose of acetaminophen is excreted unchanged within 24 hours.[7] Acetaminophen is recommended for just about every ailment we may have. Yet vitamins are a waste because they too end up in urine?

Un-metabolized vitamins are not problematic to either the person excreting them or the environment. However, urine contaminated with prescription drug spillover is a major concern. Hormones, steroids, opiates, antidepressants, antibiotics and many over-the-counter medications contribute to rising levels of pharmaceutical pollution. Drugs are designed to block or alter biological processes. Even minuscule levels have long-term risks.

The most common side effect of vitamin supplements is stomach upset and watery stool, even in cases of accidental or intentional overdose. Adverse reactions to prescribed medications cause injury or death in one of five hospital patients. Two million serious complications and 100,000 deaths are attributed to medications that were taken as prescribed every year.[8] In contrast, vitamins have been connected with the deaths of ten people in the last twenty-three years.[9]

> *Humans live through their myths and only endure their realities.*
>
> Robert Anton Wilson (1932-2007) author of cult-classic series The Illuminatus! Trilogy

Myth #3: High doses of vitamins are dangerous. High doses of anything can be toxic. Drinking too much water can be fatal. Children who eat hot dogs once a week have double the risk of brain tumors. Yet the risk for children who eat hot dogs and take vitamins is significantly reduced.[10] In truth, not taking vitamins increases the risk of disease.[11]

Vitamins are safer than any other product sold in a drugstore. High-dose vitamin therapies have been used for over 80 years. Determining the ideal dose poses little danger. The body naturally eliminates what it cannot use. It is safe to take as much as the bowel can tolerate.[12]

Naysayers emphasize *toxicity* to dissuade physicians and the public from using vitamins. The word "toxic" can erroneously imply deadly. Exceeding tolerance levels makes you feel sick for a few hours. That counts as a toxic reaction. But once the feeling of nausea passes, there are no further complications. Consider that women who take two or more aspirin a day have an 86 percent increase in pancreatic cancer, a disease that kills nearly all victims within three years.[13] That's deadly. Vitamin E decreases the risk of pancreatic cancer.[14] That's beneficial.

> "More people *live off cancer* then DIE from it."
>
> Dr. Deepak Chopra, board certified endocrinologist and holistic healer

Myth #4: Supplements do not replace a healthy diet. That's true. That's why they are called supplements and not replacements.

The concept of a balanced diet has been corrupted by food technology. Protein and sugar intake is way too high. Fruit and vegetable consumption is way too low. We need more antioxidants to balance the flood of free radicals. The standard American diet does not come close to delivering the necessary amount of essential nutrients to support wellness.

The best source of vitamins is food. But it's unreasonable to reject supplements when the diet is clearly deficient. Natural and synthetic vitamins are identical in structure. The vitamins in unprocessed plant foods do not contain trace additives (in theory; most plants are grown with pesticides). Vitamins in supplement form sometimes contain other ingredients (watch out for sugar, especially in children's chewables). Brands should be scrutinized and compared. Companies that disclose their manufacturing processes are usually high in quality. Ultimately, concerns about additives in vitamins seem frivolous when compared to the pharmaceutical contaminates in the water they are swallowed with.

Before you buy any supplement, do your homework—or look at someone else's. *LabDoor* is an independent research company that reviews accuracy, purity, nutritional value, efficacy and ingredient safety.[15] They grade brands from A+ to F. Their free,

Do your homework at Labdoor.com!

user-friendly website is a comprehensive tool that will help you get the most for your money.

The toxic medications we take for disorders do not prevent or cure disease. Side effects often sustain and increase sickness. Vitamins do not cause disorder or disease. They are proven to sustain and increase health. However, wellness doesn't sustain drug industry profits. Unfortunately, lies do.

Good Nutrition Can Subsidize Bad Decisions

When people hear me talk about my diet, they often say, "You must be so disciplined!"

I just laugh.

I am not well-disciplined. I am, however, extremely motivated. I am compelled to feel and be awesome. The truth is not complicated. I want to maximize my fun while minimizing the cost of my adventurous life.

Plants supply antioxidants. Harmful foods and medications deplete the reserves. An internal savings account stocked with an excess of micronutrients provides bonus points. A surplus can buffer the occasional vice.

Here's an example. It reads like a joke. It's a true story (though the ending doubles as a punch line).

Two women walk into a wine bar.

The first woman says, "I am exhausted! I didn't sleep well. I went to the drive-thru for lunch. I haven't even had time to pee today!" She proceeds to comfort herself with a blue-cheese-encrusted filet, a side of onion rings and a flight of white.

The second woman says, "I feel awesome! I got up early, went for a run and had veggie kabobs for lunch. I drank extra water so I won't get dehydrated by the wine." She orders, "Whatever veggies can be lightly stir-fried in a little olive oil and a flight of red, please."

They spend the next few hours laughing at each other's stories, enjoying their meal and toasting to life.

In the morning the first woman texts a meme to the second:

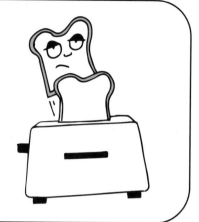

IF PEOPLE WERE MEANT TO POP OUT OF BED IN THE MORNING, THEY WOULD SLEEP IN TOASTERS.

The second woman thinks, "Fiddlee-de-dee, it's good to be me!" and pops out of bed with a smile. She swallows her vitamins, does a shot of kale and embarks on yet another Best Day Ever. She takes a selfie of her bright-eyed smile and texts her own meme in reply:

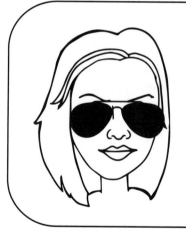

I HATE IT WHEN PEOPLE SAY, "SHE'S REALLY NICE ONCE YOU GET TO KNOW HER". THEY MIGHT AS WELL SAY, SHE'S A BITCH BUT YOU'LL GET USED TO IT.

The concept of "cheating" resonates with dieters. The good news is that it applies across the board when it comes to health. When you eat clean and avoid chemicals, you build nutritional reserves. These can sustain health when most normal people get sick, and buffer the consequences of an occasional vice. Consider that the risk of lung cancer in smokers who frequently eat green, orange and yellow vegetables can be reduced as much as 60 percent.[16] Obviously, that risk can be further reduced if they'd quit. But it's a valid point for those with more motivation than discipline.

Shift your focus from what you are giving up to what you are getting in return. Health is created one choice at a time.

Vegetables 101: Common Cooking Conundrums

If a refrigerator stocked with produce inspires you to go hungry, you are in good company. A few short cuts will make food preparation a lot easier.

Winter Squash: Many recipes instruct squash to be peeled and chopped before adding to stir-frys and soups. This method requires a vice and a chain saw. And it's totally unnecessary! Bake the squash whole (in a pan or dish as they leak). Cooking times and temps vary with size. Bake a medium squash at 400° for about 45 minutes. Be sure to remove stickers. They catch fire. After it cools, slice in half and scoop out the seeds. The skin separates without effort. Blend into soup, serve as a side or add to vegetable medleys. Acorn squash makes a delicious dairy free mac n' cheese (see recipe on page 169). Spaghetti squash doubles as angel hair pasta. Visit lifeoffthelabel.com for more recipes.

according to my friend.

Homemade Pizza: Stock gluten-free pizza crusts, organic marinara and vegan (or organic dairy) cheese. Top with frozen or fresh veggies. Sprinkle with Italian seasoning. This takes less time than ordering for delivery and costs about the same!

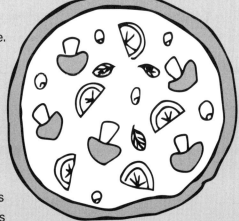

Soups as Starters: Pacific Foods, Imagine, Whole Foods 365 and similar brands offer entire lines of plant-based soups. Cream of mushroom, French onion, tomato, tortilla and many ready-to-eat varieties of soup and chili are available. Do not microwave (this reduces the living enzymes and denatures nutrients). Instead, heat in a saucepan. Transform soup into a meal by adding fresh or frozen veggies, beans, rice or lentils. Serve with green onions, cilantro, parsley, basil and thyme, or sprinkle with seasonings of choice.

Slow Roast Veggies: Season and marinate any (and all) vegetables as desired. Add a bit of water to the bottom of a roasting pan and bake for a couple of hours of at 325°. My family's favorite fall smell is slow-roasting onion, mushroom, sweet and regular potatoes, beets, carrots, peppers, and cloves of garlic. Add a few ounces of pork, beef or chicken as compliment to a primarily plant-based meal. Top with fresh or dried herbs like thyme, oregano and rosemary. Thicken a can of mushroom soup into gravy, splash with vinaigrette, or drizzle with tantalizing cashew cream sauce.

 ColleenKachmann.com/members

Seeds of Health

Normal vs Healthy

Inventory the foods you eat in a day and over the course of a week. According to the labels, should you be adequately nourished? Are you? Examine the evidence without assuming you know the answer.

How can you increase your intake of antioxidants? What foods and habits can you add (or eliminate) to counteract the formation of free radicals?

Observe the labels on the foods you eat. Can you explain the reason for, and the source of, each ingredient? Are the extra ingredients supporting or hurting your health?

Every time you consider purchasing processed food, consider what alternatives might be available. What products are you most dependent on? Why?

ColleenKachmann.com/members

PS I left this facing page blank for you.
Fill it with whatever you like. Questions, comments, to-do's, thoughts, etc.
You're welcome . . .

SEEDS OF HEALTH

CHAPTER 13

KID
FOOD
KILLS

"You can't beat the real thing."

Coca Cola

Label Lures

Food makers spend $10 billion a year to bypass the natural instincts of parents to feed their children a nutritious diet. They produce 40,000 food advertisements aimed directly at our kids. Close to 30,000 of these commercials are for candy, cereal and fast food. Children are highly vulnerable to marketing messages. These evocative appeals foster eating habits and create customers for life.[1] In contrast, only 100 commercials air each year promoting fruits and vegetables.[2] This pathetic attempt to promote healthy eating is even less effective than the congressional actions to discourage smoking.

The conveniences of today's world hold many dilemmas for modern parents. The tsunami of advertisements brainwash us, and our families, with absolute lies. I'm sorry to be the bearer of bad news, but Twizzlers do not make mouths happy. And sugar frosted flakes will never be part of a nutritious breakfast.

One cigarette is unlikely to cause lung cancer. One Big Mac does not cause heart disease. Habits do, however, have consequences. Overweight children are likely to grow up to be obese adults.[3] Obesity has been shown to reduce the length of life by an estimated five to twenty years. The lifetime risk for diabetes is now 30 to 40 percent for Americans.[4] Heart disease, kidney failure and cancer are striking people at younger and younger ages. Kid food is killing our kids. It's true when they say, that Oscar Meyer has a way with B-O-L-O-G-N-A."

Parents Just Don't Understand

It took a lot of therapy to forgive my mom for raising me to be healthy instead of normal. Each day, I was forced to bring a homemade lunch to school. Normal kids ate the school food. Granted, most of it went into the trash because, after all, it was gross. Nevertheless, I was jealous. That pizza smelled so good!

I was not allowed to wear make-up in the seventh grade. I looked twelve because I was twelve. In high school, I had to wash the family mini-van before I could borrow it. My curfew was so early that it was time to go home before I got to the party. At Christmas, Santa brought video games and boom boxes to normal kids. But my stocking was filled with oranges and the latest *Chicken Soup for the Soul.* Geeze, mom! Can a girl get a break?

My mom said I'd thank her later.

And she was right. Thirty years definitely qualifies as "later."

So, for the record, "Thanks, Mom."

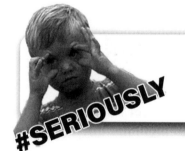

I just found a whip, a mask and handcuffs in my mom's bedroom. I can't believe it! She's a superhero.

Due to a traumatic (albeit healthy) upbringing, my single goal in life was to be normal. Of course, "normal" meant I would be like everyone else. My 16-year-old self made a solemn vow: "As God is my witness, I will never do this to my kids!" My kids would be allowed to wear make-up, stay out late and play video games. I'd serve Pop Tarts for breakfast, send money for school lunches and order pizza for dinner. My kids would be the definition of normal. And I would humbly accept my crown as The Coolest Mom in Never Never Land.

But motherhood turns brains into mush. I forgot the oath I'd made in my youth. By the time I had my first baby I was eating clean, avoiding fast food and pumping breast milk at work. I only let my son watch Sesame Street videos because I didn't want to expose him to junk food commercials. The daunting challenge was getting through the cookie aisle at the grocery without a temper tantrum.

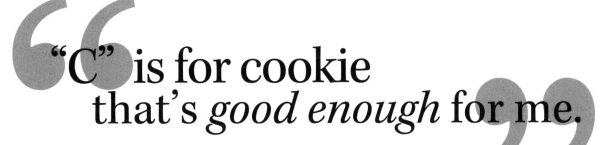

> "C" is for cookie that's *good enough* for me.
>
> Cookie Monster, Sesame Street

Well, cookies aren't good enough for my son, Mr. Cookie Monster. He's a growing boy. Next time you want to think about things that start with the letter "c," look for carrots, cantaloupe and cauliflower.

I was a diligent parent in the early years. Pre-school life is somewhat sheltered. I made my first attempt at compromise when my oldest turned four. I hosted his birthday party at Chuck E. Cheese. I intended to avoid the menu by distracting the tykes with lots of game tokens. But after the birthday boy blew out his candles, my "normal" party was exposed as a fraud.

"Where did your mom get this cake?" yelled Rude Dude over the blaring, obnoxious music. He glared suspiciously at the first piece as I offered it to my son.

"She made it," replied the birthday boy with pride. "I helped. We used real sugar instead of applesauce."

He stuck a fork in the center of his cake and attempted to shove the whole piece into his mouth. He giggled as clumps of shredded zucchini, carrot and oats crumbled back to his plate. Thin, homemade icing stuck to his flushed cheeks in the pulsating red and blue light. The other boys did not laugh on cue.

"Why is it green?" wondered Curious George. He did not mimic my son's antics and cram the cake into his face. Instead, he lifted his plate to eye level and glared in suspicion.

"What do you mean?" asked my son, looking as though the helium had just escaped from his shiny balloon.

The chaotic sounds of bells, whistles and circus music did not reduce the deafening silence that had settled over our group.

"Cakes aren't green. They are supposed to be chocolate or vanilla." Educated Eddie arched an eyebrow. "I like vanilla."

"Oh, we put *billa-stract* in it." (That's 4-year-old for vanilla extract.)

My son looked both hopeful and confused. None of his guests seemed happy. What had he done wrong?

The other mommies laughed as the rite of passage came to an abrupt end.

"It's a 'healthy' cake, boys." said Sally Sophisticate as she exchanged a condescending glance with the other moms.

"Just get a cookie from the prize counter after you win some games," Patty Pretentious instructed, as she lifted the offending plate out of her child's hands.

Great idea. The scowls turned to squeals. Arms and legs flailed. Chairs overturned as rowdy boys tumbled from the table, playfully climbing over one another like newborn puppies.

My son glanced at me over his shoulder before he ran off. The flickering strobe lights caught his expression. Time stood still as the experience crystallized in my memory. I'll never forget the look of betrayal in his eyes.

For the first time in his life, my son was embarrassed of me. (It would not be the last.) I felt bad. I was his mommy. In an instant, he was no longer a baby. A piece of his innocence was lost.

The other moms applauded my efforts but advised me to relax. Helpful Hanna pointed out, "After all, he'll only have one birthday a year."

Right, but so does everyone else. Social etiquette demands reciprocity. Birthday parties are an exchange of gifts and cake. Once a year, you give the cake and get the gifts. The rest of the year, you give the gifts and get the cake. That's a lot of cake for people with friends and family.

> *Loosen up a little.*
> America RUNS on Dunkin'.
>
> — Dunkin' Donuts

LIFE OFF THE LABEL

Food: the Gateway Drug

I tried and failed to "just relax." My attempts to resist the social pressure were frowned upon. I internalized this as rejection. I wanted to be accepted by my peers. I wanted my son to have friends. Recreational use of junk food was rewarded with praise. Healthy choices were shunned. I began to doubt my self and my ability to discern what's right. I grew dependent on the opinions of my social circle to gauge my level of normal. It seemed that eating with the crowd was they only way to make friends.

The "food fights" intensified once my kids were enrolled in school. I did not contribute the high-fructose-corn-syrup-apple-juice or artificially orange Goldfish for snacks. I requested people not give my children candy almost everywhere we went. I protested the chicken nuggets and fries that were standard lunch fair. I resorted to my mother's shameful behavior: I packed their lunches. I brought homemade food to parties and play dates. It didn't take long for me to be crowned The Food Nazi.

So much for my goal of being crowned The Coolest Mom Ever.

My kids begged for Oreos and soda pop when they went to other people's homes. Friendly moms alerted me to their intrusive behaviors and offered advice: "If you deprive them of junk food, they will crave it. Just let them have it. They won't want it anymore."

I found this notion as ridiculous as the pediatrician's advice that "any food a picky kid will eat" is better than "no food at all." That qualified hot dogs and ice cream as legitimate sources of protein and calcium.

Yet no one wanted to challenge these illogical conclusions. Friends agreed in theory but I stood alone in practice. Just because my kids want Oreos doesn't mean I have to give it to them. My desire to eat and feed my kids healthy strained relationships. Friends (and family) told me that I had an eating disorder and serious control issues.

I disagreed.

I stood my ground for almost seven years. But the battles eroded my confidence and sense of authority. I wanted to be healthy. I wanted to be normal. Apparently, I had to make a choice.

Soon after the birth of my 4th child, a federal court ruled that pizza sauce and deep-fried and battered French fries qualify as fresh vegetables.[5] Overwhelmed,

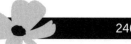

I surrendered my crusade. I accepted the antidepressants prescribed by my doctor and ordered four happy meals to go. And yes, "Supersize those banana splits. My kids need potassium and calcium. Thank you, please."

> **"Do what tastes RIGHT.** *It's better here.***"**
>
> — Wendy's

Life was soon easy and fun. We moved into Normalville and ate with the Jones. I still cooked healthy meals at home. But when things got chaotic, I went through a drive-thru or fed my kids at the movie theater or mall food court. Whatever. Wherever. My kids enjoyed their friends. They appreciated my new approach to "food fairness." Friends and I exchanged junk-food justifications for mutual validation. I swallowed my "don't worry, be happy" pills and gave up.

My pharmaceutical phase lasted about five years. It was a rollercoaster ride from hell. The medications only worked for so long. When I suffered from breakthrough bitchiness, the doctor would up my dose or prescribe something different. I would lose weight, gain weight, flip out and zone out. I needed one pill to wake up and another to go to sleep. One night I awoke in the trunk of my car (thankfully parked in my own garage). It scared me to death. Reports of nighttime driving and blackouts by fellow Ambien users were making headlines. I banned that from my list of options. But I succumbed to the belief that something was wrong with me that only doctors and drugs could fix.

What was I thinking?

I wasn't. My brain had been hijacked.

Thankfully, life intervened on my behalf. Clarity arrived the morning after I made an awful scene after my grandfather's funeral. It had been a sad day for my family. We spent the evening telling stories and toasting to his life. After several hours, much to my shame, I demonstrated why psychotropic drugs don't mix with alcohol. I was slurring and talking nonsense. A confrontation ensued. Luckily, I was confined to the safety of a hotel room. My family calmed and protected me. My mother lay with me in the bed, soothing my tears as I wept in a fog of confusion.

LIFE OFF THE LABEL

The hangover and humiliation motivated me to clean out my brain and my body. After a month of detox, the fog in my head began to clear. I felt better than I had in years. I did not feel hopeless, broken or artificially sweet. I was inspired to see beyond the boundaries of what had become a go-with-the-flow life. Once the mind-numbing drugs were out of my body I emerged from my cocoon.

As I shared in chapter one, I went to the doctor that fateful day and accepted drugs in exchange for peace, I surrendered my sense of *self* (my ego, my knowledge, my intuition) in order to survive. I thought being normal would solve the problems that overwhelmed me. Following your own path and thinking for yourself can be exhausting. Blending in with the crowd seems so much easier. And it is, but only on the surface. I can happily report that being healthy and happy is far more fun than fitting in and feeling normal.

Once the drugs were out of my system, I was reintroduced to my true Self. And she's not broken or guilty. She's healthy. And awesome.

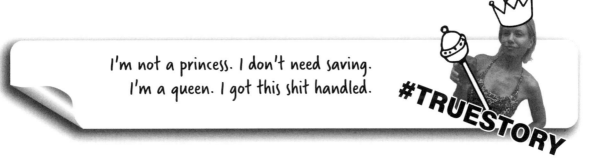

SAVE THE HOSTAGES

Anyone who has ever fed a child knows that no matter what you feed them, they are going to resist. From the first taste of a new formula, the introduction of each new smell, flavor and texture is an arduous process. Initial attempts usually include spitting, gagging and maybe even vomiting.

So we create routines and comfort around eating. We sing songs and offer rewards. We oversell our efforts like cheap car salesmen. One day, apple oatmeal in a Dora bowl with a Superman spoon on a Mickey Mouse placemat is the magical formula for all three meals. A week later, the same approach invokes a temper tantrum worthy of YouTube, and we're back to playing airplane with strained bananas.

Many factors dictate a child's mood-swinging appetite. Teeth (or lack thereof), taste buds, texture, growth spurts, television commercials and past experiences all have a place at the table. The least significant factor is the actual compatibility of the food with the child's palette.

I've heard that a food must be introduced seven times before a child accepts it. But 18 years of anecdotal evidence indicates that is a severe underestimate. Getting kids to eat anything new requires Nobel Peace Prize-worthy ingenuity and patience. SWAT-team-level negotiation skills, and intelligence training in manipulation and subterfuge also come in handy. At any given meal, the victory goes to the smartest, richest and most stubborn.

You may be well prepared to win the battle, but innocent tears can be deceiving. And exhausting. The taste of defeat is bitter and best paired with a dry Merlot.

My first approach to the vegan diet was to transition the children gradually. I limited animal products, processed foods and snacks. I encouraged them to "just try" my meals. That did *not* work. They had no interest (i.e. motivation) to eat the food I was cooking. They would sneak a peanut butter sandwich, eat a freezer pizza or blow through a box of cereal when I wasn't looking.

My next idea was to stop buying all the extras. I told them to call the 1800-NOT-FAIR hotline. But calls to the complaint department were suspiciously low. A flourishing black market for contraband developed in our home. There was hidden food, secret codes, barters for favors and cash for candy. Strange, unmarked packages arrived via UPS. I was impressed with my little band of mobsters.

Now, I get wary when they stop arguing with me. Sibling rivalry that dissolves into teamwork is a Big Red Flag. I know they are up to something when hand-signals and positive attitudes replace insults and eye-rolls. I feel like Alice (the housekeeper) in an episode of The Brady Bunch Visits the Twilight Zone.

I alternate between looking the other way and beating them at their own game. I go through phases where I stop buying bread, peanut butter and oatmeal. There are no chips, cereal or frozen pizzas. When the pantry is barren, hunger pains improve the chances my children will eat what I make. But it is a balancing act. I cannot control everything, especially when they are at school or in other people's homes. And there are days when (gasp!) my own life takes priority over what they are eating.

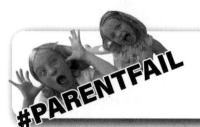

#PARENTFAIL You're making it difficult to be the parent I thought I would be.

I also fight fire with fire by indoctrinating them through documentaries and books. They aren't the only ones with stubbornness in their DNA. After all, I am their mother.

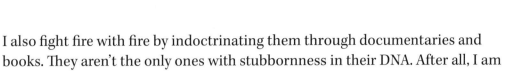

See my list of favorites on page 135.

> **Silly Rabbit, *Trix are for kids.***
>
> — Trix Cereal

THE CRAFTY CONTRACT

Every year, when the kids bring home their science fair assignments, it's a truckload of work dumped in my lap. I am the designated project manager for four separate teams. While I appreciate the opportunity to participate in my children's education, it's just as much work for me as it is for them. It would be easier to just do it all myself.

One year, I used the science fair to sneak in a bit of awareness about how important food choices are, even for kids. My girls, third and fifth graders at the time, didn't stand a chance against my devious scheme. I suggested an experiment in diet.

I offered to let them eat junk food or whatever they wanted for an entire month. We would survey their perceptions and school performance. In exchange, my 9-year-old would adopt a gluten-free diet and the 11-year-old would eat only unprocessed foods. They signed up without reading the fine print: the healthy diet would also last an entire month.

Yeah. I'm a tricky, mean mom.

We developed self-assessment forms, which they filled out three times a day. A 5-point scale, ranging from -2 to 2 (with zero being neutral) measured everything for attention span, attitude, motivation, tummy and headaches, skin issues and emotions. Two adults evaluated them each day, usually a teacher at school and then me or their dad.

For two months, I reminded them daily to fill out their forms. I showed them how to collect outside research. I helped prepare their food. Actually, I only had to do that for the good-for-you-food month. The second month was a free-for-all. This provided extra time so that they could input all of the information into an Excel spreadsheet and graph the data. (Just kidding; I did that.)

It became obvious to all involved, especially my daughters, that diet affects everything. They felt so good they seemed a little disappointed when the first month ended. For the sake of the project, they ate extra crap just to see how bad they felt. If they had been smart, they would have eaten cleaner so the contrast would not have been so dramatic. But kids don't grasp consequences. Indeed, the results proved to be of statistical significance. I calculated Σ (standard deviation) and helped them make conclusions.

I expected the project to earn national attention. I thought it was a mistake when the only award bestowed was for participation. Indeed, the feedback from the judges was glowing and complimentary. But my involvement was crystal clear and the judges were duty-bound to put the fair after science.

I conducted an awards ceremony anyway, complete with 1st place ribbons (I ordered them on-line). My daughters earned a valuable lesson. They learned that food choices have consequences for kids too. They still eat junk food when they can get away with it. They are too young to care about their grades, budding figures or even bad moods. That's still my job. But the science fair project left a memorable impression. A seed was planted. It will flourish . . . in time.

COOKING WITH KIDS

Teach kids about high quality food. First you gather high quality food. Involve them in meal planning. My kids help plant the garden. I take them with me to the grocery store and farmers markets. I let them pick the produce. I invite each to join me one-on-one to assist in meal preparation. I show them how to "sneak" more veggies into the meal. Conspiracy brings us together. When they participate in the process, they appreciate the end result.

It's important to sit down as a family for meals (even if a few members are missing). Discuss the foods you make. Share your opinion. (I don't always like what I make—though sometimes, I feel like I deserve an award for Top Chef.) Blend analytical observations of taste and texture with the sensual experience of satiety. Hit the nutritional highlights of what the food has to offer. Entertain their ideas for alternative preparations. Encourage them to help make improvements the next time.

A few hours after a meal, inquire as to how they feel. This is also an effective tactic after a junk food binge. When my kids complain of headaches and bellyaches, I don't offer them medication. I ask them what they've eaten. They roll their eyes but it works every time. No sympathy for you! Children who understand that food choices affect their entire life will become conscious eaters.

During meals, I'm fine if a kid picks around an offering. I encourage them to try a few bites but I'm pleased with what they have learned to like. Also, a little hunger goes a long way. Stubbornness does not cause starvation. Kids in third world countries stand in line for hours just to receive a small portion of bland rice or mush. When it comes to food, pickiness stands in direct proportion to choice.

It is also important to parent as a team. Kids can spot a weak link in the chain of command a mile away. They will divide and conquer parental units like little Napoleons. Don't let them. Decide on the rules and stand firm on each other's behalf.

Cooking at home is hard enough. Eating in the outside world requires Olympic talent and dedication. To get more good food into your kids than bad, you need playbooks, diversion tactics and contamination drills standardized and running on all cylinders. It is exhausting. That's why most people don't do it.

I talk to my kids about food every day. I encourage them to eat as many vegetables and as little junk as possible. My lectures seem to translate into "Blah-blah-greens-blah-blah-vitamins-blah-blah-good-for-you." But there are glimpses of hope when they choose something healthy without any direction from me. I try not to let them see me smile.

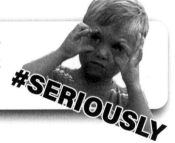

When I was little, my dad had me convinced that the ice cream truck only played music when they were sold out. Well played Dad. #SERIOUSLY

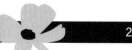

Treats for Kids

Kids want cookies and freezer pizzas. So do their friends. These "treats" are the official definition of "kid food." I let my kids have as much as they want (with a caveat, of course). I purchase gluten-free and organic baking ingredients. When they indulge, they must make it themselves.

This introduces them to cooking with recipes and reduces impulse eating. It also makes a mess of the kitchen. All too often, the counters are left sticky and the pans and dishes dirty. I don't get mad (unless I do). I just nag them until the kitchen is restored to its former state of clean (assuming it was). Eventually, this strategy will motivate them to do it right the first time. In the event that it becomes easier to finish the job myself, the offending child is assigned dinner dishes for as long as it takes to realize that cleaning the kitchen doesn't hurt.

Middle School: Bad Attitude, Bad Grades and Bad Diet

My son struggled for several years with his grades. By the time he was in middle school, I was used to seeing bad report cards. There had been many changes in his life that provided easy excuses. He had been in six different schools over a four year period. We moved three times. But despite poor grades, he had tested into the gifted program with a high IQ. So I tried not to worry. (I just dreaded parent/teacher conferences.)

One morning, the summer before my son entered seventh grade, was I pin-balling through the house: cleaning, organizing and gathering laundry. I found him reading. I had yet to remind him 37 times, so it caught me off guard. The I'm-So-Proud-of-You-Speech was interrupted when something odd grabbed my attention. He was reading the book upside down—the exact same book he'd been (not) reading for the last three summers.

My bubble of confidence imploded as reality set in. OMG! My little wannabe engineer couldn't read. Or worse, he was a conniving liar who refused to read. He was faking it to earn video game time and make his siblings look bad.

Thank God there was no nanny-cam to record my outburst. Frustration welled from deep pools of emotion. Kids are a lot of work; a fact not disclosed in the glossy *Joys of Being a Parent* brochure. "Why is everything a fight?" I yelled.

I ripped up the book. I had a meltdown that would have left a two-year-old embarrassed.

After I took a time-out (moms need them too), I had a heart-to-heart discussion with my son. It became clear that he was struggling, not rebelling. I wanted to help, not punish.

I took him to a doctor of integrative medicine who prescribes diet and lifestyle changes rather than symptom control via pharmaceuticals. He charges out-of-pocket. We paid out-the-nose. Natural medicine can be quite expensive and is not usually covered by health insurance. It is sad to note that it's cheaper and easier to go to a "normal" doctor. The problem is that a 15-minute visit, a prescription and low co-pay rarely result in wellness.

A blood test suggested my son is sensitive to gluten. Analogous to the pain scale, his intolerance was estimated at four. Full-blown celiac disease tops the chart at ten. That may not sound significant, but I was screaming for an epidural when I hit three in early labor. At the very least, gluten sensitivity could reduce his ability to concentrate.

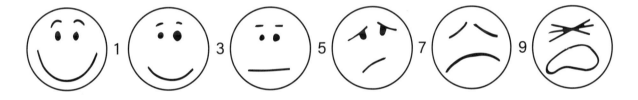

The doctor recommended a gluten-free diet—to a middle school, preteen male. The suggestion was overwhelming. How would I ever convince that dude to eat his vegan veggie burger without a bun? But I had to try. So I did what any desperate mother (vegan or otherwise) might do. I offered him meat, cheese and gluten-free junk food. He took the deal and agreed to try the diet for the remainder of the summer.

I created a special shelf in the pantry that was just for him. It was filled with gluten-free breads, pizza crusts, chips and cereals. I bought as much meat and cheese as he could swallow. He ate whatever junk food he wanted as long as it was "gluten-free."

Summer reading efforts resumed. I gave him the first *Harry Potter*. Four weeks later, he had finished all seven books in the series. He reported that he hadn't realized there had been a constant pain in his stomach (until it stopped hurting). He didn't know that his brain was in a fog of confusion until it cleared. Gluten-free, he felt free. He stuck to his diet like someone with a shellfish allergy. He even survived a week of camp where the only healthy options were the water fountain and Peanut M&Ms. I sent his special food. The camp accommodated his diet. My son thrived.

I'd love to say "the end," but that summer would only be the first chapter. His father and I announced our divorce. By Christmas, he wouldn't eat a gluten-free cracker to save his life. There comes a point where a boy becomes a man by experiencing the consequences of his choices. Rejecting the gluten-free diet gave my son a sense of control as he struggled with painful changes.

The only thing I can do for my man/boy at this point is to love him without conditions. I am still his mom, so I do retain a bit of authority. He must use his own money to buy sugary breakfast cereals and I throw away anything I find that is not organic. I offer advice and give lectures. (I've podcasted the repetitive ones to save time.) I barter documentaries for video games. I do shots of kale with him. When he struggles, I remind him of that gluten-free summer. But I've placed the responsibility of his success on his shoulders. I have no doubt he will rise to the challenge.

Picky People Pick Pizza

I talk with my kids about food until I'm sick of hearing my own voice. I trick them into science fair projects and bribe them with organic junk food. I include them in the kitchen and spend time showing them how to cook. I don't keep medications in the house. When cold and season arrives, I make miso soup, juice greens, cut up oranges, offer oregano oil and serve glasses of detox clay. Sometimes they opt out. Increasingly, they opt in. I teach by example. Each time one of us avoids an illness, it reinforces that wellness is a consequence.

Eating whole and unprocessed foods requires cooking and to some extent, gardening. I have a natural talent in the kitchen, but I was not born with a green thumb. The knowledge and know-how required to grow herbs, greens and vegetables requires more than just "knack." Each summer's efforts are a potpourri of success and failure. I read and experiment. I learn from my mistakes. I salvage what I can and start over when necessary. I have come to embrace the process. The joy is in the creative effort, not the fruits of my labor (or lack thereof).

My kids are less enthusiastic. The excitement of planting food in early spring evaporates with the sweat (and tears) of summer-long weeding and watering. By September they don't want to pick, pluck or pull the peas, peppers and potatoes, if only because they'll be asked to help chop them for dinner.

Healthy food is the foundation for a high quality life. But homegrown vegetables are not the treats that children in our culture have come to expect. When my kids see me preparing the proceeds of my daily harvest, the whining ensues. They just want pizza. I hear the echo of my own childhood disappointments. "Why can't we eat like normal families?"

Gardening has taught me that the forces of nature are too strong to resist. Parenting has taught me that persistence is most effective when coupled with strategy. I do understand their desires. Often I say, "No problem. I'm not in the mood for a fight. Pizza it is!"

I appear resigned and start chopping as they run off to play. They fail to notice the smirk on my face. Really, darlings, have we met? Do you think my evil plot to save the planet with vegetables can be foiled by a simple request for pizza?

Not a chance.

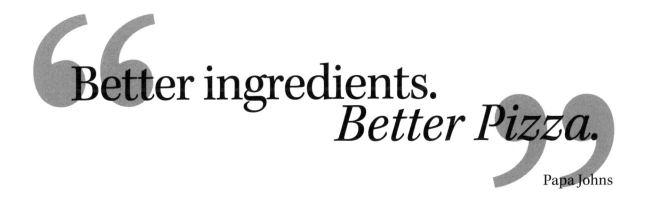

"*Better ingredients. Better Pizza.*"
— Papa Johns

Bright green kale, juicy red tomatoes, orange and yellow bell peppers, and a sweet Vidalia onion land in my large cast iron skillet. I chop a few cloves of garlic, add a pinch of sea salt, drizzle with olive oil and heat on low until colors peak in brightness. The sauté is transferred to the blender, along with fresh thyme, basil, oregano, a tablespoon of organic sugar, and about 1/2 cup of nutritional yeast flakes (these add a mild pungency similar to Parmesan cheese).

If the color is too green to pass for marinara after a whirl in the blender, a can of tomato paste adds authenticity (a small amount of bright red beet also works). I test the flavor and season until it will pass for "not homemade."

The sauce smothers two gluten-free (store-bought) crusts. One pizza is topped with 1/2 cup of organic mozzarella. A little compromise with dairy cheese creates an alibi for my deceit. The other pizza (mine!) is served with vegan cheese and drizzled with cashew cream (see the cashew cream recipe on page 50).

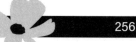

Fragrant aromas summon the kids into the kitchen. A harmless looking, gooey cheese pizza is cooling on the stove. I have also blanched fresh green beans and flavored with a balsamic glaze. The kids know their mother would never serve pizza without forcing an obligatory side of vegetables.

They are right about that.

Recipe for Balsamic Glaze

- ½ cup balsamic vinegar
- ¼ cup maple syrup
- ¼ cup olive oil
- 2 Tbsp. soy sauce (optional: great for Asian flavor)
- pinch of garlic salt (optional)
- 1 tsp. cornstarch (optional: will thicken if heating.)

Whisk all of the ingredients except the cornstarch. Taste and adjust flavor to preference. Use as a salad dressing or a marinade. To intensify the flavor, create a reduction by bringing mixture to a boil and adding cornstarch (or equivalent thickener such as arrowroot or agar). Stir and simmer until desired consistency is reached.

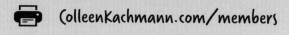
ColleenKachmann.com/members

The Cupcake Conspiracy

When other kids at the ballpark are given money for hot dogs and cotton candy, I am given the cold shoulder. My kids cry "foul" and "no fair." They still fight the word "no" because once upon a time, the answer was often "whatever." I must own that.

There are a lot of food bullies in the world. Middle school intimidation tactics are alive and well amongst grown-ups. When one parent sets a limit another does not, relationships become strained. If your decision is outside the bounds of "normal," the pressure to make an exception is fierce. In a group setting, each parent's choices affect other people's children. This triggers negative emotions on all sides. It is important to be ready to face these challenges. They have the right to say, "yes." And you have the same right to say, "no."

My son's soccer team celebrated a weekly holiday known as Cupcake

Wednesday. Every parent was expected to contribute during the season. When I reserved my date, I noted that I would be contributing a variety of chopped fruit.

The response was frightening. It was akin to what one might expect if I had offered to serve an active strain of the Ebola virus. I got hate e-mails from mad mommies and disturbed dads. They expressed concern that the boys would be traumatized by my refusal to provide the obligatory "treats." I was harassed with:

"But it's a special occasion!"
"They expect cupcakes!"
"They'll be so disappointed!"
"They deserve a treat after a hard practice!"

It was another round of normal versus healthy. Let the games begin.

Monkey Balls

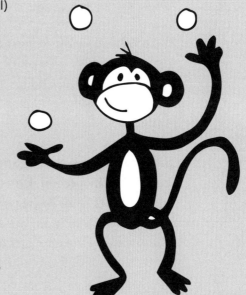

- 4 ripe bananas, mashed
- 4 Tbsp. nut butter: peanut butter, almond butter, or sunflower seed butter
- 2 Tbsp. black-strap molasses or honey (optional)
- 1 Tbsp. vanilla
- 2 tsp. cinnamon
- 4 Tbsp. shredded unsweetened coconut
- 2 Tbsp. ground flax seed
- 4-6 tsp. cocoa powder
- 1/2 cup chocolate chips
- 1 cup cooked pumpkin
- 3 cups cooked quinoa
- 1/2 cup nuts: chopped almonds, walnuts, cashews, peanuts, hazelnuts
- 1/2 cup seeds: sunflower, pumpkin, hemp, sesame, chia seeds
- 1-2 cups dried fruit: raisins, figs, dates, apricots, cranberries or Gogi berries

Mash bananas (potato masher), stir in remaining ingredients. Scoop mixture into mini muffin tins. Place muffin tins in freezer until frozen. Remove "Monkey Balls" from muffin tins and store in freezer bags. Can be eaten frozen or slightly thawed.

 ColleenKachmann.com/members

Growing athletes don't deserve to be fed poison after a job well done. These "treats" are filled with HFCS, trans fat and petroleum-based dyes. A peace-seeking parent volunteered to bring cupcakes to compliment my "thoughtful" gesture. I was polite when I declined the offer. I followed through and delivered enough juicy, sweet fruit to feed a small army. The army ate it. In fact, they loved it. Each boy, including the coach, made a point to thank me for the special effort. Several parents did as well. Others sulked at my nerve to buck tradition. Regardless, I stood my ground.

We must stop fighting each other and start fighting back.

Candy is found in classrooms, churches and pediatricians offices. Party food is always pizza and cookies (unless it's hot dogs and chips). Team fundraisers are held at fast food restaurants. School socials serve ice cream bars. The PTA sells donuts and greasy popcorn. Concession stands peddle nachos with cheese and cotton candy. Even fine-dining restaurants offer separate "kid" menus filled with junk. Halloween candy appears in August. Christmas candy goes on sale at Thanksgiving. Valentine's Day is now a season that opens after New Years. The Easter Bunny lays jellybeans and Cadbury eggs. We celebrate our independence with red, white and blue desserts. Not to mention all the birthday parties on the calendar in between.

Enough!

The producers of junk food have inserted their products into every corner of our lives. And we are voluntarily consuming our own health, one bite at a time. As parents, we must take a stand if we want our kids to survive and live well. Muffins with Mom and Donuts with Dad are not gatherings that strengthen families.

The great news is that fighting back doesn't require violence. Just stop buying and eating the poison. Don't make exceptions. There is never a good reason to justify bad food. Bring your own food to events. Yes, people will notice and talk. But wellness is as contagious as illness. Your actions will inspire others to follow suit. Be the change you want to see. Create a new normal that is healthy.

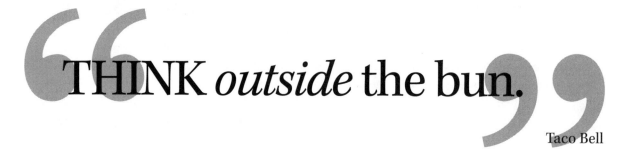

"THINK *outside* the bun."

Taco Bell

The Parable of Responsibility

A condensed version of Charles Osgood's *A Poem About Responsibility*.

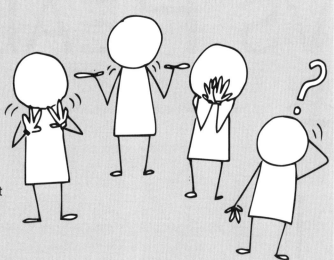

This is a story about four people named Everybody, Somebody, Anybody, and Nobody. There was an important job to be done. Everybody was sure that Somebody would do it. Anybody could have done it, but Nobody did it. Somebody got angry because it was Everybody's responsibility. Everybody thought that Anybody could do it. Nobody realized that Everybody wouldn't do it. It ended up that Everybody blamed Somebody when Nobody did what Anybody could have done.

Kale Chips: Better than Popcorn

Cut the stems off a bunch of kale (or two—it cooks down a lot). Cut or rip leaves into big pieces. Even easier, grab a bag of pre-washed chopped kale from the produce section at the grocery store.

Spread a thin layer over a cookie sheet. Massage leaves with olive oil (or other favorite) and a little salt. Get creative with flavor. Experiment with organic seasoning packets, yeast flakes, balsamic vinegar, cashew cream and more.

Bake at 400° for about 15 minutes, until the edges start to turn brown. Turn over with a spatula and continue to bake to desired tenderness. The crispier they are, the more they literally melt in your mouth (though chewy is good too). Watch them carefully in the last few minutes as crispy turns to burnt fast.

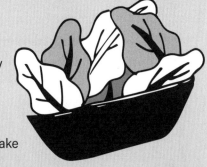

Note: Leftover kale chips are great snacks and salad toppers. Take them for lunch, sporting events and movies. Kids love them!

ColleenKachmann.com/members

Normal vs Healthy

Your children are offered poison everywhere they go. What is your strategy to reduce their exposure?

Children see. Children do. How are you modeling wellness for your children?

What advertisements and slogans capture your children? How can you counteract these messages?

A constant barrage of marketing messages presents bad food as normal, convenient and healthy. Deprogramming your family requires intention, time and effort. What strategies might work in your home?

 ColleenKachmann.com/members

PS I left this facing page blank for you.
Fill it with whatever you like. Questions, comments, to-do's, thoughts, etc.
You're welcome . . .

Chapter 14

Afford the Best on a Budget of Less

"Too many people spend money they haven't earned to buy things they don't need to impress people they don't like."

WILL ROGERS (1879-1935) ACTOR AND SOCIAL COMMENTATOR.

DOLLARS AND SENSE

Time and money seem to be limiting factors when it comes to lifestyle changes. Budgets are tight. Stress is high. Life is overwhelming. Careers, kids, and daily responsibilities consume our energy. The pressure to do more with less comes from all directions.

Ready for some fantastic news? Living off the label doesn't cost more time, money or energy. In fact, it returns them. Yep. That's right. You, my friend, are about to get a refund! Normal isn't healthy; it's expensive and exhausting.

I haven't washed my hair with anything but water for two years. The only thing I use on my face (besides a bit of organic make-up) is coconut oil. It fills fine lines and wrinkles better than anything I've tried. I also use coconut oil to shave my legs, make homemade deodorant, clean leather bags, and condition wood floors. I don't waste time reading labels at the drug store or grocery. I keep a few inexpensive ingredients stocked in my home that work for almost everything.

I have changed the way I shop. I spend less money on food than I did before I switched to an organic and unprocessed diet. (Accounting software confirms this fact.) I order high-quality produce and ingredients on-line. This eliminates impulse buys at the grocery store. I purchase in bulk whenever possible. I save both time and money because I am not consumed with hunting for bargains and waiting for items to go on sale.

I use homemade laundry detergent. I make a year's supply in 30 minutes at a tenth of the cost. And I can whip up a gourmet dinner from scratch in the same time it takes to idle through the drive-through or call for carryout. This requires forethought and having the right ingredients on hand. I've developed (and tested) strategies for this. I will share them with you in this chapter.

The perception of convenience is an illusion. Convenience is only a concept that leads to the purchase of products we do not need.

Consider the dishwasher. Even low-budget apartments dedicate cabinet space to this basic "necessity." The appliance costs $500-$1,000. A month's supply of detergent is between $5 and $10. Yet the gadget does not reduce much (if any) elbow grease. Clean outcomes require a thorough pre-rinse. The strategic arrangement (and rearrangement) feels like a game of Tetris. Wash cycles range one to two hours. If a child loads the dishwasher, the inevitable cemented food must be scrubbed. The dishes must be put away. Why do we perceive this to be convenient?

I have bad dishwasher-karma. Leaks, broken racks, and clogged drains require costly repair. On the other hand, maybe I just have bad kid-karma. As a parent, I am obligated to insist they help with the dishes. This makes for more trouble than it's worth. Recently, I've asked them to wash things by hand. Interestingly, there have been less hassles. Turns out, the best dishwashers have two hands and are not sold in stores.

We're being sold a bunch of crap. The good news is that you don't have to buy it.

Advertisements create a perception of need. Artificial demand keeps us running to the store. If your grocery cart is filled with laundry soap, cleaning supplies, beauty products, and other household "necessities," you have more money than you think. Extend the organic and unprocessed approach to all areas of life and free yourself from the cycle of consumerism. There are cheap, healthy, and safe alternatives to most commercial products.

"The new slavery is *consumerism*."

Bryant McGill (1969-) American author and human rights activist

CREATE YOUR OWN BRAND OF CLEAN

Laundry detergent is mandatory, especially if you have messy children. Cheap laundry detergent isn't worth the discount when stains or funky smells ruin clothing. Unfortunately, the good stuff is expensive. But why? The chemistry of detergents is not alchemy: it's basic soap and water. The new high-efficiency machines call for low-sud formulas that cost even more. They shouldn't. The bubbles we've come to associate with clean are only added for psychological appeal. Manufacturers are betting that if you can afford a fancy machine, you can afford the premium on fancy detergent.

The "secret patented formulas" made by brands we trust actually double as addictive aromatherapies. That's right. Patented fragrances are addictive. Think about it. The olfactory nerve is located near the amygdala, which controls our emotions and memory.[1] We associate memories with scent. Detergent fragrances are cleverly concocted to transform the labor of laundry into sentiments of love. They are as habit-forming as your favorite flavor of ice cream. Comfort food. Comfort chores. Same appeal. Neither provides any real comfort. We just think they do.

A friend gave me a baggie of her homemade laundry detergent. It worked just as well as any detergent I'd ever tried, if not better. But I struggled with the idea of making it myself. I assumed it would be complicated. If it was easy, wouldn't I already be doing it? And the lye-scented memories of my own mother's homemade soap were not pleasant. I preferred the artificial outdoor fragrance of my favorite formula of Tide. I used the last of my gifted trial and replaced it with the $20 box of Normal (If it's got to be clean, it's got to be Tide).

The friend who had given me the free trial followed up with the tenacity of a door-to-door sales person. I made the standard excuses: I didn't have time; I didn't know where to get the ingredients; I didn't know if my food processor was up to the task. She became so frustrated with my reluctance that she volunteered to drive the four hours that separate our homes. She would help make my first batch in exchange for a full-course vegan meal.

I agreed only because I looked forward to her visit.

I planned the menu. She loaded her car with supplies. Game day arrived. The experience was anti-climactic. We made a year's worth of laundry detergent in less than half an hour.

I was embarrassed by how easy it was and excited by the success. In an instant, I was a DIY (Do It Yourself) addict. I wanted to tackle another project immediately.

We ran a short victory lap around the house. There was potential everywhere. I spotted a near-empty box of Cascade and Googled for DIY dishwasher soap recipes. The ingredients were basically the same with a few additions that would be cheap and easy to find. We went to the store to replenish provisions. After dinner, we loaded the machine and gave it a try. The results sparkled with inspiration.

Regardless of my ability to afford name brand detergents, I avoid buying them. It is so damn easy to make them at home that it is an unconscionable waste of money. It takes less than half an hour to supply my family for a year. I even make extra as gifts and starter packets for high-maintenance friends with DIY anxiety disorder. If you do the money-math on a standard name brand option and adjust for accurate portion sizes, it costs about 40 cents to wash a full load of clothes. That expense can be reduced to less than 4 cents per load using three simple ingredients.

And we are doing away with the penny?

Try making your own detergent. Watch the instructional video on my *Colleen Kachmann* YouTube channel if you want a visual demonstration (or just a good laugh).

> "A rich man has money. A wealthy man has *time*."
>
> W.C. Fields (1880-1946) American comedian, writer and the common man's philosopher

Homemade Laundry Detergent

- 1 cup Borax
- 1 cup Arm & Hammer's Super Washing Soda
- 1 bar Fels Naptha/Kirk's Castile bar soap

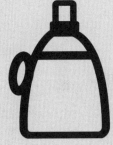

Cut soap bar into chunks, blend ingredients in a food processor. Use 1 Tbsp. per load. An occasional addition of ½ cup white vinegar to the machine's bleach container will keep the washer fresh.

 ColleenKachmann.com/members

Homemade Dishwasher Detergent

- 1 cup borax
- 1 cup Arm & Hammer's Super Washing Soda
- ½ cup citric acid (double if dishes are cloudy or you have hard water)
- ½ cup kosher salt
- 1 gallon white vinegar (separate to 1 cup per use)

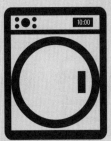

Stir the dry ingredients together and pour the mixture into a wide mouth container. Use 1 Tbsp. of mixture for each load. Splash about ½ cup of vinegar into the bottom of the machine before you start the wash cycle.

The wide mouth container is necessary, as the dry mix gets clumpy with moisture. You can also add about 1 Tbsp. of rice or use a knife to loosen a portion.

 ColleenKachmann.com/members

Do Almost Everything for Only $3

 Liquid Drain Cleaner: Pour equal amounts of baking soda and white vinegar into the drain. Enjoy the volcano-effect. Leave for 30 minutes. Flush with hot water.

 Window Cleaner: Mix a 50/50 solution of white vinegar and water. Use black and white newspaper to scrub windows and mirrors.

 Oven Cleaner: Mix ¾ cup baking soda, ¼ cup salt and ¼ cup of water to create a thick paste. Apply damp to oven walls and let it sit overnight. Rub gently with steel wool on tough spots.

 Toilet Bowel Cleaner: Pour ¼ cup baking soda and 1 cup vinegar into toilet. Allow it to set for a few minutes before scrubbing. If grime builds up between cleanings, drain the toilet bowl and scrub with hydrogen peroxide.

 All-Purpose Cleaner: Mix ½ cup vinegar and ¼ cup baking soda into ½ gallon water. Use to clean shower, chrome fixtures and tile. A micro-fiber cloth can help eliminate streaks. Make a Scouring Powder paste by pouring hydrogen peroxide into baking soda. Use a toothbrush to scrub grout and around faucets.

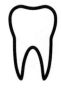 **Mouthwash/Teeth Whitener:** Dilute hydrogen peroxide with a swig of water, swish-swish. Don't swallow. Dissolve baking soda in water to neutralize garlic breath or create a paste to brush teeth.

 Acne and Pimples: Dab hydrogen peroxide directly to blemishes. Massage with coconut oil to treat dryness without clogging pores.

Life off the Label

Ear Wax: With head on a pillow (use a towel), fill ear canal with hydrogen peroxide and allow it bubble for a few minutes. Turn head to drain. Repeat for chronic buildup.

Stain Removal: Hydrogen peroxide is very effective on blood, grass, and red wine stains. Use it to pretreat clothing before washing. Dilute for dark colors and rinse immediately. (Spot test first.) Add a cup of vinegar to the washer for white loads.

Deodorizer: Acids and bases are usually the source of unpleasant odors. Acidic odors include sour milk, rotten eggs (sulfur), sewage (methane), garlic, onion, pickle and sauerkraut. Basic (alkaline) odors include spoiled fish, ammonia-filled urine and compost (nitrogen). Baking soda eliminates odor by neutralizing and buffering pH levels. Sprinkle over carpets before vacuuming, make a paste for scrubbing and keep an open box in the refrigerator.

Wound, Infection and Fungus Care: Start with a 50 percent dilution (1 to 1 ratio) of hydrogen peroxide and water. Apply directly to the affected area. If no skin irritation occurs, use full strength in subsequent applications. Rinse with water.

Disinfectant: Mix two parts water and one part each of hydrogen peroxide and white vinegar. Use on cutting boards, countertops and contaminated surfaces. Wash meat and vegetables to inhibit rot. Rinse with water.

Produce Spray: Mix equal parts water, hydrogen peroxide and white vinegar. Spritz and rinse with cold water.

Fire extinguisher: Baking soda releases carbon dioxide and produces water when it's heated. This both smothers and cools a fire. It is very effective for grease and electrical fires.

COCONUT OIL CURES

Coconut oil is my new favorite addiction. I seriously can't get enough of it. I use it all over my body, including my face. There are no body lotions or beauty creams on the market that work better on my skin, regardless of cost. I've even stopped using the self-tanning lotion that I once coated my body with from head to toe every day. I no longer see the need. My skin is supple and soft. (This claim has been substantiated by peer-review.)

Coconut oil has awesome medicinal properties, both inside and out. It inhibits opportunistic bacteria, viruses, and fungus and has multiple benefits to our immune system. It also facilitates the absorption of minerals such as calcium and magnesium in teeth and bones.[2] Unlike many other natural oils, it absorbs easily into the skin without leaving a greasy residue.

Coconut oil is also a great source of non-carbohydrate fuel. It contains medium chain fatty acids that are easy to digest and immediately available as energy. (The medium chain fatty acids account for the lack of greasy residue.) It assists in the absorption of fat-soluble vitamins. It is also ideal for baking as it can withstand higher temperatures without denaturing. So add it to your smoothies or use it to make popcorn. It's delicious and nutritious.

Coconut oil also serves as a makeup remover, shaving lotion, and facial and body moisturizer. It's the only cream that actually fills in fine lines and wrinkles around my eyes. It keeps connective tissues strong and exfoliates dead skin cells. You can add it to your tub to moisturize dry and itchy skin, apply it to your lips as a balm, and mix it with baking soda to create toothpaste.

When coconut oil is mixed with several essential oils, it is 10 times more effective than DEET against mosquitos.[3] Full disclosure, I still seem pretty tasty to the little suckers regardless of the toxicity of my protection. My personal approach is called a screened-in porch, but I do use this recipe when I'm in the woods or watching the sunset on the patio.

Another off-label use for coconut oil is an Ayurvedic practice for detoxification called oil pulling. Developed thousands of years ago in India, Ayurveda is one of the world's oldest holistic healing systems. Candida and streptococcus collect in the mouth and contribute to plaque formation and tooth decay, as well as illness and inflammation throughout the entire body. These microorganisms are covered with a lipid (fat) membrane, which serve as their skin. When these cells come into contact with the coconut oil, a fat, they naturally adhere to each other. Like dissolves like.

Insect Repellent Recipe

- 4 oz. rubbing alcohol or witch hazel
- 4 oz. coconut oil
- 1 Tbsp. vanilla extract or Madagascar vanilla
- 10 drops of one or a combination of essential oils: lemon, eucalyptus, catnip, neem, citronella, geranium, clove, lavender, cedar leaf, turmeric, rosemary

Directions: Mix ingredients together in a small spray bottle with a tight lid. Carry in a sealed plastic baggie. Shake well before applying. Apply to clothes and exposed skin.

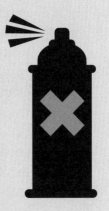

ColleenKachmann.com/members

Fluoride-Free Toothpaste

The United States is one of the only developed countries that adds fluoride to drinking water. As there is no increase in tooth-decay for countries that don't, it's time to ask the question: why? Fluoride has been linked to brain damage, lower IQ in children, and mulitple health problems.[4] It is a known endocrine disruptor that affects bones, brain, thyroid and pineal glands and even blood sugar levels.[5]

You can't avoid all of the fluoride in our water, but you can get it out of your toothpaste. Make your own.

- 3 Tbsp. each of coconut oil and baking soda
- 2 tsp. stevia or erythritol (adjust for sweetness)
- 25 drops peppermint oil (adjust for taste)

Mix ingredients. Store in a wide mouth jar with a lid.

ColleenKachmann.com/members

Swish a tablespoon of coconut oil in your mouth for 20 minutes. The best time to do this is when you first wake up (before brushing your teeth), when bacteria, viruses, and fungi levels are most concentrated. Yes, it's a little gross to walk around with a mouth full of oil, but not as gross as blowing chunks of green snot because you get sick. Don't swallow the oil because it will be loaded with the toxins and debris pulled from of the gums and tongue. Spit into the toilet, as the oil may clog the sink drain. Rinse your mouth with water.

Coconut oil soothes and inhibits inflammation caused by athlete's foot, ringworm, cold sores, ear infections, chicken pox and skin rashes, bug bites and bee stings, hemorrhoids, and even head lice. Healing remedies often call for coconut oil to be mixed with essential oils such as oregano, tea tree, and lavender. Consult homeopathic guides for specific recipes.

Just a word of caution to fellow over-achievers: coconut oil is oil. The first time I substituted it for my after-shower moisturizer, I applied it quite liberally. It felt and smelled great. But an hour later, my eye makeup was on my cheeks, my t-shirt was plastered to my skin and socks would not stay on my feet. I needed to fine-tune my application strategy. I tried applying it while in the shower. Bingo. Now, it doubles as shave gel and hair conditioner. The excess wipes off with my towel when I am done.

Coconut oil also serves as the base for my homemade deodorant. I've been using it for two years and love it. Stay tuned for the recipe later in this chapter.

Organic coconut oil is available in bulk and easy to find online. I pay $27 for 87-ounces at Costco. That's five times cheaper than the 12-ounce jar sold at Whole Foods. I suggest you stock up. Once you see and feel what this versatile oil can do for you, you won't want to run out.

LIFE HACK: COCONUT OIL MAGIC

- Remove makeup, use as a shaving lubricant, condition skin, lips, and hair.
- Use in insect repellent, deodorant, and toothpaste recipes.
- Reduce fungal, bacterial, and viral infections.
- Substitute for vegetable oil and butter when baking and cooking. To avoid the subtle coconut flavor, look for refined varieties.
- Clean, condition, and soften leather goods like shoes, furniture, and car interiors.
- Lubricate squeaky wheels and sticky mechanisms in place of WD40.
- Clean and condition wood furniture and floors. (Test a small area first.)
- Remove chewing gum from virtually anything, including carpets and hair.
- Polish metal. (Test it first.)
- Clean soap scum. (Apply with a damp cloth, spray with white vinegar and wipe with a dry cloth.)
- Remove oil-based paints from hands and paintbrushes in lieu of mineral spirits.
- Clean and add a glossy finish to broad-leaf indoor plants.

 ColleenKachmann.com/members

THE NO-POO DO

My brother is a big-wig financial adviser (or so he claims). He travels a lot, and often has the inside scoop on the latest trends. After a business trip to Hollywood, he called to tell me that he has stopped washing his hair. Evidently, the sexiest of the sexy people don't use shampoo. It's called the "No-Poo" movement. He advised me to hop on the bandwagon.

I responded with sarcasm. "No-poo? No shit! That's the tip-of-the-year from the fancy-schmancy-consultant? Thanks, bro." I hung up on him.

Several months later, I received a call from a friend who lives on the west coast. She blurted out, "I haven't washed my hair in two months!" I rolled my eyes and tried to hang up. I accidentally pressed "speaker' instead of "end call." She rambled on about her hair as I fumbled with my phone. The sincerity in her tone caught my attention.

Her hair is a lot like mine. It's thick but fine, damages easily, and is often greasy. A haphazard ponytail requires more primping than either of us will admit. After a few months of washing with only water, her hair was so thick that it was difficult to manage. Like me, budget-blowing conditioners and volume enhancers are required just to leave the house. Now, her silky, shiny locks required few, if any, products.

I found this impossible to believe.

She sent a selfie of her fabulous new style. I was suspicious that it was a screen-shot of her celebrity-double. She looked amazing. But anyone can edit a photo these days.

She went on to tell me that the key is vigorous brushing. This distributes the oils. In the shower, it must be thoroughly rinsed. She uses dry shampoo when it feels oily. Her bouncy hair looks professionally styled. She told me to try it so I could see for myself.

I am naive by nature. She knew she had me at "hello."

The first few days were awful. I brushed, rinsed, and repeated, ad nauseam. I tried dry shampoo. Regardless, by the end of the second day, oil was seeping through the brim of my hat. I sent my friend a screen-shot of Jeff Daniels in *Dumb and Dumber* and the middle-finger emoji. Frustration mounted. Four days in and I couldn't even leave the house. The trial seemed destined to fail. But my stubborn nature rose to the surface. I am not friends with defeat.

I know when to cut my losses, however. If I couldn't go out in public after the next water-wash, I would lather in sudsy failure and move on. Greasy hair will not get me into the sexy club. I decided to try rubbing baking soda into my scalp and submerging my head underwater in my final attempt. I massaged my head as I soaked. I brushed against the roots as I blew it dry. It felt thick in lieu of clean. I analyzed the results.

I could hardly believe my eyes.

VINTAGE IS SEXY

The beauty advice of my grandmother's generation included brushing hair "100 strokes per side every day." Once upon a time, the "I-have-to-wash-my-hair" excuse was totally legit. Nobody shampooed more than once a week. The process was an event. My grandmother maintained her coif between trips to the salon by sleeping on her back in uncomfortable curlers secured by a tight headscarf. The supine position also kept the green cold cream from gluing her face to the pillow. In addition, she wore a girdle, did housework in heels and washed nylons in the sink.

Feminists rebelled against these cruel and unusual punishments in the "Oh, Hell No!" movement.

Daily shampooing became the norm in the 1970s. The trend coincided with an increase in television, radio, and magazine commercials. Super-models selling over-priced hair products flaunted lustrous, sexy-smelling locks. A child of this era, I grew up believing I needed the most expensive shampoo I could afford. Quality brands were only available in exclusive salons. Free samples of rejuvenating eye creams and wrinkle-reducing serums hooked us in to spending more.

What if these beauty products are actually the source of our beauty problems?

Hair follicles contain natural oils that are essential to healthy locks. Frequent washing strips these oils and stimulates the sebaceous glands to release more oil. Harsh chemicals create the suds we associate with "clean." They leave hair susceptible to damage, especially when styled with high-heat hair dryers and flat irons.

Like dish soap and laundry detergents, shampoos and conditioners come in fragrances designed to entice our senses. We are not consumers buying products. These products are consuming our money. We supply the profits for the companies selling empty promises. Chemical-laden merchandise doesn't enhance our beauty or keep us young. They addict us to ensure we buy more.

I couldn't believe my eyes when I looked in the mirror on the fourth day of my "no-poo" adventure. I saw progress. My hair looked good enough to venture into public without a hat. Over the course of the next year, my hair went through several phases of detox. At first, my scalp's oil production kicked in to overdrive. Baking soda kept it under control. But as weeks turned to months I noticed that my fine hair was too dry. Instead of using baking soda to counter an oily scalp, I needed coconut oil to condition my ends. I discovered that baking soda makes an excellent root boost. The effect is similar to the expensive cement texturizers that dirty up freshly shampooed hair to enhance shape. I rub a little into my crown and BAM! Hello hottie.

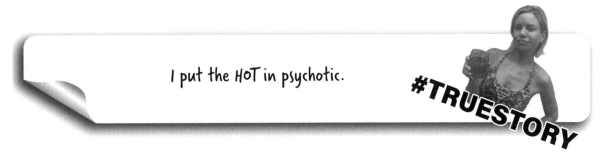

I put the HOT in psychotic.

#TRUESTORY

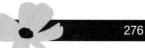

RACE FOR THE CURE—
RUN FROM THE CANCER

As I settled into life without shampoo, my focus shifted to my armpits. Not because I was stinky—in fact, I was always powder fresh. I used commercial antiperspirants without concern. I exercise daily. I sweat a lot. I never tried natural deodorants because it's common knowledge that they don't work. The stench of body odor makes me gag. I accepted the unknown chemicals in hygiene products as a necessary evil. Many days, a second application was needed. I was grateful for the chemistry that kept me fresh. The fact that everyone uses antiperspirants was comforting. It feels safe in the normal crowd.

Breast cancer is the most common cancer diagnosis in women. One in eight of us will be diagnosed at some point in our life.[6] We are taught how to do self-examinations once a month to make sure we catch it early. I don't want to catch it at all! I know the chill of terror upon discovering a painful lump. It's happened twice. I was lucky both times. Medical exams identified them as plugged ducts. But the experiences were still close calls. I wondered if I would be so lucky the next time. I assumed that, in all likelihood, there would be a next time.

I ran across a recipe for homemade deodorant while doing research on coconut oil. I disregarded it with a flippant "whatever." Coconut oil cannot possibly be that awesome. But the potential tugged at me.

Over a short span of time, three women I know were diagnosed with breast cancer. They were each healthy, vibrant, and under forty. One did not survive. If cancer can happen to them, I thought, I might be next.

I decided to investigate the research, if only to be *sure* my Secret was worth the compromise.

I was terrified by what I found. Yet again, a product we use every day is filled with toxins. Yet again, we are told by those charged with protecting us that, "the FDA does not have any evidence or research data that ingredients in underarm antiperspirants or deodorants cause cancer."

Right. But where's the evidence that it *doesn't* cause cancer? There isn't any. "Because studies of antiperspirants and breast cancer have provided conflicting results, additional research is needed to investigate this relationship and other factors that may be involved."[7]

Notice the contradiction. If there is no evidence, how is there conflicting evidence? I believe this translates to, "We are doing our best to invalidate the inconvenient and unprofitable information.

Remember that the FDA does not require companies to test personal products for safety. Patent holders are obligated to submit evidence of harm, not proof of safety. Antiperspirant manufacturers are currently hiding behind a population-based study that claims there is no cause for concern. In 2002, a study compared the hygiene habits of breast cancer patients with a control group of women who did not have cancer. This is a curious approach. Why not compare cancer rates in women who use antiperspirants with populations who don't use them? The study found no connection between antiperspirants and breast cancer. Their conclusion dismisses the "rumors circulating the Internet" as "unfounded."[8]

But a lack of data is not proof of safety! A 2003 study published in Europe surveyed breast cancer survivors. The connection is clear. The more often women shaved and used antiperspirant, the earlier the age of cancer onset.[9] Regardless, the researchers dared only to conclude that antiperspirants *might* play a role in breast cancer. Since then, scientists around the globe have cited major concerns about the effects of long-term, low-dose exposure to antiperspirants. The call for more research is loud and urgent.

Fifteen years later, we are still waiting. Safety concerns of antiperspirants have been dismissed because no one can prove beyond a shadow of a doubt that they foster disease. Life keeps going (for most of us). We mourn the dead, celebrate the survivors and get yearly mammograms. Every October, pink ribbons plaster every product and event. We slather our armpits with toxins that might play a role in cancer as we Race for the Cure. But at least we don't stink, right?

Wrong. There is no lack of information on the harmful ingredients in antiperspirants. There is no official study on the products because the unofficial study is too lucrative. The United Kingdom, Australia, and Northern America have the highest incidence of breast cancer in the world. Noncommercial, third-world countries have the lowest cancer rates. Certainly, diet and environment are factors. But hygiene habits cannot be overlooked.[10] Denying the truth does not reduce its impact.

Parabens are found in antiperspirants. They are also found in 99 percent of breast cancer tumors.[11] There is no concrete proof that they cause cancer, but it's clear that one fuels the other in some way. The EPA (Environmental Protection Agency) links the class of parabens used in antiperspirants to metabolic, developmental, hormonal, and neurological disorders, as well as various cancers.[12]

Aluminum is used in antiperspirants to block sweat ducts. It reduces the amount of sweat that reaches the skin's surface. Sweat glands must absorb the aluminum for it to be effective. This confirms that it penetrates skin, tissues, and blood stream. Indeed, the aluminum in antiperspirants can be detected in the urine 15 days after application.[13] It mimics the effects of estrogen and is an endocrine disrupter. It can alter DNA and cause mutations in gene expression. Aluminum is a neurotoxin that inhibits more than 200 biologically important functions. It crosses the blood-brain barrier and accumulates in a semi-permanent manner. Aluminum is also associated with Lou Gehrig's disease and Alzheimer's.[14]

The evidence is overwhelming. To claim antiperspirants are safe because there isn't proof they are not is ass-backwards. To race for the cure, you must run from the cancer.

Aluminum Free Deodorant

The reason we perspire is to regulate body temperature and expel waste. Sweat itself doesn't stink. Skin bacteria feeding on the sweat produce the odor. Sweat is similar to urine in that it contains water, ammonia, urea, sugars, and body salt. The more concentrated the contents, the more microbes have to eat and the more pungent the result.

Holding in urine leads to bladder and kidney infections. When you "gotta go," go! We wipe and flush to avoid the odor of stagnant urine. Proper hygiene supports urinary tract health and maintains a sense of dignity.

Clogging the sweat glands inhibits essential internal detoxification processes. Byproducts of bodily processes must be released, we need to sweat just like we need to use the bathroom. Again, proper hygiene is important. Cleanse the skin with soap and water when odor threatens.

I started with a simple coconut oil and baking soda recipe. These two ingredients keep my "no-poo" hair fabulous. I hoped their magic would work in my armpits. Indeed, they prevented odor effectively. I did not stink. The only drawback seemed to be an occasional rash after vigorous exercise. The baking soda (a natural odor absorber) is abrasive. Still, I was surprised and excited that my first try worked as well as it did.

I researched alternatives to baking soda and played around with other ingredients. I have used homemade deodorant everyday for two years. I love it. My teenage sons even offered to try it. (Just kidding. I paid one with cash and blackmailed the other.) They begrudgingly applied it before school, the gym, and sport practices. They reported back that it works "fine."

That's a ringing endorsement and far more reliable than FDA approval!

Everyone's body chemistry is different. Do not be discouraged if the ratio of ingredients in my recipe is not ideal for you. Expect to experiment. Start with small batches. It helps to understand the purpose of each option.

- **Coconut oil** inhibits the bacteria that produce odor, acts as an emollient, and is the key ingredient in most recipes.
- **Baking soda** neutralizes acids and bases, the most common source of odor. It is the best natural deodorizer.
- Raw, unrefined **shea butter** contains vitamins A and E and essential fatty acids that are easily absorbed by the skin. It has anti-aging and anti-inflammatory properties and can counteract eczema and dryness.[15]
- Organic **beeswax** is a skin softener that counteracts the abrasiveness of baking soda. It seals in moisture without clogging pores. It thickens, emulsifies (keeps oil and water from separating) and is a natural bactericide. Beeswax keeps ingredients firm and prevents settling.[16]
- **Bentonite clay** adsorbs (bonds to) toxins so they are not reabsorbed into the skin. See *Detox with Bentonite Clay*—page 281 for more information. Other commercial clays can work as well.
- **Essential oils** such as lavender, tea tree, and lemon have subtle healing properties with unique and specific benefits. They also allow you to create a personalized scent. Many combinations of essential oils smell fantastic.

An unexpected bonus of using homemade deodorant appeared in summer. My preferred daily uniform is a crisp white t-shirt. I used to buy them in bulk because yellow pit stains limited their life span. Evidently it's the aluminum that leaves the stain, not the sweat. Disposable t-shirts are a thing of the past.

Detoxification of antiperspirant chemicals takes time. In the first few weeks, it's common for the armpits to turn a scaly brown. The dead skin easily exfoliates in the shower. Also, occasional chafing can be soothed with Aloe Vera, camphor or pure coconut oil. You may get "pity" in the first few months (sweaty, with a chance of stink). Stick it out. The temporary inconvenience of changing your shirt a few times pales in comparison to cancer. It took my body a full year to adjust. Now, I only sweat during exercise. I don't ever smell of body odor, even on days that I don't get a shower.

Antiperspirants interfere with the body's natural ability to regulate temperature. If you've used commercial products since puberty, give your system time to adjust. Aluminum antiperspirants do not solve hygiene problems; they create them. My detoxification system is much lower maintenance now that my sweat ducts aren't plugged with toxins.

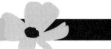

A few practical problems are easy to avoid. Coconut oil melts at 74 degrees and can be a leaky mess in the summer. Store deodorant in a small jar with a screw-top lid and use fingertips to apply. When traveling, keep it sealed in a plastic baggie. If the baking soda leaves you chafed, try substituting with arrowroot or food grade silica. Until you are confident with your recipe, keep wipes and a small container of baking soda or natural talc-free powder on hand. Cleanse and dust skin to avoid a hygienic emergency.

Aluminum Free Deodorant

Ingredients:

- 4 Tbsp. coconut oil
- 2 Tbsp. baking soda
- 1.5 Tbsp. beeswax
- 1 Tbsp. shea butter
- 4 tsp. bentonite clay
- 10-20 drops of essential oils

Melt the beeswax, coconut oil and shea butter on VERY low heat. Whisk often. Once it is liquid, remove from heat. Add the clay, baking soda and essential oils of choice (optional) until thoroughly combined.

Transfer to a wide mouth 2-4 ounce jar with a screw top lid.

Place in the freezer. Stir (or shake) every few minutes until it appears consistent. It will set within 10 minutes. Apply daily with your fingers. Store upright at room temperature.

If you tend to get "pitty" on busy days (sweaty, with a chance of stink), dust armpits with baking soda using a powder brush. I keep a small jar in my bathroom and a small container in my purse. For occasional oil residue on clothing, pretreat with a drop of dishwashing liquid.

For a visual demonstration and helpful hints on locating the ingredients, watch the instructional video on my Colleen Kachmann YouTube channel.

 ColleenKachmann.com/members

Detox with Bentonite Clay

Detoxification is essential to healing and staying well. Purified volcanic ash clay has been used by medicine men for thousands of years to neutralize toxins and restore health.

Viruses, bacteria, and impurities cause rashes, acne, oily skin, eczema, and psoriasis. Bentonite clay is a negatively charged alkaline that attracts and binds with these toxins. The clay pulls toxins through the skin when applied externally and pushes them through the digestive tract when taken orally. Chronic conditions don't often disappear overnight. But regular use can reduce and eliminate symptoms that afflict our bodies.

Internally, the clay acts similar to the activated charcoal used to treat poisonings and overdoses. Activated charcoal, however, is manufactured from coal and petroleum and infused with other harsh acids, bases or salts. It is not effective on many toxins that contaminate our food and environment.[17] In comparison, bentonite clay is safe for daily use and does not induce constipation or dehydration. It doesn't interact with the body chemically; instead it serves as a magnet to which toxins hang on for a free ride out of your system.

Bentonite clay contains trace minerals that are key in cellular functions. Conventionally grown foods are deficient in micronutrients. Modern farming depletes trace minerals and fills the soil with toxic chemicals. Nutrition 101 teaches that vitamin B_{12} is essential, but most of us have no idea that cobalt is critical for B_{12} absorption. The clay also contains selenium, which supports the thyroid, neutralizes free radicals, and supports the immune system. Chromium helps to control blood sugar and regulate metabolism. Copper, zinc, magnesium, manganese, and boron are additional minerals often missing from an overly processed diet.

Dissolve bentonite clay in eight ounces of water and drink for an internal detox. Add water to make a paste for facemasks, armpits and muscle pain.

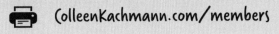

ColleenKachmann.com/members

BEAUTY IS MORE THAN SKIN DEEP

Skin is the largest organ of the body. Reconsider the safety of any hygiene and beauty product you wouldn't eat. Chemicals penetrate the skin and are absorbed into tissues. Protect yourself with a no-risk assumption that everything applied on the outside has an effect on the inside.

The average adult uses nine personal care products each day that contain 126 different chemicals. Ninety percent of ingredients have not been evaluated for safety. Women can absorb five pounds of chemicals per year from makeup alone. That doesn't include body lotions, deodorants, shampoo, and other personal care products.[18] We use products without thinking, unwittingly exposing ourselves to toxins.

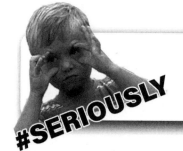

#SERIOUSLY — Maybe you should eat some make-up so you can be pretty on the inside.

The FDA's official policy won't surprise you.

"Cosmetic products and ingredients are not subject to FDA premarket approval authority; with the exception of color additives ... Cosmetic firms are responsible for substantiating the safety of their products and ingredients before marketing."[19]

Hmm ... Where have we seen that approach before? The exact same policy applies to genetically modified foods.

It is difficult to avoid the obvious poisons in personal care and cleaning products. "Organic" food labels are far more restrictive. In fact, some "organic" beauty products contain only a single-digit percentage of organic ingredients.[20] The Organic Consumers Association found the presence of a carcinogenic contaminate (1,4-dioxane) in 47 percent of "all-natural" products.[21] The chemical isn't listed on the label because it is an accidental by-product of a process used to make harsh ingredients milder. This reminds us that good intentions don't always produce healthy outcomes.

We ingest, inhale, and absorb thousands of chemicals. Many of these chemicals accumulate in our body. Long-term exposure to small amounts (thought to be safe) has cumulative effects. This means the impact over our lifetime has yet to be determined.

As awareness of problematic chemicals increases with consumers, manufacturers respond with alternatives. But often the replacement is as bad as the original. For example, "BPA-free" products often contain BPS, a similar chemical that also disrupts hormones. And when PCBs were banned in 1977, the flame-retardant industry replaced them with PBDE. When this was discovered to be just as toxic, new chemicals were used that are now linked to heart disease, obesity, and cancer. It's a toxic game of whack-a-mole. The solution is not to replace one dangerous substance with another, but to stop using them all together.

Sodium and/or Ammonium Laureth Sulfate (SLS, ALS, SLES)

Any ingredient that ends in -eth has been through ethoxylation. This process creates a surfactant that allows substances like oil and water to dissolve in one another. Nitrosamines are a byproduct. Unintended byproducts are not listed as ingredients on the label. Nitrosamines (the same carcinogen found in processed meats and cheese) are known irritants to the skin, lungs, and eyes. They can cause organ toxicity, neurotoxicity, DNA mutation, and cancer.[22] Shampoos with laureth sulfates can render more cancer-causing nitrates to the body than eating a pound of bacon![23]

Polysorbates

Polysorbates are used to dissolve oily residue from the hair. Remnants disrupt the natural pH of skin. They bind with the natural oils that serve as protective barriers for the hair and skin. This perpetuates the cycle of excess oil production and disrupts the flora of microbes that live in mucous membranes and the intestines.[24]

Parabens

Parabens are preservatives that prevent the growth of bacteria, mold, and yeast. They also have estrogen-mimicking properties associated with an increased risk of breast cancer. Parabens are easily absorbed through the skin and used in many products, including makeup, body washes, deodorants, shampoos, and facial cleansers. It is alarming that over 99 percent of breast cancer tumors contain parabens.[25] The EPA (Environmental Protection Agency) links parabens to metabolic, developmental, hormonal, and neurological disorders, as well as various cancers.[26]

Plastic: PVC (polyvinylchloride), BPA (bisphenol A), Phthalates

- PVC is used to make water pipes, inflatable swimming pools, pacifiers, plastic wrap, containers for toiletries, and cosmetics, and more.
- BPA is found in water bottles, canned foods, and beverages and on printed sales receipts.
- Phthalates are found in clothing, footwear, medical equipment such as IV components, surgical gloves, breathing tubes, ink, children's products, and product and food packaging.

These chemicals impair hormone functions and are linked to many of the health problems and diseases on the rise in the United States. Nearly all Americans have blood levels above those known to cause harm in laboratory animals.[27,28]

Poly- and Perfluoroalkyl substances (PFAS)

Non-stick cookware; flame, stain and water repellant clothing; fast food and carryout wraps; pizza boxes and microwave popcorn bags—even dental floss—contain dangerous toxins. They accumulate in the body. It takes four years for levels to go down by half even if no more is taken in. They cause neurobehavioral problems, high cholesterol, tumors in multiple organs, hypothyroidism, inflammatory bowel disease (IBD), and liver dysfunction and toxicity.[29]

> How *old* would you be if you didn't know *how old you are?*

Satchel Paige (1906-1982) legendary pitcher in Major League Baseball

Synthetic Fragrance and Colors

When you see "fragrance" listed as an ingredient, read it as, "hidden chemicals that may be hazardous to your health." Patented "secret formulas" can hide nearly 3,000 chemicals under this term.[30] Many are associated with allergies, asthma, dermatitis, respiratory distress, and have negative effects on the reproductive system. Some of them cause cancer.[31] "Fragrances" are listed among the top known allergens. They are designed to create brand loyalty because scents influence emotion and memory.

Triclosan

Triclosan is found in most hand sanitizers and antibacterial soaps, as well as deodorants and toothpaste. It is a known endocrine disruptor (especially to thyroid and reproductive hormones), interferes with muscle function, and irritates the skin.[32] Triclosan accumulates in the body and has been detected in 75 percent of urine samples in a broad sample of the U.S. population.[33] It has been shown to be no more effective than soap and water.[34] The unregulated use of triclosan, despite the evidence of danger, shows a blatant disregard for the health of the American people.

Propylene Glycol

Propylene glycol is used as a skin-conditioning agent. Examples are petroleum jelly, mineral oil and glycerin. It is used to treat skin irritations, despite being classified as an irritant and skin penetrator.[35] It can cause dermatitis as well as hives, especially in people that already have eczema and other skin allergies. Side effects appear to be related to the quantity and frequency of use.[36]

Formaldehyde

Funeral parlors and taxidermists are not the only industries that make good use of formaldehyde. It is found in nail polish, shampoo, soap, fabric softener, hair straightener, and even baby products. It is added in products to prevent bacterial growth. Surprising new evidence (surprising to whom?) links formaldehyde to several types of cancer including leukemia. It causes allergic skin reactions and may also be harmful to the immune system.[37]

Every exposure to a toxin is a drop in your bucket of health. How much can your bucket hold? It's impossible to know until it overflows. Check out the Environmental Working Group (EWG) website (www.ewg.org) or download their app for more information on specific cosmetic and personal care products.

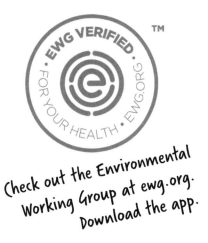

Check out the Environmental Working Group at ewg.org. Download the app.

THE FOUNTAIN OF YOUTH

The more commercial products I cut out, the better I look and feel. As you experience the same, the motivation to clean house intensifies. It's fun to find alternatives that work. Leftover bottles of shampoo, detergents, and cleaning products become reusable containers filled with ingenious concoctions. Every label you notice offers a challenge: is this necessary and what are my options?

Time invested to rid your life of labels will add quality years to your life. Invest the money you save into eating and living well. Instead of declining with age, you'll brighten. Freedom from the Corporate Hunger Games allows you to set and achieve goals. Independence is sexy.

Living off the label is neither expensive nor difficult. Change feels different until new habits feel normal. Wellness feels good. Life off the label is awesome. Make no excuses. Have no regrets.

> *Everyone should know the "WAR on CANCER" is largely a fraud.*
>
> Linus Pauling (1901-1994) pioneer in orthomolecular (vitamin) therapy

STARVING CANCER

Our body produces 50 million new cells every second. The rate of error during replication is about two percent. This means that every day, there are one million cancerous cells in your body. A healthy immune system destroys mutations before they proliferate. Cancer is not detectable until billions of cells are out of control.

The body is designed to heal itself. This capability is the core of cancer treatment. Chemotherapy, radiation, or surgery cannot destroy every cancerous cell. They get rid of what they can. However, these treatments also destroy good cells, including immune agents that fight and repair further mutations. The rationale is to hope the healthy cells are stronger than the cancer.

Traditional treatments damage tissues and organs, and introduce toxins that stress the kidneys, liver and immune system. Individuals are very susceptible to infection and complications. Drugs that break down that body must be countered with treatments that heal. Supporting the immune system and detoxification process with nutrient-dense food, vitamins, and supplements is essential. The environment that fostered the proliferation of cancer must be repaired. If the cause of the cancer is not addressed, it will move to another part of the body or metastasize in the lymph system.

Cancer thrives on:

- **Sugar**. Sugar feeds cancer.[39] Every bite is a setback when fighting disease. Healthy people should limit sugar to unrefined sources such as fruit, pure maple syrup, and local honey. Cancer patients should avoid all added and unnecessary sugars. View food as medicine. Healthy fat and protein, colorful vegetables, nuts and seeds, green tea, probiotics, high doses of vitamin C, and nutritional supplements filled with antioxidants, omega-3 fatty acids and minerals will restore health.
- **Mucous**. Milk and dairy products create congestion. The mucous stagnates in the sinuses, lungs and intestines. Cancer thrives in these environments.
- **Acid-Forming Foods**. Processed foods, artificial sweeteners, soda, meat, and dairy products increase acid levels of the blood. Pathogens and tumors flourish in acidic environments. Cancer cells have a tough protein wall. When digestive proteins are depleted by an onslaught of these foods, the immune system (housed primarily in the gut) has fewer resources to "digest" mutant cells.
- **Poor Oxygenation**. Daily exercise and deep breathing provide extra oxygen to keep cellular replication processes running smoothly.

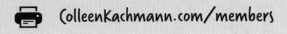 ColleenKachmann.com/members

Normal vs Healthy

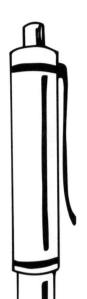

As you contemplate change, what do you perceive to be your most limited resource? Money? Time? Energy?

What resources do you have? How can you use them to compensate for resources that are limited?

Examine the ingredients in your beauty, bathroom, laundry and cleaning products. Are they necessary? Are they problematic? What are the alternatives?

Decreasing the chemicals in your life will improve your health. What "low-hanging fruit" in your life provides the easiest place to start?

ColleenKachmann.com/members

LIFE OFF THE LABEL

PS I left this facing page blank for you.
Fill it with whatever you like. Questions, comments, to-do's, thoughts, etc.
You're welcome . . .

CHAPTER 14B

INVEST THE REST

"Have you ever read a book that changed your life? Me either."

JIM GAFFIGAN, COMEDIAN, ACTOR AND AUTHOR.

SUBSIDIZING SERENDIPITY

This book will not change your life. Only you can do that. The desire to change won't do much either. So what's the good news? Action is the antidote for stagnancy.

Act well; be well.

It's normal to feel overwhelmed once you realize that your lifestyle must change. But don't give up before you start. When taken one decision at a time, wellness is rewarding and thus sustainable. As you become well, you'll want to stay well. You'll protect the investments you make in yourself. The motivation for further improvements will naturally appear when you are ready for the next change.

Do you want to be well? If so, that goal must become your new number-one priority. Wellness is the foundation for all success, if only so that you can reap the rewards of other endeavors. If you are not first and foremost well, nothing else you do will matter (for long).

To get where you want to be in life, you need to know where you are. Elevators that stop at 14B do not actually bypass the fearsome 13th floor. The common misnomer keeps everyone comfortable. But you can't break barriers and defy limitations inside your comfort zone. Be honest with yourself. What changes do you need to make? What normal behaviors are not creating health? What does your future hold if you continue to live as you are?

The only reward for believing in setback is camaraderie with people doing the same. When a friend understands how we feel, our problems have merit. But validation can breathe life into any illusion. It's critical to foster relationships that have positive value. Don't waste time complaining and commiserating. Invest your energy in planning and expanding.

Do you spend more time on social media and binge-watching Netflix than you do creating memories for yourself? Do the lives of others seem more interesting than your own? Why? Who deserves your attention more than you? If you aren't proud of yourself, it's easy to fall into the trap of watching instead of doing. And that's ok. If you are stuck on the 13th floor, honor your location. Stop referring to it as 14B. Find the stairwell, look at the map, and pinpoint "you are here." The following 14 steps will take you in the right direction.

> "I would never belong to a club that would have ME as a *member*."
>
> Groucho Marx (1890-1977), comedian

#1: Change the Culture in Your Kitchen

It will surprise you how much time and talent it *doesn't* take to cook. Making a home-cooked meal requires no more time than idling in the drive-thru or waiting for take-out. Put on music. Light candles. Turn off the little and big screens. Invite people in. Keep your space clean. Make the kitchen the preferred meeting place in your home (as opposed to the couch in front of the television).

Even if it's not completely from scratch, a home-cooked meal is still better than fast food. When you are overwhelmed and tired (and cooking elicits Thelma and Louise-like fantasies), call in the troops. Everyone who eats should contribute in some way. It takes effort to "train" kids and spouses to help, but future generations will reap the rewards. Teaching others to cook reduces pressure on you and pays the gift forward.

Preparing a meal requires planning. So does agreeing on a restaurant and collecting orders. Cleaning up after dinner doesn't take long if everyone helps. If you aren't a servant, don't act like one. Don't whine. Don't apologize for delegating tasks as though your time is less valuable than anyone else's. Set clear expectations. Hold everyone accountable. Be generous with compliments. Make requests instead of criticisms. Positive energy attracts more of the same.

#2: Purchase a Good Knife

Actually get two. It's nice to have one large chef knife and one petite. This allows two people to work in unison. There is a lot of chopping involved in the preparation of unprocessed food. You can't run a marathon in a cheap pair of shoes. Hacking at vegetables with a dull butter knife is no fun. Cooking is creative and artistic. The right tools are essential.

If you think of cooking as a chore, it will be. Instead, think of cooking as an opportunity to spend time by yourself, with your spouse, or a child. Chopping is a great stress reliever. Daily frustrations are transformed into happy, healthy meals. Slice and dice your troubles away. Just be careful for the sake of your fingers!

#3: Use a High-Speed Blender

Blenders make more than margaritas. Fibrous plant foods are transformed into culinary works of art in high-performance machines. Frozen bananas whip into velvety ice cream, and cashews into buttery Alfredo sauce. An extra serving of spinach is easy to conceal in a protein shake. With juice bars all the rage, these machines allow you to make your own, far less expensive versions at home.

If you already have a blender, use it. Hardier brands can handle the demands of frozen foods, nuts, and even laundry detergent. High-speed blenders start at about $150. The investment will pay for itself if you use it to make more than smoothies. It's "cheaper" to purchase a higher quality machine than to replace inexpensive ones that burn up grinding peanuts into fresh peanut butter. I learned this the hard way. My appliance graveyard got two blenders and a food processor in one year. I finally forked over the cash for a Vitamix and have used it every day since I bought it. (The Ninja now offers comparable quality at half the price.)

Find whole food cookbooks that offer unique recipes for blenders. It's quite amazing what these machines can do. Do your homework, however. Before you buy, ensure the appliance you purchase offers a satisfaction guarantee, comprehensive warranty, replacement parts, and customer support.

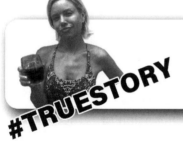

#TRUESTORY How can you tell if someone owns a Vitamix? Don't worry. They'll tell you.

#4: Find a Source of Fresh Organic Produce

I would love to spend my Saturday's squeezing juicy melons and smelling fragrant herbs at the local farmers markets. But Saturdays are busy with soccer games, cleaning, laundry, and yard work. Most grocery stores stock organic produce. Several national chains now source from local farmers in various communities. It is critical to add your own demand for these supplies.

On-line services that provide access to local produce and quality pantry items are expanding across the country. I shop from my office once per week. It takes 5 minutes. Food is delivered to my doorstep in insulated containers. Look for companies like Green B.E.A.N. Delivery, Peapod, Fresh Direct, Door to Door Organics, food cooperatives, and CSAs (community supported agriculture). As you peruse available options, remember that good food is not cheap. But illness is more expensive. Distribute funds accordingly.

7 Time Saving Tips

1. Chop up veggies and fruit before you put them away. This makes it easy to make salad and snacks during a busy week. Store them in airtight containers or "green" bags that can be rinsed and reused.
2. Shop online. Grocery and produce delivery services are available in many communities. Don't let premium prices scare you. Look for good deals. Realize that you save money every time you don't go to the store. Sales items, impulse purchases, and clever marketing gimmicks are budget busters. Analyze overall cost and savings. Find organic pantry items online as well. Free shipping on minimum orders is often available. Before you check out, search "promo codes" for the website. There are many coupons available when you take the time to look or sign up as a member.
3. Double or even triple your recipes. Think beyond the next meal. Chop all the vegetables at once. Store in sealed containers. Make extra meat for quick tacos, chili, and spaghetti later in the week. Eat leftovers for lunch, redesign them into additional meals or freeze.
4. Save scraps. Don't put stems, peels or produce that are about to go bad in the trash or compost. Keep designated containers in your freezer. Separate fruits and vegetables. Add to soups, smoothies and stir-frys. Or cover with water and blend. Simmer and season into a nutritious broth.
5. Stock the pantry. Organic soups, broths, gluten-free pastas, rice, pre-cooked lentils, quinoa, and beans are invaluable starters. Include frozen or leftover vegetables to the mix or serve them on the side. Dinner can be ready in 20 minutes or less.
6. Insist that kids participate. Teach them to chop, wash dishes, stir the pot, and put away leftovers. The more they are included in meal design and cooking, the more likely they are to appreciate the result.
7. Reusable grill and baking mats make clean up simple. Avoid the scrubbing!

ColleenKachmann.com/members

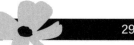

#5: Honor Thy Veggies

You wouldn't throw a $20 steak on the grill without first tenderizing, marinating, and seasoning it with desired flavors. Give vegetables the same respect! Soften the flavor and texture of eggplant by tenderizing it with salt. Soak onion and broccoli in lemon water to reduce bitterness. Marinate sweet peppers and mushrooms with olive oil and fresh herbs. Grilled cauliflower brushed with sweet butter and buffalo seasoning trumps greasy chicken wings every time.

Cook vegetables at the lowest possible temperature to retain micronutrients and soften fiber (for easier digestion). A good rule of thumb is to steam/sauté/roast/grill until colors are at peak brightness. Veggies that are a little crunchy are healthiest. If kids don't like the crisp texture, a quick whirl in the blender creates a sauce. Toss vegetables with a bit of oil to maximize fat-soluble vitamins and mineral absorption.

#6: Eliminate Distractions

Modern life is filled with distraction. Rabbit holes of mindless information splinter our attention and diminish our ability to set and achieve goals. If we don't direct our focus with specific intention, it will be directed for us.

Smart phones, tablets, televisions, and computers give us access to unlimited information. The digital information age has the potential for unbelievable productivity. Yet all too often, the tools we use to control our life end up controlling us.

Do you tend to watch programs, buy products and use services based on advertisements? If so, computerized algorithms designed to generate profit are directing your attention and money. How would life be different if you didn't have these distractions?

Find out.

The agendas of others are not designed to enhance your life. Don't allow technology to consume you. Instead, consciously design a strategy for the future. What do you want your life to be? Cut the leash that is your phone. Put it on the charger in another room; go places without it. Turn off the television. Let your mind wander; foster your sense of curiosity. Marinate the details of important world events in your own brain—don't take on the opinions of talking heads that are written for the benefit of corporate sponsors.

Define clear boundaries for your space, time, and energy; spend them in service to your own personal agenda. The borders of your life will expand with awareness.

#7: Cook in a Cast-Iron Skillet

Cast-iron may appear to be a relic of the pioneer days, but they are good for more than campouts. Cooking in cast-iron increases the amount of iron available in many vegetables.[1] Skillets are non-stick and can be used for sautéing, baking, and grilling. Dutch ovens can handle anything.

A few words of advice: Season the skillet before its first use (especially if it's vintage). Heat it on the stove top until it's smoking hot, rub oil into it, and let it cool. Repeat this a few times to create a non-stick coating, and then periodically to maintain it. The more you use it, the less maintenance it requires. Before storing it, dry thoroughly, and coat with a bit of oil. When residual water leads to rust, scrub and re-season.

Cast-iron cookware is expensive, but it can last for lifetimes. Shop in attics and antique stores and give new life to a forgotten treasure.

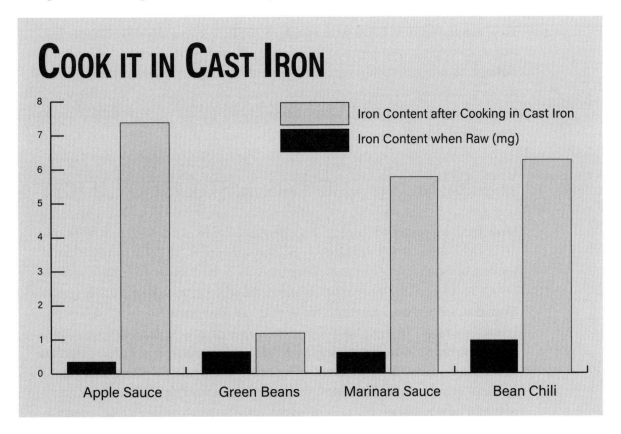

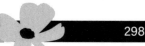

#8: Connect with Yourself and Others

Set goals and keep them in plain view. Get an old-school notebook, binder, cork or magnetized white board. Fill it with pictures and ideas that motivate you in times of stress.

- Collect recipes, quotes, and information. Pin inspiring images of the life you are daring to live next to reminders of what you are leaving behind.
- Make note of your obstacles. Identify possible solutions. Have confidence in your ability to live free.
- Take time each week to evaluate your progress. Set new goals on a regular basis. Take corrective action when efforts seem to cost more than they are worth.
- Write a letter to the "normal" version of you. Describe the healthy version of you emerging with change. Review for encouragement in times of frustration and stress.
- Design an "emergency happiness" kit that contains songs, images, and activities that will raise your spirits and reignite your passion to live and be well.

Finally, make connections with *real people*. Surround yourself with positive influences; share your passion to live and eat well with others. Challenges are difficult to navigate when you face them alone. Look for support and camaraderie. Being healthy will soon feel normal. At some point, you'll be the one with the experience and helpful advice. Life off the label is the proverbial "road less traveled." But it is on the map.

#9 Remove the Biggest Offenders

Stop drinking soda pop. Stop using chemical-laden condiments. Stop taking OTC (over-the-counter) medications. Buy only non-GMO and organic varieties of processed food. Stop watching television. Reduce the time you spend on social media. Don't peruse magazines filled with tempting advertisements from Corporate Headquarters. Think and live for yourself.

When I stopped mindlessly viewing all of the digital screens, I found the time to write a book. What endeavors will you pursue with extra time and mental space? Consciously replace each old habit with a new one. Identify your talents and find new hobbies. Try new physical activities; schedule regular exercise into your week. Write, paint, cook, design, garden, dance, sing, play—create! Repeat until your new version of normal is exactly what you envisioned.

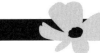

A Lemon a Day Keeps the Doctor Away

Add half of a lemon (rind included) to warm water or hot tea. Drink first thing in the morning on an empty stomach. Refill all day. The benefits are remarkable.[2]

- Lemons contain potassium, calcium, and magnesium. These electrolytes are essential for proper hydration.
- Lemons contain citric acid, which enhances digestive enzyme action and regulates bowel movements.
- Lemon cleanses the liver and stimulates the production of detoxifying enzymes.
- Lemons have anti-inflammatory properties and ward off infection in the tonsils, throat, and respiratory tract.
- Lemon is a powerful antioxidant that protects the body from free radicals and strengthens the immune system.
- The high potassium content in lemons improves symptoms of depression and anxiety and supports function of the nervous system.
- Lemon cleanses blood, blood vessels, and arteries. A lemon a day can reduce blood pressure by 10 percent.
- Lemons dilute uric acid, the build up of which leads to pain in the joints. This raises the pH of blood, which blocks the proliferation of pathogens that thrive in acidic environments. Numerous studies have found that cancer cannot thrive in an alkaline environment.
- Lemon relieves heartburn and can help dissolve gall bladder, kidney, and pancreatic stones and other calcium deposits.
- The pectin fiber in lemon suppresses hunger, reduces cravings, and raises metabolism.

 ColleenKachmann.com/members

#10 Understand Detox

If you have been eating S.A.D. (Standard American Diet) for a long period of time, toxins are hiding in your fat cells—even if you are not overweight. The release of these toxins from the body is not a feel-good process. Embrace the discomfort as a sign that you are healing. Take care of yourself during this experience. (See *Tips for Surviving Detox* on page 58.)

Consult a functional or integrative doctor if symptoms are prolonged or unbearable. Just don't give up. You are worth the effort. The harsher the symptoms, the better you are going to feel.

#11: Stop Using A Microwave

Microwaves zap living enzymes that aid in digestion. Use the stovetop or oven to prepare meals. Yes, real cooking requires more time. This is a bonus that will decrease the amount of junk food you (and your kids) eat. Remove the instant from the gratification. The anticipation of good food tingles the senses. It's foreplay! The intensity of flavor, fragrance and visual appeal will increase. And if the cuisine is not quality, the subtle differences between hunger and appetite will be easier to discern. Real hunger doesn't appreciate artificial ingredients. You'll be hungry before you should because your body craves nutrients. Don't refuel with crap.

#12: Become a DIY-er

(Pronounced "do-it-yourself-er" or "D-I-Y'er")

Don't let the words that come from your mouth define what you believe. "I can't cook" can easily be challenged with a box of organic rice pilaf and a set of directions. If you can read and tell time, you can cook.

Start small. Tackle one change at a time. Make your own deodorant, laundry detergent or cleaning supplies. Grow herbs, sprouts or plant a small vegetable garden. Learn to make yogurt. Mix organic seasoning blends from a recipe. Put together a delicious marinara from scratch. Try fermenting sauerkraut. Doing things for yourself will become just as quick and easy as running to the store. Convenience is a marketing concept that creates profits, not health.

Macro-Warning on Microwaves

There is an effective way to increase the quality of micronutrients in every food you choose to eat, even processed foods. Stop using the microwave. At least use it as little as possible. Stand at least a foot away when it is running and remove food from all packaging.

Microwaves cause water particles to resonate at a very high frequency. This rapid heating process provides convenience. But radiation damages protein molecules and denatures micronutrients. Up to 97 percent of the antioxidants in broccoli are destroyed after being microwaved.[3] Even worse, amino acids and enzymes are disabled. Carcinogens and free radicals form in their place.[4]

Microwaves destroy the DNA of whatever they penetrate. Even the safest models emit some radiation. Damage over a lifetime is cumulative. Long-term, low-level exposure has equivalent effects to short-term, intense exposure.[5] Microwaves also cause plastics and toxins to leach into food. Notice that even paper packages are coated with colors and sealants. This adds to the onslaught of chemicals that bombards our bodies.[6]

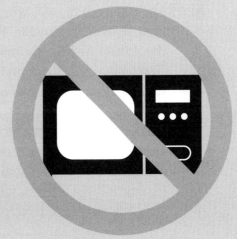

Before freezing foods, separate portions so that you do not have to deal with huge chunks and bundles. Think ahead and pull out dinner ingredients in the morning or thaw overnight in the refrigerator. Drop frozen meat into a bowl of hot water. It can be grill-ready as fast (if not faster) as using the defrost setting on the microwave.

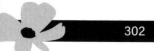

#13 Remove Your Obstacle Opinions

Normal excuses undermine healthy results. Here are the most common thoughts and words that make it difficult to create new habits.

"I'll have just one piece."

Maybe. But that one piece is served over a precipice. Addictions are triggered by the first bite. Cravings for bad foods will go away if you nourish yourself with satisfying foods. The longer you avoid unhealthy options, the less you'll want them.

"It's a special occasion!"

Why is unhealthy food synonymous with special occasions? There are far more exceptions than rules when it comes to bad food. When two or more are gathered, refusing low quality food can be perceived as rude. We collectively accept the status quo because rejecting it makes others uncomfortable. When you say "no thank you," an option is exposed. That's not cool on free-for-all Fridays. But saying, "no thank you" to bad food is a "yes, please!" to your health.

Participating in the problem is not the answer. Some people will view your choice as an indictment against their own. But it's not personal. There is no need to be concerned with someone else's issue. Anger and resentment appear in passive aggressive statements like, "I'm sorry this food isn't good enough for you." You are not obligated to reply.

"Everyone expects meat."

Who is everyone? What people say and do reveals their character. Don't mistake the opinions of others as a reflection on you. If someone criticizes your efforts, they are rude. That's to their embarrassment, not yours.

"I can't afford to buy good food for that many people."

That's okay. But contributing bad food to a gathering for the sake of budget is bad karma. If it's not good enough for you, don't serve it to others. Consider these options:

- Buy and bring less. No one will starve.
- Skip the expensive, pre-washed, sliced and diced produce. Prepare it yourself. Save money with time and effort.

- Take hummus and carrots, apples and peanut butter or a bean medley with salsa and crunchy lettuce dip-strips. Serve iced water with lemon or cucumber and mint.
- Don't bring anything. Again, no one will starve. We all "forget" from time to time. No excuse required. No food is better than bad food.

> **People are convinced by observation, *not* argument.**
>
> Will Rogers (1879--1935) Comedic actor, social commentator

"I could never give up cheese."

I loved cheese. So I didn't give it up. I replaced it. I started with dairy free alternatives (Daiya and Follow Your Heart are my two favorite brands). But when I discovered cashew cream, the substitutes were no longer needed.

Pizza is much better now that I don't feel sick after I eat. A stone-baked, crispy-thin, gluten-free crust, brushed with olive oil and freshly chopped garlic is the foundation of perfection. Homemade marinara, seasoned veggies, and fresh herb toppings leave nothing to be desired. Drizzle with cashew cream and a masterpiece emerges from the oven.

Have I mentioned cashew cream enough? Because I can say it again. Cashew cream. (see page 50)

"There were no other options."

Failure to plan is planning to fail. Unless you are confident that your preferred foods will be available, eat before you go anywhere. Or bring a meal from home. Be bold and make no apologies. Bring organic condiments and desired ingredients to restaurants. Peruse menus for options and order a customized stir-fry. Take veggie burgers to cookouts. Call ahead to catered events and ask if your dietary restrictions can be accommodated. Always be polite and don't complain when the answer is "no." Thank servers for their candor and prepare accordingly.

Keep a can of nuts in the car for emergencies. Pack food in your bag. Worst-case scenario: remember that only breast-fed babies need to eat every three hours. You can't die of hunger, only starvation. Hunger symptoms include impatience, however. Try to remain civil.

#14 Choose to Snooze

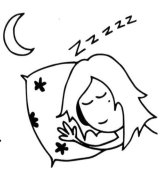

The body restores and repairs itself during uninterrupted rest. Your abilities to focus, solve problems and manage stress all require sleep.[7] People who sleep only six hours a night on a regular basis are the cognitive equivalent of being drunk.[8] Your quality of life depends on sleep. You cannot thrive physically, emotionally, or mentally when you are sleep deprived. If you are not getting 7-8 hours of sleep per night, you are putting yourself at a disadvantage.

New habits require discipline. All too often, we simply forget about our intention and time gets away from us. Set an alert on your phone for one hour before your ideal bedtime: "Hey Sexy! It's called beauty sleep for a reason. Go get some. You'll be even more awesome tomorrow."

The Beautiful Truth

Does your state of health reflect the beauty of your inner spirit? If not, do something different. It's never too late and you're never too old to be the main attraction in your life. What you see in the mirror is a reflection of yesterday. What you feel in your heart is potential for tomorrow.

If your external body does not reflect your internal image, make some changes. Identify your passions and pursue them with determination.

There is a fascinating dichotomy in the way we approach change. We make resolutions, read self-help books, and go to therapy. Each year, vision boards are filled with good intentions. We buy into the next New-Year-New-You!-trend and hope that momentum sustains us. But predictably, serendipity doesn't strike for most of us. It's easier to believe that "most people never change." The odds are against us. Unconscious beliefs manifest in self-fulfilling prophecy.

Defining our flaws preserves their existence. Consider how easy these words roll off our tongue:

- "I'm awful with numbers."
- "I have social anxiety."
- "I have a terrible sense of direction."
- "I have bad knees."
- "I don't have enough time."

- "I'm too old to do that."
- "I can't dance."
- "I've always been overweight."

Inevitably, we mess-up the math, avoid social situations, do the same thing we did yesterday and repeat mistakes. We don't make the time or have the energy to expand our comfort zone. When weaknesses define our normal, we don't question their validity. Habits hold us back.

Unless . . .

We approach our shortcomings as challenges. Words followed by action have unlimited potential. Consider:

- "Brain teasers have improved my math skills. I get better all the time."
- "Whenever I meet someone new, I try to learn three things about them."
- "I pay close attention to landmarks so that I don't get lost."
- "I strengthen my knees with exercise. A fast walk feels better than running."
- "Time management and organization allow me to accomplish my goals."
- "I love being the oldest one in the room. Wisdom is beautiful."
- "My dance moves are quite unique. Watch and learn."
- "I don't eat processed foods. I am losing weight."

The beautiful truth is that change is not driven by chance. Change is driven by you. God doesn't work for you. He works through you. Support hope and prayer with plans and action. Don't wait for an invitation to your own life. It's already there. It's yours. Take it and run.

> **"Unless someone like you *cares a whole awful lot*, NOTHING is going to get better. *It's not.*"**
>
> — Dr. Suess, *The Lorax*

BE A POLITE PARTY POOPER

Newsflash: What you eat is not anyone else's business. And what other people think about what you eat is not *your* business.

When faced with social eating, avoid confrontations. The less you say, the better. Do not engage in a discussion about why you are not eating what someone else is. This creates a challenging emotional dilemma. People will feel bad, argue in their own defense or submit to your "rightness" and put down their fork. This is not beneficial to relationships you wish to keep. Of course, if you are looking to burn a bridge, light up the conversation with "I can't believe you are eating that crap."

Maneuver buffet bullies with short explanations. Avoid commentary about the evil options. If someone is genuinely interested in your diet, offer to discuss it later. Heated discussions taint the group dynamic in social situations. Wiggle out of conflicts with a simple response and change the subject.

- "I'm doing a 30-day cleanse (or challenge) because I've been feeling so sluggish."
- "I'm on a diet."
- "How's your mom?"
- "Hey! Is that a squirrel?"
- "I'm training for a (5k, 10k, Cancer Walk, bike race, triathlon). I am so excited."
- "I've had (insert health concern) so I am cutting (pick a poison) to see if I can avoid (reference a medical intervention)."

ColleenKachmann.com/members

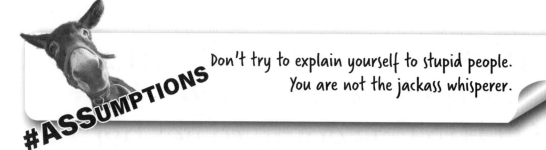

#ASSUMPTIONS Don't try to explain yourself to stupid people. You are not the jackass whisperer.

DIY
Homegrown Sprouts

Sprouts offer all of the essential amino acids that our bodies can't synthesize. They are a "complete protein," similar to the egg (without the cholesterol). Sprouts have the highest amount of micronutrients you can get in a single bite of food. Quality concerns are legitimate as grocery store varieties can carry listeria. Growing them at home is safe provided that you rinse them each day.

Instructions:

- Soak about 2-3 Tbsp. of sprout seeds in water for 24 hours.
- Transfer to a glass jar.
- Rinse every 12 -24 hours or so. A screen colander (or screen lid) makes this easy.
- Store jar on a windowsill or counter top. Sunlight enhances the nutrition.

Early sprouts appear within two days. You can begin to eat them as soon as they are tender. They flourish through about day six. Seal and store them in the refrigerator to extend shelf life beyond a week. Counter the early signs of rot with a vinegar rinse. Toss them in salads, smoothies or stir-fries.

Sauerkraut Recipe

Fermented foods like yogurt and sauerkraut are essential to gut health. Commercial brands are pasteurized, which kills the probiotic microbes. In less than 30 minutes, you can make a supply that lasts up to six months.

You will need a ceramic crock and a pestle. The inside of a slow cooker or Dutch oven can be used as a crock. A heavy meat hammer can serve as the pestle. Shred or finely chop three large or four small green cabbage heads for a two-gallon batch. Add two inches of cabbage to the crock. Sprinkle the layer with two pinches of sea salt and one pinch of caraway seeds. Smash with the pestle until the leaves are covered in their own juices. Repeat with additional layers. Churn with your hands and cover with several layers of wrap. Churn and re-seal every few days.

It is essential to keep the kraut sealed during fermentation because oxygen rots the cabbage. Use several layers of plastic wrap and a rubber band to secure the top seal. Some recipes say to wait a month before eating. I found it edible (and belly-friendly) within 7-10 days. I eat a few bites medicinally every day and encourage my family to do the same. If it starts to rot, it's obvious. If you wonder if it's bad, then it probably is.

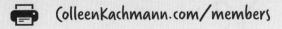 ColleenKachmann.com/members

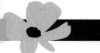

Normal vs Healthy

Look at your life from the perspective of someone less fortunate than you. What advantages do you take for granted?

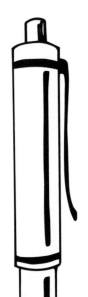

What talents and resources do you already have that will support the changes you want to make? What do you still need?

Normal excuses must be exchanged for healthy habits. What excuses do you make? What habits need to change?

Think of the most successful people in history. If they stepped into your body, how would they overcome your challenges?

 ColleenKachmann.com/members

PS I left this facing page blank for you.
Fill it with whatever you like. Questions, comments, to-do's, thoughts, etc.
You're welcome . . .

INVEST THE REST

CHAPTER 15

CREATE YOUR OWN BRAND OF HEALTH AND HAPPINESS

"Happiness is a choice that requires effort at times."

AESCHYLUS (525-456 BC) IS KNOWN AS THE FOUNDER OF THE GREEK TRAGEDY

BONDAGE BROKEN

I was sinking in desperation after the birth of my fourth child. (Chapter 1 begins with this story.) My daughter was born premature and had colic. An inconsolable infant is overwhelming. Simultaneously managing my home and three other children was grueling. I had very little space and time to myself. Daily chores exhausted me. Chronic pain intensified my stress. I was eating fat-free diet foods, trying to lose the baby weight. I didn't know I was malnourished. I was tired all of the time. I drank large amounts of caffeine to counter the fatigue. The stimulant left me (and my breastfed baby) deprived of sleep. The cycle perpetuated itself.

I sought help from my family doctor. His approach was to manage my ailments with pharmaceuticals. He prescribed several medications. I accepted them without scrutiny. Citalopram did suppress my tears. It did not diminish the tedium of daily responsibilities. Ativan quieted my brain. It did not reduce the overwhelming chaos that created the anxiety. Pain pills allowed me to continue the heavy lifting required of full-time mothers without taking the time to heal. Ambien knocked me out but failed to remedy the reasons I couldn't sleep.

In hindsight, the medications enabled me to continue the harmful habits that precipitated their demand.

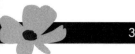

About a year into my "pharmaceutical phase," a cherished girlfriend approached me with a concern. I was drinking too much. I made no secret (only jokes) that night-night time was the new happy hour. I appreciated her honesty. But I didn't' really care (drug-induced apathy has pros and cons). It was years before I learned that anti-depressants intensify cravings for alcohol in casual drinkers and can lead to alcohol abuse. The liver cannot metabolize both simultaneously.[1] The enhanced buzz is pleasant and intoxicating. To be fair, there were clear warning labels advising that alcohol not be consumed. But drugs that soothe concerns also inhibit caution.

Intervention arrived dressed in vanity. I was gaining weight. Dry white wine pairs nicely with a fresh bag of crisp, salty potato chips. The dark circles under my bloodshot eyes were impossible to conceal. I went to my doctor and told him the truth. The emotion-disabling drugs blunted my shame, but the confession took courage nonetheless. Hidden in the haze was a sincere desire to be well. I expected that outpatient rehab would be recommended. I was prepared to attend AA meetings. To my surprise, alcoholism was not diagnosed. Instead, medication to "calm the cravings" was prescribed. I tried it and hoped for the best. The cure didn't come.

I countered weakness with intelligent strategy. I committed to evening activities and exercise to bypass temptation. I made plans with friends so that social pressure ensured moderation. Beyond that, I drank alone and hid the evidence. The downward spiral was slow but steady. I am grateful that I fell into the safety net of my mother in the hotel after my grandfather's funeral. My confidence was shattered but I was motivated to take action. I removed alcohol from my home and began to wean myself off the pharmaceuticals.

The detox off the drugs was excruciating. Neurons misfired, sending currents of electricity through my head and down my spine. My pupils ached; even low light was too bright. Small sounds mutated into shrieks. Tissues prickled. Muscles throbbed. I was in a constant state of agitation.

But the intense pain served its purpose. To heal, I had to feel. For way too long, I had muted the visceral sensations in my body. I had suppressed my own needs because they interfered with my perception of the needs of my family. But I was done numbing myself so that I could ignore myself. I was ready to exchange my self-denial-cleverly-disguised-as-over-indulgence habits for real empowerment. After a month of detox, my body and mind were clean and clear. I felt in control, fearless, and had more energy than I knew what to do with. The experience taught me a valuable lesson: pain is not to be ignored.

Life's a bitch like that. It gives you the test first. The lesson follows.

HEALTHY BECOMES NORMAL

The first step to becoming healthy (and happy) is to admit that you are not. A map is useless until the "You are here" point is identified. If you purchased this book, you answered "yes" to at least one of these questions:

- Do you eat low-fat and reduced-calorie foods, yet struggle with weight?
- Classify seasons by allergies, asthma, colds and flu?
- Take yourself and your kids to the doctor as often as you do your elderly parents?
- Feel overwhelmed by stress and mental health issues?
- Dread getting older as disease and painful deterioration seem inevitable?
- Struggle between what is socially acceptable and doing what's right for your family's health?

My mission in writing Life Off the Label is not to scare you with everything that is wrong. But the education is necessary if you want to make it right. The advice of Big Pharma, Big Food and Big Government serves them, not you. Stories of misadventures and my strategies for success can provide you with a framework for your own new beginning. Once you see that the labels in your life are optional, your own brand of health and happiness will develop a persona to your liking. Momentum will carry you from the illusions that have restricted your potential. Each change that you make will lead to another. As you experience your own power, it will expand.

Have you ever met someone who thinks they can do whatever they want? Maybe you've only watched them on T.V. Does it frustrate you when people dare to do as they please, and then dare to get away with it? If so, this reveals your first challenge. The way you view the world determines your place in it. Whatever you think becomes your truth. If you think you can't, you won't. If you know you can, you do. Any plan can fail. But people aren't failures unless they believe they are. Successful people appreciate the lessons that come with the good *and* the bad.

If you perceive yourself at a disadvantage, you are. If you see the abundance of life, you manage unexpected shortages with intelligence. Life happens to everyone; it's how you react that counts. Every problem begins with a question: Are you a victim or a survivor?

How will you answer?

Profit From Your Pain

Albert Einstein is best known in popular culture for his mass–energy equivalence formula, $E = mc^2$. The equation reveals that energy has weight, and mass has energy. This important truth helps us make sense of the mind–body connection. We must understand that energy matters.

We perceive emotions to be figments of our imagination. A broken leg requires medical attention. A broken heart is something to "get over." But emotions are neurochemical. They are as real as bone, blood and muscle. Drugs that alter levels of dopamine and serotonin in the brain affect the sensations we feel in our body. Thoughts generate chemical reactions that influence our health. Positive thoughts lead to wellness. Negative thoughts create dysfunction in our nervous, cardiovascular, hormonal and immune systems. Neurochemicals are the bridge between the mental and physical worlds.

Energy is measured by its ability to cause things to happen. Matter is anything that has mass and takes up space. Emotions are both energy and mass. Einstein's law applies. Energy is transferable, thus joy and fear are contagious. Energy performs work, thus optimism improves productivity. Stress manifests as a knot in the neck or wrench in the back—it has mass that is palpable. Thoughts of gratitude and enthusiasm generate "feel good" endorphins; anger enzymes are acidic and corrosive. Emotions impact both the mind and body.

Thoughts and feelings influence the way we interact with the world and the way the world interacts with us. Indeed, energy matters.

We all experience pain from time to time—it's part of life. Anger, shame, loss and fear are unavoidable. But internalizing these feelings keeps them intact. Negative emotions are the result of negative thoughts. The only way to change the way you feel is to change what you are thinking about. The desire to move forward must be stronger than the inertia holding you back. Positive actions will nourish and heal.

> **Education is not *learning the facts*, but training the mind *to think*.**
>
> — Albert Einstein (1879-1955)

To heal, you must feel. Admit when you are hurt. Feel the embarrassment of being wrong. Cry when you feel sad. But don't dwell on the thoughts that led to the sensation. Ruminating on cyclical issues keeps sad stories alive. Acknowledge the pain and then shift your focus to something that lifts your spirits. Whatever you pay attention to will grow. Whatever you neglect will die.

People who are happy and healthy act that way. Their behavior creates their reality. You cannot live in the caves of misperception, bound by normal views, and also live in freedom. You are now equipped with the knowledge that will allow you to redesign your fate. If you want to be happy and healthy, all you must do is act like a happy and healthy person. Apply what you have learned. Your life is the consequence of your actions. Take responsibility for each one.

Anger is like Poop

All humans have emotions. Deep breathing has a calming effect on both the mind and body. Thoughts breathe life into anger, corroding the brain of the person who feels it. I explain the anatomy of anger to my kids with an analogy.

Everybody poops. The toxins and waste in our bodies must be released. Don't be embarrassed when you have to poop. Be discrete. If the poop is stinky, light a candle. Turn on the fan if you need to pass gas. If you don't feel clean, use a wet wipe to prevent skid marks on your underwear. Flush the toilet when you are done.

The urge to poop arises when waves of muscle contractions move waste through the digestive tract. Sensations of anger arise when waves of energy bring problems into focus. Poop and anger must be eliminated before they can serve a purpose. Poop removes toxins. Anger removes apathy. Poop composts into fertilizer. Anger fuels corrective action.

Everybody gets angry. The negative energy must be released. Don't be embarrassed by your feelings. Be discrete. Anger is a byproduct; it is neither the problem nor the solution. Negative reactions sustain problems. Positive actions sustain solutions.

Energy is contagious. Bad moods, good moods, silliness and sappiness are enhanced or squelched by interactions with others. Relationships are energetic; people can bring us down or lift us up. We can't change the words and actions of other people. But how we respond has a powerful effect that ripples through our body and out into the world. If you snap at the waitress, she may be rude to the next customer. That customer pays it forward to their child, who kicks the dog. Why should a dog suffer because you were in a bad mood? Poor dog.

When you feel good, you behave well. Your interactions with others are positive. The world responds in kind. When you smile, dogs you have never met wag their tails. Do you see how energy manifests? It is your sole source of power. Optimism, confidence and productive behaviors influence the entire world.

The good news is both liberating and frightening. Do you know why some people are able to do whatever they want with no restrictions applied? Because they believe that they can. And so can you. You can do whatever you want. But you must *do* it. Freedom is not a gift—it is a challenge. You. Can. Do. Anything.

Freedom Earned

I have struggled with eating disorders and obsessive–compulsive food issues my entire life. Close friends contend that my vegan journey appears to be a new manifestation of the old issues. They are right. The caveat is that I have harnessed the hysteria. The cyclical thought patterns are still there; so I've put them to good use. The brain is a powerful weapon that can create or destroy.

When I began writing about my plant-based adventures, I discovered that the flip side of insanity is passion. I filled my website with recipes, anecdotes and strategies. The list of topics I wanted to research and explore expanded in all directions. I entertained the idea of turning my adventures into a book.

When I entered the divorce process, I needed a job, not a hobby. I was a teacher by trade but my license had expired. Requalifying myself for a job with the age group I avoided between 8 a.m. and 3 p.m. was not the fresh start I envisioned. I am intelligent and hard working. But I had been a homemaker for 15 years. My kids were old enough to manage alone before and after school, but I love being around when they arrive home to tell me about their day. Unfortunately, my job as a mother no longer included a paycheck and health insurance. I needed a career for my sake and theirs.

I wanted to pursue my passion. I just didn't know how to turn a little blog into a profitable website in a short period of time. I did not want to peddle products or turn off my readers with pop-up ads for products I'd never endorse. I did not want to sell my time doing one-on-one kitchen consultations or teaching cooking classes to small audiences. I knew the key to a sustainable income was to write a book. Only a book could establish my authority as an expert and provide a tangible product I could sell.

The clock was ticking. I had to make a choice. Do I write the book or a resume for the job I didn't want?

It was 8:45 a.m. on a Thursday when I made the decision. I got my kids to school. I turned off my phone. I shut off email notifications. I logged out of Facebook. I didn't start the laundry, look at the stack of bills, write a grocery list or go for a run. I sat down in front of my computer and seat belted my butt to the chair.

"Screw it." I told my dogs. "I'm going to sit here and write until some tangible force drags me out of this chair. I am not *going* to write a book. I am writing a book. I do not want to work for myself. I work for myself. Starting today."

The only actual obstacle facing me was my own fear. I was not being kicked out of my home (yet). My children were not going hungry. There was no obligation to be anywhere. The opportunity was mine to pass or take. I had everything I needed. Except for one minor detail: clarity.

Chronic digestive issues, hair loss and the complications of vegan ideals had to be acknowledged. How could I write a book about the health benefits of a vegan diet when my body seemed to be falling apart?

I couldn't. I wouldn't. I was determined to tell the truth. So I let go of the allegiance to my labels and forged ahead. This decision transformed problems into potential and breathed life into my stories. Rich material lay in my personal failures and contradictions. I embraced them both. The setbacks propelled my progress.

Well, That Didn't Work
An Autobiography

#SERIOUSLY

Brand New You

Look at the optical illusion. Do you see the young woman or an old hag? You can shift your focus from one to the other, but you can't see both at the same time. Life is the same way. All situations are a matter of perception. What's important to realize is that there's always another point of view.

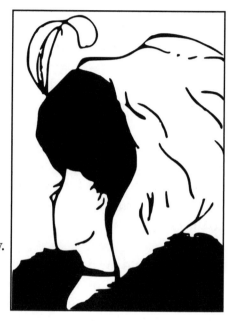

I am the old haggard woman. I have foul moods and ugly outbursts. I throw pity parties no one attends. I am also the beautiful young woman filled with confidence and joy. I am both crazy and sane. I am ahead and behind. I'm doing it right and messing it up. Yep. All true stories.

Regardless of what you see at first glance, you have the ability to shift focus. No circumstance is intrinsically good or bad. Every situation offers advantages and disadvantages. Victims and survivors face the same challenges. Look at yourself and your life. What do you see at first glance? What other possibilities can be seen from a different angle?

I am not happy or healthy all of the time. I know that chronic stress is a disorder of thought. Yet overwhelming responsibility is not a figment of the imagination. I will not renounce my children or let my home fall apart. My own needs do not negate my commitments. Life has a rhythm of two steps forward, one step back. Bad days are part of the Cha-Cha. Life is a dance.

Do you have an inner badass? Is there a version of you that exists in an alternate universe? We all have secret dreams and desires. What would you do if you could do anything? The realization that you are free may be more terrifying than exhilarating. If the chains that bind you are imaginary, you've been stuck for some reason. And that reason will have to be dealt with. Your inner badass has some work to do.

Are you ready for a better life? If shitty food and avoidable disorders are holding you back, why are you indulging them? Maybe you can't do what you want today, but what about tomorrow? Or next year? Feel the yearnings in your soul. Passions are not delusions; they are divine inspiration. Why are you here? What were you meant to do? Are your actions laying the foundation to fulfill your life's purpose?

Daring to be different takes a lot of courage. You are leaving the illusions of bondage and accepting the invitation to live in freedom. It may feel as though others are to blame for your circumstances. But this is true only if you want it to be. The permission to move forward can only come from you. Don't feel guilty and don't blame others for your current state of being. Unlock your chains, stand up and walk out of the cave into the sunlight. This will require you to leave fellow prisoners behind. Leave the guilt behind as well. Freedom is available to everyone willing to act on the invitation.

There is no shortage of love, money or time. Love comes from within and money can be made. There are 24 hours in every day regardless of who you are. Many of us think that sacrificing our own happiness will provide happiness for someone we love. Noble endeavors don't work that way. You feel happy when you make a worthy sacrifice. If you are not happy, the surrender is in vain. The ripple effect applies to both sadness and satisfaction. Sorrow begets sorrow. Joy begets joy.

Trusting your gut is terrifying—especially when it bloats with evidence that you're doing something wrong. Respecting the body and taking care of one's self is hard work. But investing in health and happiness is far more rewarding than the inevitable pain of neglecting to do so. Why do we exchange our potential for a piece of cake or bag of chips? Why do we accept the heaviness of weakness when strength is so invigorating? It may seem easier to be unhappy than to be radiant. That's a lie you must stop believing. Feeling awesome is not the norm. But the norm isn't healthy. Leave it behind.

You now know the truth. Packaged products are filled with chemicals. Food addictions make us fat and sick. Our kids are being poisoned. Conventional farming is destroying the environment as well as our health. Symptom suppressants ignore inflammation and perpetuate disorder. Disease is the result of malnourishment, not a lack of medication. These facts affect us all.

But fate is flexible. There is an option to "opt out" of the insanity. Will you take it? Are you willing to clean out your mind and your body? Illness is created with food and marinated in the brain. Disease and disorders can be reversed —not with drugs that cause more dysfunction, but with foods that nourish and heal. Our thoughts limit or empower us—we can choose to be a victim or a survivor.

Wellness is not a blessing. It is a way of life that requires effort. You will be healthier the moment you decide to act healthy. Your internal attitude will manifest in time. Examine all of the labels in your life. Look beyond food and products. Ingrained beliefs about who you are and what you are capable of are labels that must also be removed. Take notice of everything that goes into your body and comes out of your mouth. Is your brand of health and happiness what you want? If not, what needs to change? Remember that God works through you, not for you. Take responsibility for yourself. Act today how you want to feel tomorrow. Have faith in yourself. You can do this.

Whatever you decide, there is no right or wrong. There is what you do, what you don't do and how that works out.

> "You have *brains* in your head. You have *feet* in your shoes. You can steer yourself *any direction* you choose. You're on your own. And you know *what you know*. And YOU are the one who'll decide where to go."
>
> Dr. Suess, *Oh the Places You'll Go*

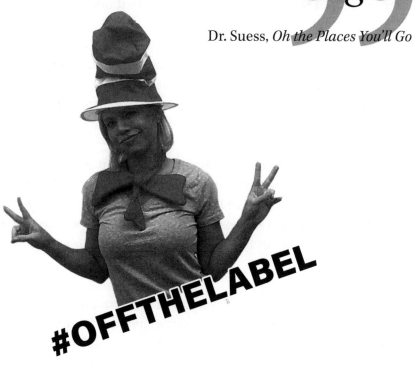

Life off the Label

Response-Ability

If truth isn't negotiable, what assumptions are holding you back? Willpower won't foster lasting change until negative beliefs are exposed and challenged.

Identify the truths of your life. Title a new journal, "My Life As It Is." Inventory the following starting points. Leave a few pages between each to allow room to journal.

- I am (your weight) pounds. My feelings about my body are . . .
- I take (list of medications, both daily and occasional).
- Throughout the year, I suffer (list specific symptoms, frequency and intensity of symptoms and illnesses).
- I consume (list specific fast and processed foods) when (frequency and location)
- I am stressed out by (routines, situations, obligations, limitations).
- I do (list specific activities, routines and habits that are unhealthy and/or stressful).
- I do not (list specific activities, routines and habits that would be beneficial to you).

After each answer, write the word "Why." This will expose the thoughts and stories that create your life as it is. Note only the first thoughts that come to mind. Do not over-analyze or take a lot of time. (For example, I take antacids several days a week. Why? Because spicy foods and stress give me heartburn.)

Tackle each "Why" on a new page with the Downward Arrow Technique. This may take days, weeks or a lifetime. Identify the story or thought. (Spicy foods and stress give me heartburn.) Ask, "If this is true, what does it mean?" (I shouldn't eat spicy foods. But I can't control the stress.) Ask again, "If this is true, what does it mean?" (I love food more than my body. Stress is not my fault.) Ask again. (I prefer instant gratification to long-term wellness. I am reactive to problems, not proactive with solutions.) Ask again. (I don't want to take responsibility for my life.) Ask again. (I'm afraid of ridicule and failure.)

You will probably discover that many "Why" beliefs reduce to the same subconscious fears. But identifying the fear is much easier than letting go of it. Fear may seem to protect us. In truth, fear is a prompt—a call to action. Analyze each fear with three questions. 1) How has this fear served me? 2) What has this fear cost me? 3) What is my call to action?

Fear is overcome when you accept response-ability[2] (the ability to respond wisely regardless of fear). If you are happy with the current direction of your life, make no changes. If life could be better, make it so. Remember, you can do anything you want—if you are willing to do it.

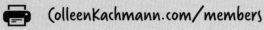

NORMAL VS HEALTHY

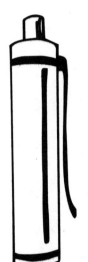

How are you different from the person who bought this book?

NORMAL

What new habits and perspectives will sustain your transformation from "normal" to "healthy?"

HEALTHY

How have misperceptions about your self and the world limited your life to this point?

NORMAL

How does it feel to be a person who believes they can accomplish anything they set their mind to?

HEALTHY

 ColleenKachmann.com/members

PS I left this facing page blank for you.
Fill it with whatever you like. Questions, comments, to-do's, thoughts, etc.
You're welcome . . .

CREATE YOUR OWN BRAND OF HEALTH AND HAPPINESS

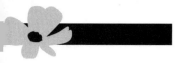

INDEX

A

acetaminophen 125, 130, 233
acid
    Acid-Forming Foods 287
    acid reflux .... 55, *See also* GERD
acne 98, 163, 195, 268, 281
activated charcoal 281
addiction 8, 9, 19–23, 26, 36, 37, 41, 64, 87, 302, 319
adipose fat 67
advertisements . 7, 10, 45, 59, 86, 110, 158, 160, 241, 264, *See also* marketing
Agent Orange 92
aging 42, 65, 67, 212, 230
alkaline 212, 299
Allegory of the Cave, The 175
Allegory of the Coin, The 13
Allegory of the Television Set, The 180
allergies . 10, 43, 56, 98, 148, 163, 175–187, 209, 210, 284
    allergic reactions 69, 71, 124, 127, 178, 184, 185
    allergy medications 189, 210
    allergy symptoms 163, 177, 179
    healing 188, 209
all natural 7, 70, 72, 74, 142, 148, 282
Ally 32
aluminum 59, 62, 278
    aluminum free deodorant 280
Alzheimer's 65, 68, 101, 278
Ambien 246
American Cancer Society 82, 94
American Heart Association 70, 79
anger 163, 205, 314–315
antibacterial soaps 114, 285
antibiotics 114, 116, 122, 126, 127, 130, 139, 146, 151, 159, 167, 189, 347
anti-fungal medications 43
anti-inflammatory 116, 122, 125, 299
    medications 116, 124, 200
    processes 186
    properties 177, 201
antioxidants 10, 48, 71, 186, 228, 234, 301
antiperspirants .... 276–280, 285, *See also* deodorant
anxiety .. 10, 43, 65, 71, 163, 185, 193, 195, 205, 299
appetite .... 22, 23, 31, 41, 45, 66, 300, *See also* cravings
artificial
    colors 68, 71, 146
    ingredients. 8, 21, 47, 55, 57, 68, 70, 72, 80, 179, 188, 300
    sweeteners 26, 31–38, 212, 287
aspartame 32, 36, 72, 212
aspirin 125, 126, 234
asthma 6, 10, 56, 71, 99, 125, 126, 163, 174–187, 209, 210, 284
    attacks 179
    symptoms 125, 177–178
Attention Deficit Hyperactivity Disorder (ADHD) 43, 56, 195
Au Bon Pain 153
autism 56, 101
autoimmune, *See* disease
    disorders 99, 122, 195, 196
    response 43, 59, 200

B

bacteria 49
    beneficial .... 103, 112, 126, 130, 134, 219–220, *See also* microflora
baking soda 14, 142, 270, 274–275, 278–279
bananas 25, 140, 257, 294
Barnouin, Kim 35
bean burger 229
bees 96, 97
    beeswax 279–280
    colony collapse disorder 97
beneficial bacteria, *See* microflora
bentonite clay 58, 188, 279, 281

BGH (Bovine Growth Hormone)........... 90
BHA...................................... 69
BHT...................................... 69
Big Food. 8, 9, 19, 22, 23, 67, 79, 90, 92, 146, 313
Big Pharma................... 8, 59, 92, 313
Big Tobacco 8, 9, 23, 67, 71, 79, 82, 87
bioengineering.......................... 119
biotechnology 88
biotin................................... 126
birth control........................... 201
bloating ...43, 134, 163, 185, 195–197, 212, 319
bloodletting 27
blood pressure...........67, 209, 211, 299, *See also* hypertension
    medications....................... 189
blood sugar...23–24, 26, 41, 51, 57, 64, 66, 211, 271, 281
BPA (bisphenol A) 73, 284
brain
    chemistry.......................67, 216
    fog................. 43, 55, 163, 196, 197
BRCA gene 117
British government 71
Brown & Williamson..................... 87
Bt protein 96
bullies........................ 11, 256, 306
Butylated Hydroxyanisole and Hydroxytoluene 69

C

caffeine........................... 27, 37, 159
CAFOs, *See* concentrated animal feeding operations
calcium.............49, 124, 158–160, 164, 212
Canada...............................94, 96
    Health "Gaps Analysis" 95
cancer... 10, 36, 40, 49, 67–71, 87, 94, 103, 160, 209, 210, 227, 276, 283, 284, 287
    breast.............. 94, 117, 220, 276, 277
    colorectal 68
    lung..................... 82, 87, 94, 236
    pancreatic 68, 234
    prostate............................. 94
candy.........................67, 98, 241, 258
capitalism 81, 82
carbohydrates 15, 23–25, 47, 48
carotenoids.............................. 49
casein 161, 165, 168
cashew cream 15, 50, 75, 166, 169, 237, 303
cast-iron............................221, 297
CDC (Centers for Disease Control) ..59, 62, 63
celiac, *See* disease
Certified Organic 142, 144–147
chickenpox vaccination 131
chickens....................... 140, 213, 220
Chipotle 153
chiropractic medicine............... 195–198
cholesterol 68, 101, 116, 117, 127, 209, 211, 218
cigarettes............... 21, 33, 80, 82–88, 177
Cochrane Collaboration................... 62
coconut oil 263, 270–273, 279, 280
colony collapse disorder, *See* bees
commercials...............132, 158, 182, 241
commodities 158, 213
concentrated animal feeding operations (CAFOs) 167, 212
congestion............. 57, 129, 146, 163, 287
consumerism . 6–7, 102, 111, 146, 264, 275, 296
conventional agriculture97, 140, 141–143, 146, 167, 281
cooking... 25, 237, 250, 251, 252, 254, 293, 295, 297, 300
cosmetics....................... 69, 282, 284
cows 93, 94, 140, 165, 167, 212, 219
cravings .. 8, 20, 23, 26, 31, 41–45, 64, 140, 146, 200, 201, 231, 299, 302, *See also* appetite

D

dairy ... 9, 90, 129, 139, 157–169, 158, 162, 179, 184, 188
    industry.................... 90, 158, 167
    intolerance.......................9, 168
    sensitivities 163, 178, 188, 201
deodorants .... 114, 273, 276, 285, *See*

also aluminum free deororant
depression.... 10, 43, 55, 65, 193, 195, 230, 299
dermatitis 120, 284, 285
detoxification. 40, 44, 57, 58, 130, 270, 278, 279, 281, 287, 300, 312
diabesity................................. 21
diabetes . 10, 21, 23, 31, 56, 67, 68, 70, 116, 124, 209, 211, 218, 241
diet
    industry...........................19, 31
    soda 31, 36, 37, 72
digestion 40, 41, 47, 98, 123, 126, 184, 188, 193–195
digestion (con't)
    digestive system 10, 49, 162, 163, 178, 189, 198, 218
disease 56, 68, 74
    autoimmune.............43, 59, 122, 209
    celiac 6, 56, 74, 195, 253, 334
    Lou Gehrig's.......................65, 278
    Parkinson's........................65, 68
    prostate............................. 68
divorce 198–200, 217, 316
DIY...................... 265–266, 300, 307
DNA. 9, 48, 59, 68, 88, 89, 96, 103, 117, 125, 227, 278, 283, 301
doctors.............................. 43, 62, 86, 114, 130, 132, 158, 167, 182, 183, 195, 197, 210, 216, 220, 230, 232, 247
Downward Arrow Technique.............321
DPT vaccination.........................61
dressings 50, 67, 75, 123, 227, 256
drugs....114–117, 120, 122, 167, 177, 188, 210, 233, 287, 312, 314
    over-the-counter (OTC) 124–126, 189
    prescription..116, 122, 125–126, 189, 198, 211, 246

E

ear
    infections 128–130, 163, 272
eczema......... 43, 98, 163, 195, 279, 281, 285
electrolytes 49, 212, 299
emotions 10, 45, 71, 163, 193, 194, 199, 200, 203, 205, 265, 314, 315
Environmental Protection Agency (EPA)...97, 277, 283
Environmental Working Group (EWG) ...285
ephedrine 32
erectile dysfunction................. 116, 117
essential oils..................... 270, 272, 279
European Commission.................... 97
European Union 71, 94
EVOS....................................153
exercise..19, 40, 71, 115, 116, 171, 199, 227, 287

F

factory farmed.................... 93, 140, 141
fast food..........21, 69, 70, 74, 153, 241, 284
fat........7, 39, 44, 48, 57, 64–69, 140, 164, 179
    cells 8, 26, 44, 57, 114, 212, 300
    fat-free foods....................5, 26, 32
    trans fat.................68–70, 142, 179
fatty acids 127, 201, 279, 287
fiber.....................48, 66, 70, 211, 218
fibromyalgia.........................43, 196
fish................................ 151, 212
flavonoids 49
flu
    flu shot 59, 62, 109, 110, 111
    symptoms...................... 115, 125
fluoride.................................271
folate.................................... 58
folic acid...........................58, 124
food
    "food fights"................. 10, 44, 245
    intolerances........... 184, 194–195, 201
    labels 90, 99, 100, 118, 142, 282
    safety 70, 88–103
Food and Drug Administration (FDA) . 57, 63, 68, 71, 72, 89, 92–96, 103, 129, 142, 167, 277, 282
formaldehyde.......................36, 285
fortified food ... 10, 49, 118, 166, 211, 216, 230

fragrance ... 265, 275, 284
frankenseeds ... 88
Frank Statement ... 86
free radicals ... 10, 48, 125, 227, 228, 234, 281
fructose ... 22, 66–67, 115
fungicide ... 100

G

Gardasil ... 60
garlic ... 58, 115, 129, 130, 268
gastro-esophageal reflux disease (GERD) 124, 195
gastro-intestinal ... 124, 163
generally recognized as safe ... 68
genes ... 89, 114, 117, *See also* DNA
    gene expression ... 117, 278
Genetically Modified Organisms (GMOs) 9, 68, 88, 90–103, 146, 179
    corn ... 96, 101, 139, 212
    crops ... 88–90, 99–103
    soy ... 97, 98, 101, 220
genetics ... 71, 117, 183, 231
global warming ... 140
glucose ... 66, 226, *See also* blood sugar
glutathione ... 125
gluten ... 165
    gluten free diet ... 179, 249, 253
    sensitivity ... 253
glycemic index ... 23–25, 70
Glyphosate ... 101, 103
greenhouse gases ... 140
growth hormones 72, 90, 93, 139, 146, 167, 211, 213
Guillain-Barré syndrome ... 110
gut ... 67, 96, 103, 319
    dysfunction ... 195
    flora ... 42, 49, 112, 126, 134, 178, 201, 218

H

H1N1 virus ... 62, 109–110
Haiti ... 99, 100
hand sanitizer ... 114
Happy Cow ... 153
Harvard School of Public Health, The ... 68, 70, 160
healthcare ... 19, 80, 132, 150, 232
Heart-Check Meal Certification ... 70
heart disease ... 10, 23, 70, 82, 99, 124, 209, 230, 241, 283
heavy metals ... 166, 228
hepatitis C ... 103
herbicides ... 89, 98, 103
high fructose corn syrup (HFCS) ... 22, 66, 67, 146, 179
histamines ... 125
HIV ... 103
homemade deodorant ... 263, 279
homemade dishwasher detergent ... 267
homemade laundry detergent ... 264, 267
hormone
    dysfunction 69, 73, 103, 114, 212, 283–285
    imbalance ... 43
hydrogen peroxide ... 115, 142, 268
hypertension ... 124, *See also* blood pressure

I

IGF-1 (Insulin-like Growth Factor) ... 94
immune system ... 42, 47, 89, 112, 122, 125–127, 127, 178, 186, 196, 281, 285, 287
    dysfunction, *See* autoimmune disorders
immunity ... 112, 115
indigestion ... 200
indoor plants ... 188
inflammation 9, 10, 42, 43, 55, 67, 120, 122, 126, 176, 177, 178, 179, 186, 198, 200
inflammatory bowel disease (IBD) ... 6, 56, 101, 284
influenza pandemic ... 110, *See also* H1N1 pandemic
insecticide ... 96
Insect Repellent ... 271
insulin ... 22–24, 57, 64, 66, 199

integrative medicine 253
       doctors 300
iodine 221
iron 214–215, 221
irritable bowel syndrome (IBS) 55, 195

J

Jason's Deli 153
Journal of Orthomolecular Medicine (JOM),
       The 231–232
juicing.................................. 46

K

kale chips.............................. 259
kidneys 58, 69, 96, 115–116, 124, 210, 212
       stones 165, 212
Kraft 79–80

L

LabDoor.......................... 134, 234
labels... 65, 67, 71, 86, 90, 93, 99, 100, 104, 118,
       142–145, 147, 164, 282, 319
       label law 102
Labels 147
lactose 161, 165, 168
leaky gut............. 126, 194–196, 200–201
Lemonade 153
lemon(s)............... 58, 64, 115, 201, 299
leukemia 285
lignins.................................. 49
liver 58, 69, 96, 116, 125, 130, 299
livestock...................... 140, 141, 213
lobbying 19, 59, 67, 68, 102, 146
lobotomies 27
lunch meat 70, 72
       processed meat 212, 283
Lyfe Kitchen 153
lymph

nodes 115, 129
system 40, 287

M

mac & cheese........................... 169
macronutrients....................... 47, 48
Marine Stewardship Counsel (MSC) 151
marketing ... 70, 168, *See also* advertisements
McDonalds 21, 70, 143
medication 9,
       10, 114, 120, 125, 132, 134, 166, 175, 176,
       179, 183, 184, 200, 209, 210, 233
Medline 231
mercury (thimerosal) 59, 62, 151, 166
metabolism.......... 39, 41, 124, 227, 232, 299
microflora 42, 49, 115, 126, 134, 219, 283
micronutrients ... 8, 10, 39, 46, 47, 48, 66, 178,
       188, 211–212, 214, 301
microwave..................... 49, 300, 301
migraines.................... 36, 65, 71, 163
minerals.................... 49, 142, 159, 230
miso....................... 75, 121, 123, 134
Monosodium Glutamate (MSG) 64–65, 68, 74,
       98, 142, 146, 179
Monsanto 89, 90, 92, 93, 97, 99, 102, 103
       Protection Act 102
mucosa................................ 201
mucous.................... 196, 204, 283, 287
mucus.............................. 57, 129
mullein (clove) oil....................... 129
Murray, Tomas.......................... 160

N

Nabisco................................. 79
National Vaccine Injury Compensation Pro-
       gram....................... 59, 61
neonicotinoids 96, 97
Neti Pot............................... 115
neurochemicals........................ 314
neurological

damage 166
disorders 69, 209, 277, 283
problems 36, 110, 116
neurotoxin 36, 59, 65, 278
niacin 231
nicotine 21, 23, 34, 87, 159
NIH (The United States National Institute of Health) 232
Ninja, The 294
nitrates 68, 72, 142, 179
nitrosamines 283
Non-GMO certified 68
non-steroidal anti-inflammatory drugs (NSAIDs) 125–126, 130, 189, 201
Noodles and Company 153
No-Poo Do, The 273, 275
NSAIDs, *See* non-steroidal anti-inflammatory drugs (NSAIDs)
nutritional deficiencies .10, 179, 196, 210, 216, 230–231

O

Obama, Barack, *See* President Obama
obesity .. 5, 21, 23, 65–67, 79–80, 179, 241, 283
obstacle opinions 302
oil pulling 270
Olestra 32
olfactory nerve 265
omega-3 fatty acids 151, 201
oregano oil 115, 254
organic
brands 147, 152–153
certification 142–145
dairy 93, 146, 166
farms 146
food 9, 75, 139, 142–146, 150, 294–295
orthomolecular medicine 230, 231
osteoarthritis 124
osteoporosis 124, 159–160, 165, 210
oxidative stress 227, 228

P

pain 116, 120–122, 124–133, 159, 186, 202, 312, 314
Panera Bread 153
parabens 277, 283
Parable of Responsibility, The 259
Parkinson's, *See* disease
pathogens 112, 115, 117, 122, 126, 134, 159
PCBs 92–93, 151, 283
pesticides 88, 99, 140, 143, 146
pharmaceutical ...... 59, *See also* Big Pharma
industry 231
pollution 233
Philip Morris 79, 82
Phoenix Organics 144, 145
phthalates 284
physicians, *See* doctors
phytonutrients 49, 211, 220
pigs 140, 213
plant-based diet ...10, 170, 209–210, 214–216, 221
plant milks 166–167
plants 48–49, 166, 188, 211, 226, 228
plastic 72–73, 188, 284, 301
PVC (polyvinylchloride) 284
poly and perfluoroalkyl substances (PFAS) 284
polysorbates 283
prebiotics 130, 134
premenstrual symptoms 140
President Obama 90
probiotics .. 44, 58, 115, 130, 134, 201, 219, 221
processed food .. 6, 11, 21, 22, 42, 44, 48, 64, 68, 71, 117, 200, 201
profits 6, 55, 67, 68, 79, 133, 146, 168, 176
promoter genes 89
propaganda 10, 102, 218
propylene glycol 285
protein 21, 47–48, 164, 229
animal 159
dairy 161, 165
plant 166, 214, 218
supplements 98, 165

psoriasis 43, 195, 281
puberty 139

Q

Quick, Bill 145

R

radioactive drinks 27
rBST 93, 94
Recommended Dietary Allowances (RDA) 230
restaurants 69, 74, 153
rotation diet 188
rotavirus 60
Roundup 98, 101, 103

S

salad dressing, *See* dressings
sauerkraut 307
Searchlights on Health 82
seasonings & dips 75
shampoo 188, 273, 283, 285
shea butter 279
shopping 14, 263, 295
side effects 116, 119, 120, 125, 133, 188, 210, 231, 235
skin . . . 43, 69, 149, 162, 177, 182, 195, 270, 278, 282, 283
Skinny Bitch 35
slavery 27
sleep 115-116, 116, 179, 304
SmartFresh 143
smoking 21, 33, 82-87, 94, 179
social eating 306
soda pop 31, 34, 67, 159, 212
Sodium and/or Ammonium Laureth Sulfate (SLS, ALS, SLES) 283
soy 68, 97-98, 101, 220
sprouts 307

statins 116, 189, 211
steroids 122, 124, 201
stress . . 10, 71, 117, 179, 184, 193, 194, 198, 199, 200, 202, 205, 216, 219, 227
subsidies 67, 143-146, 158
Subway 21, 70
sucrose 66
sugar . 7, 22-23, 26-27, 31, 42, 66, 115, 160, 179, 199, 226-227, 287
 alcohols 32, 51
sunscreen 149
supplement(s) . . 58, 98, 130, 134, 165, 188, 201, 211, 221, 230-234
Surgeon General 79, 86
sustainably grown 143, 144
sweat 115, 276-280
 glands 278
swine flu . . . . 109, 110, *See also* H1N1
synergistic effects 9, 57, 71, 72
synthetic fragrance and colors . . . . 284, *See also* fragrance

T

tapeworms 27
Taylor, Michael 89, 90, 91, 157
terminator genes 88
texturized vegetable protein (TVP) 74
thimersol, *See* mercury
threshold of toxicity 56, 62-65, 72, 90
thyroid 6, 43, 189, 271
 function 73, 114, 285
 medication 159
tobacco industry, *See* Big Tobacco
Tobacco Industry Research Committee (TIRC) 86
toothpaste 270-271, 285
trace minerals 49, 281
trans fats 68, 142, 179
triclosan 114, 285
turkey 140
TVP, *See* texturized vegetable protein (TVP)

U

United Nations Food and Agricultural Organization (FAO) 213
United States Department of Agriculture (USDA) 26, 143, 145, 157, 158, 160
    USDA Certified Organic 142–145
urinary tract infections...................212

V

vaccines 58–65, 72, 110, 111, 116, 133
vegan.. 10, 74, 170, 210, 214, 218–219, 221, 231
    diet 161, 210, 248
vegetables 210, 211, 218, 225, 236, 237, 296
    benefits.. 10, 115, 134, 188, 211–212, 228, 236, 287
    consumption................170–171, 210
    cruciferous................14, 58, 130, 171
    glaze..............................227
    nutrient absorption 164, 184, 219
    preparation ... 15, 227, 237, 256, 295–296
vitamin(s) . 48, 58, 115, 188, 211, 221, 230, 231, 232, 233, 234, 287
    A 49, 165–166, 279
    B................... 49, 127, 165, 216, 231
    B_6..............................58, 124
    B_{12}....................58, 124, 221, 281
    C 49, 58, 165, 215, 231, 287
    D 49, 124, 151, 158, 166, 186, 216, 221, 231
    E........ 49, 58, 98, 166, 186, 215, 234, 279
    K 49, 126–127, 165–166
    therapies..........................233
Vitamin Water............................27
Vitamix................................294

W

whey 161, 165
Wigand, Dr. Jeffery.......................87
withdrawal 21, 36–37

World Cancer Research Fund (WCRF), The 70

X

Y

yeast 42–43, 126, 142, 188
    infection 43
    nutritional yeast flakes 50, 169, 227
    overgrowth 43–44, 115, 200, 201

Z

zinc 115, 124, 201, 231, 281

Endnotes

Chapter 1—Awareness is Freedom

1. "Nearly 7 in 10 Americans Take Prescription Drugs, Mayo Clinic, Olmsted Medical Center Find." *Mayo Clinic.* June 19, 2013. http://newsnetwork.mayoclinic.org/discussion/nearly-7-in-10-americans-take-prescription-drugs-mayo-clinic-olmsted-medical-center-find/?_ga=1.6760370.1440752329.1405534487
2. Hayes, Jeffrey. 2015. *Bought.* Bobby Sheehan Film. Working Pictures. United States.
3. Adams, Jefferson. "Celiac Disease Rates Skyrocket: Up 400% in Last 50 Years." *Celiac.com.* Celiac Disease and Gluten Intolerance Research. July 7, 2009. http://www.celiac.com/articles/21859/1/Celiac-Disease-Rates-Skyrocket-Up-400-in-Last-50-Years/Page1.html
4. Cosnes, J. Gower-Rousseau,C. Seksik, P. Cortot, A. "Epidemiology and natural history of inflammatory bowel diseases." *Gastroenterology.* May 2011; 140(6): 1785-94. http://www.ncbi.nlm.nih.gov/pubmed/21530745
5. Moss, Michael. *Salt, Sugar, Fat: How the Food Giants Hooked Us.* New York: Random House, 2013. Print.
6. "Ice cream make you happy, say Unilever Scientists." *Food Navigator.* May 4, 2005. http://www.foodnavigator.com/Science/Ice-cream-makes-you-happy-say-Unilever-scientists
7. "The Gut-Brain Connection." *Harvard Health Publications.* Harvard Medical School. http://www.health.harvard.edu/healthbeat/the-gut-brain-connection

Chapter 2—The Reality of Food Addiction

1. "Nearly 7 in 10 Americans Take Prescription Drugs, *Mayo Clinic.* Olmsted Medical Center Find." *Mayo Clinic.* June 19, 2013. http://newsnetwork.mayoclinic.org/discussion/nearly-7-in-10-americans-take-prescription-drugs-mayo-clinic-olmsted-medical-center-find/?_ga=1.6760370.1440752329.1405534487
2. Reisner, Rebecca. "The Diet Industry: A Big Fat Lie." *Bloomberg Business.* 2008.
3. Munro, Dan. "Annual U.S. Healthcare Spending Hits $3.8 Trillion." *Forbes.* February 2, 2014. http://www.forbes.com/sites/danmunro/2014/02/02/annual-u-s-healthcare-spending-hits-3-8-trillion/
4. Hyman, Mark, MD. *The Blood Sugar Solution: 10-Day Detox Diet.* New York, NY: Hachette Book Group, Inc. 2014. Page 8.
5. *Diabesity* is a registered trademark of Shape Up America! April 28, 2006.
6. Jones, Val, MD, MA. "The Diabesity Epidemic: Let's Rehabilitate America." *MedGenMed.* 2006; (8): 34.
7. http://usatoday30.usatoday.com/money/industries/food/2004-04-15-mcd-active-meals_x.htm

8. http://www.boxtopsforeducation.info
9. https://www.marketday.com
10. Hyman, Mark, MD. *The Blood Sugar Solution: 10-Day Detox Diet*. New York, NY: Hachette Book Group, Inc. 2014. Page 31.
11. Belinda Lennerz, David Alsop, Laura Holsen, Emily Stern, Rafael Rojas, Cara Ebbeling, Jill M Goldstein, and David S Ludwig "Effects of Dietary Glycemic Index on Brain Regions Related to Reward and Craving in Men." *American Journal Clinical Nutrition*. September 2013; 98: 641-647. http://ajcn.nutrition.org/content/98/3/641
12. Rettner, Rachael. "Is Sugar a Drug? Addiction Explained." *Livescience*. October 28, 2013. http://www.livescience.com/40749-addiction-drugs-sugar.html
13. Hyman, Mark, MD. *The Blood Sugar Solution: 10-Day Detox Diet*. New York, NY: Hachette Book Group, Inc. 2014. Cites: Lenoir M, Serre F, Cantin L, Ahmed SH "Intense Sweetness Surpasses Cocaine Reward." *PLoS ONE (Public Library of Science)*. 2007; 2(8): e698. http://journals.plos.org/plosone/article?id=10.1371/journal.pone.0000698

CHAPTER 3—FOOD IMPOSTERS AND FREE-FAT CALORIES

1. Guy Fagherazzi, Alice Vilier, Daniela Saes Sartorelli, Martin Lajous, Beverley Balkau, and Françoise Clavel-Chapelon "Consumption of Artificially and Sugar-Sweetened Beverages and Incident type 2 Diabetes." *The American Journal of Clinical Nutrition*. 2013; 98(10): 249-50. http://ajcn.nutrition.org/content/98/1/249.full
2. Fowler, SP. Williams, K. Resendez, RG. Hunt, KJ. Hazuda, HP. Stern, MP. "Fueling Obesity Epidemic? Artificially Sweetened Beverage Use and Long-Term Weight Gain." *Obesity (Silver Spring)*. August 2008; 16(8): 1894-900. http://www.ncbi.nlm.nih.gov/pubmed/18535548
3. Iyyaswamy, Ashok. Rathinasamy, Sheeladevi. "Effect of Chronic Exposure to Aspartame on Oxidative Stress in the Brain of Albino Rats." *Journal of Biosciences*. September 2012; 37(4): 679-688. http://www.ias.ac.in/article/fulltext/jbsc/037/04/0679-0688
4. Levitsky, D. Halbmaier, C. Mrdjenovic, G. "The freshman weight gain: a model for the study of the epidemic of obesity." *International Journal of Obesity and Related Disorders*. 2004; 28(11): 1435–1442. http://www.nature.com/ijo/journal/v28/n11/pdf/0802776a.pdf
5. Sheilds, J.W. "Central Lymph Propulsion." *Lymphology*. 1980; 13: 9-17.
6. Gustin, Mike. Ullmann, Breanna. Myers, Hadley. Chiranand, Wiriya. Lazzell, Anna. Zhao, Quiang. Vega, Luis. Lopez-Ribot, Jose. Gardner, Paul. "Inducible Defense Mechanism Against Nitric Oxide in Candida Albicans." *Eukaryotic Cell*. June 2004: 715-723. http://ec.asm.org/content/3/3/715.full.pdf
7. Gates, Donna. "The Largely Unknown Health Epidemic Affecting Almost All Americans." *Body Ecology* 2015. http://bodyecology.com/articles/unknown_health_epidemic.php

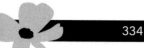

8. Vazquez-gonzalez, D. Perusiquia-Ortiz, A. Hundeiker, M. Bonifaz, A. "Opportunistic Yeast Infections: Candidiasis, Cryptococcosis, Trichosporonsis and Geotrichosis." *The Journal of German Society of Dermatology.* May 2013; 11(5): 381-93; quiz 394. http://onlinelibrary.wiley.com/doi/10.1111/ddg.12097/abstract

9. Humiston, John. "Candida Symtoms." *CandidaMD.* January 11, 2011. http://www.candidamd.com/candida/symptoms.html

Chapter 4—A Culture of Chemicals

1. Asthma Statistics." *American Academy of Allergy Asthma & Immunology.* 2015. http://www.aaaai.org/about-the-aaaai/newsroom/asthma-statistics.aspx

2. CDC's *Vital and Health Statistics.* "Summary Health Statistics for U.S. Children: National Health Interview Survey, 2012. Series 10, Number 258. http://www.cdc.gov/nchs/data/series/sr_10/sr10_258.pdf

3. CDC's *Vital and Health Statistics.* "Summary Health Statistics for U.S. Adults: National Health Interview Survey, 2012." Series 10, Number 260. http://www.cdc.gov/nchs/data/series/sr_10/sr10_260.pdf

4. SN Visser, RH Bitsko, ML Danielson, R Perou. "Increasing Prevelance of Parent-Reported Attention-Deficit/Hyperactivity Disorder Among Children—United States, 2003-2007." *MMWR.* Nov 12, 2010; 59(44); 1439-1443. http://www.cdc.gov/mmwr/preview/mmwrhtml/mm5944a3.htm

5. http://www.cdc.gov/ncbddd/autism/data.html

6. http://www.cdc.gov/nchs/data/databriefs/db10.htm

7. Adams, Jefferson. "Autoimmune Diseases on the Rise." *Celiac.com.* August 30, 2012. http://www.celiac.com/articles/23013/1/Autoimmune-Diseases-on-the-Rise/Page1.html

8. http://www.worldhealth.net/news/one_in_three_us_children_born_in_2000_wi1

9. Moynihna, Julie. Villiger, Maggie. "Do Diets Work?" *PBS.* January 13, 2004.

10. Kresser, Chris. "The little known (but crucial) difference between folate and folic acid." *Chris Kresser.com.* March 9, 2012. http://chriskresser.com/folate-vs-folic-acid

11. Green, RJ. Murphy, AS. Schulz, B. Watkins, BA. Ferruzzi, MG. "Common tea formulations modulate in vitro digestive recovery of green tea catechins." *Molecular Nutrition and Food Research.* September 2007; 51(9): 1152-62. http://www.ncbi.nlm.nih.gov/pubmed/17688297

12. "Everything Added to Food in the United States (EAFUS)." U.S. Food and Drug Administration. http://www.fda.gov/Food/IngredientsPackagingLabeling/FoodAdditivesIngredients/ucm115326.htm

13. http://articles.mercola.com/sites/articles/archive/2010/11/04/big-profits-linked-to-vaccine-mandates.aspx

14. CDC Vaccine Schedule 2014. http://www.cdc.gov/vaccines/schedules/downloads/child/0-18yrs-schedule.pdf

15. Gerber, Jeffrey. Offit, Paul. "Vaccines and Autism." A Tale of Shifting Hypothesis." *Clinical Infectious Diseases.* February 15, 2009; 48(4): 456-461. http://www.ncbi.nlm.nih.gov/pmc/articles/PMC2908388/

16. Hayes, Jeffrey. 2015. *Bought*. Bobby Sheehan Film. Working Pictures. United States.
17. Malone, Kevin. Hinman, Alan. "Vaccination Mandates: The Public Health Imperative and Individual Rights." *Centers for Disease Control*. http://www.cdc.gov/vaccines/imz-managers/guides-pubs/downloads/vacc_mandates_chptr13.pdf
18. "Nearly 400 Medicines and Vaccines in Development to Fight Infectious Diseases." *Medical News Today*. September 12, 2010. http://www.medicalnewstoday.com/articles/200689.php
19. Beckel, Michael. "U.S. Chamber Dominates Third Quarter Lobbying as Large Health, Energy Companies Also Continue to Spend Big." *OpenSecrets.org*. October 21, 2009. http://www.opensecrets.org/news/2009/10/us-chamber-dominates-third-qua/
20. Statista. "Global Vaccine Market Revenues in 2005, 2009 and 2015." http://www.statista.com/statistics/265102/revenues-in-the-global-vaccine-market/
21. Finn, Patricia. "Emergency Injunction Stop Shots Now." 9/20/2014. http://pfinnblog.weebly.com/blog/archives/07-2014
22. Courthouse News. "Court Uphold Mandatory Vaccinations in New York." *Sleuth Journal*. January 11, 2015. http://www.thesleuthjournal.com/court-upholds-mandatory-vaccinations-new-york/
23. Malone, Kevin. Hinman, Alan. "Vaccination Mandates: The Public Health Imperative and Individual Rights." *Centers for Disease Control*. http://www.cdc.gov/vaccines/imz-managers/guides-pubs/downloads/vacc_mandates_chptr13.pdf
24. Centers for Disease Control. "Notice to Readers: Updated Recommendations From the Advisory Committte on Immunization Practices in Response to Delays in Supply of Influenza Vaccine for 2000-01 Season." *MMWR*. http://www.cdc.gov/mmwr/preview/mmwrhtml/mm4939a3.htm
25. Centers for Disease Control. "CDC's Advisory Committee on Immunization Practices (ACIP) Recommends Universal Annual Influenza Vaccination." February 24, 2010. http://www.cdc.gov/media/pressrel/2010/r100224.htm
26. Jefferson, T. Rivetti, A. Di Pietrantonj C. Demicheli, V. Ferroni, E. "Vaccines for Preventing Influenza in Healthy Children." *Cochrane*. August 15, 2012. http://www.cochrane.org/CD004879/ARI_vaccines-for-preventing-influenza-in-healthy-children
27. Alber, Erwin. "Flu Shot for Pregnant Women? CDC Covers Up Influenza Vaccine-Related Fetal Deaths." *Health Impact News*. March 26, 2015. http://healthimpactnews.com/2014/press-release-cdc-covers-up-influenza-vaccine-related-fetal-deaths/
28. Shaw, Christopher. "Aluminum in the Central Nervous System (CNS): Toxicity in Humans and Animals, Vaccine Adjuvants, and Autoimmunity." *Immunologic Research*: Impact Factor: 3.53. April 2013. http://www.researchgate.net/publication/236266138_Aluminum_in_the_central_nervous_system_(CNS)_toxicity_in_humans_and_animals_vaccine_adjuvants_and_autoimmunity
29. Hernandez-Bautista, R. Alarcon-Aguilar, F. Del C Escobar-Villanueva, M. Almanza-Perez, JC. Merino-Aguilar, H. Fainstein, M. Lopez-Diazguerrero, N. "Biochemical Alterations During the Obese-Aging Process in Female and Male Monosodium Glutamate (MSG)-Treated Mice." *International Journal Molecular Science*. June 27, 2014; 15(7): 11473-94. http://www.ncbi.nlm.nih.gov/pubmed/24979131
30. Totheroh, Gailon. "You're Brain's Biggest Enemy." Three-part series *CBN News Health and Science*. http://www.cbn.com/cbnnews/107774.aspx

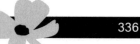

31. "Biochemical Alterations During the Obese-Aging Process in Female and Male Monosodium Glutamate (MSG)-Treated Mice. *International Journal Molecular Science.* 2014 Jun 27; 15(7): 11473-94. http://www.ncbi.nlm.nih.gov/pubmed/24979131
32. Baylock, Russell. *Excitotoxins: The Taste That Kills.* Albuquerque, NM. Health Press NA Inc., 1997.
33. Totheroh, Gailon. "You're Brain's Biggest Enemy." Three-part series *CBN News Health and Science.* http://www.cbn.com/cbnnews/107774.aspx
34. Mercola. "Startling New Evidence: Too Much Soda Consumption Causes Your Neurons to Stagnate for 20 Minutes." *Mercola.com.* http://articles.mercola.com/sites/articles/archive/2011/02/28/new-study-confirms-fructose-affects-your-brain-very-differently-than-glucose.aspx
35. Levi, Boaz. Werman, Moshe. "Long-Term Fructose Consumption Accelerates Glycation and Several Age-Related Variable in Male Rats." *The Journal of Nutrition.* Sept 1, 1998; 128(9): 1442-1449. http://jn.nutrition.org/content/128/9/1442.full
36. http://drhyman.com/blog/2011/05/13/5-reasons-high-fructose-corn-syrup-will-kill-you/
37. Kershaw EE, Flier JS; Flier. "Adipose tissue as an endocrine organ." *Journal of Clinical Endocrinology & Metabolism.* 2004; 89(6): 2548–56. http://www.ncbi.nlm.nih.gov/pubmed/15181022
38. Fields, Scott. "The Fat of the Land: Do Agricultural Subsidies Foster Poor Health?" *Environmental Health Perspectives.* October 2004; 112(14): A820-A823. http://www.ncbi.nlm.nih.gov/pmc/articles/PMC1247588/
39. Hyman, Mark, MD. *The Blood Sugar Solution: 10-Day Detox Diet.* New York, NY: Hachette Book Group, Inc. 2014. Cites: Lenoir M, Serre F, Cantin L, Ahmed SH (2007) "Intense Sweetness Surpasses Cocaine Reward." *PLoS ONE* 2(8): e698. http://journals.plos.org/plosone/article?id=10.1371/journal.pone.0000698
40. Warshaw, Hope. "High-fructose Corn Syrup." *The Washington Post.* June 18, 2013. http://www.washingtonpost.com/lifestyle/wellness/high-fructose-corn-syrup-vs-sugar/2013/06/18/fdbedb90-c488-11e2-914f-a7aba60512a7_story.html
41. Nothilings, Ute. Wilkens, Lynne. Murphy, Suzanne. Hankin, Jean. Henderson, Brian. Kolonel, Laurence. "Meat and Fat Intake as Risk Factors for Pancreatic Cancer: The Multiethnic Cohort Study." *Journal of the National Cancer Institute.* October 5, 2005; 97 (19). http://jnci.oxfordjournals.org/content/97/19/1458.full.pdf
42. Micha, Renata. Wallace, Sarah. Mozzaffarian, Dariush. "Red and Processed Meat Consumption and Risk of Incident Coronary Heart Disease, Stroke, and Diabetes Mellitus: A Systematic Review and Meta-Analysis." *Circulation*, online May 17, 2010. http://www.hsph.harvard.edu/news/press-releases/processed-meats-unprocessed-heart-disease-diabetes/
43. "Our Cancer Prevention Recommendations." *World Cancer Research Fund.* http://www.wcrf.org/int/research-we-fund/cancer-prevention-recommendations/animal-foods
44. Lesser, Lenard. Kayekjian, K. Velasquez, P. Chi-Hong, T. Brook, R. Cohen, D. "Adolescent Purchasing Behavior at McDonald's and Subway." *Journal of Adolescent Health.* October 2013; 53(4): 441-445. http://www.jahonline.org/article/S1054-139X(13)00119-5/abstract
45. "SUBWAY® Restaurants Become First in the Industry to Meet and Receive the American Heart Associations Heart-Check Meal Certification." Press Release from Subway Franchise

World Headquarters, 2012. http://newsroom.heart.org/news/american-heart-association-s-new-234696

46. "Shining the Spotlight on Trans Fats." *Harvard School of Public Health.* http://www.hsph.harvard.edu/nutritionsource/transfats/

47. Sebedio, Jean Louis. Christie, William. "Metabolism and Physiological Effects of Trans Monounsaturated Fatty Acids from Partially Hydrogenated Vegetable Oils." *The AOCS Lipid Library* (American Oil Chemists' Society). 2009. http://lipidlibrary.aocs.org/OilsFats/content.cfm?ItemNumber=39223

48. "Butylated Hydroxyanisole. Report on Carcinogens, Thirteenth Edition." *National Toxicology Program. U.S. Department of Health and Human Services.* http://ntp.niehs.nih.gov/ntp/roc/content/profiles/butylatedhydroxyanisole.pdf - search=Butylated Hydroxyanisole

49. Toxnet, Toxicology Data Network, U.S. National Library of Medicine. HSDB: Butylated Hydroxyanisole. CASRN: 25013-16-5. Search "BHA" in Hazardous Substances Data Bank.

50. "A Summary of the Science linking Food Dyes with Impacts on Children's Behavior." *Center for Science in the Public Interest.* April 8, 2014. http://www.cspinet.org/fooddyes/Food-Dyes-Fact-Sheet.pdf

51. Kobylewski, Sarah. Jacobson, Michael. "Food Dyes: A Rainbow of Risks." *Center for Science in the Public Interest.* 2010. http://cspinet.org/new/pdf/food-dyes-rainbow-of-risks.pdf

52. "Decoding Meat + Dairy Labels." *Environmental Working Group.* http://www.ewg.org/meateatersguide/decoding-meat-dairy-product-labels/

53. Soffritti, Morando; Belpoggi, Fiorella; Esposti, Davide; Lambertini, Luca, Tibaldi; Eva; Rigano, Anna. "First Experimental Demonstration of the Multipotential Carcinogenic Effects of Aspartame Administered in the Feed to Sprague-Dawley Rats." *Environmental Health Perspectives.* March 2006; 114(3): 379-385. http://www.ncbi.nlm.nih.gov/pubmed/16507461

54. http://www.cspinet.org/reports/chemcuisine.htm

55. Pauling, Linus and Ewan Cameron. *Cancer and Vitamin C.* Philadelphia, Camino Books. 1993.

CHAPTER 5—DANGEROUS AGVENTURES

1. Gorman, John. "Philip Morris Agrees to Buy General Foods." *Chicago Tribune.* September 28, 1985. http://articles.chicagotribune.com/1985-09-28/business/8503060172_1_hamish-maxwell-philip-morris-headquarters-in-rye-brook

2. "R.J. Reynolds Makes $4.9 Billion Offer to Buy Nabisco Brands." *Los Angeles Times.* June 3, 1985. http://articles.latimes.com/1985-06-03/business/fi-5701_1_nabisco-shares

3. Sing, Bill. "Kraft to Be Sold to Philip Morris for $13.1 Billion." *Los Angeles Times.* October 31, 1988. http://articles.latimes.com/1988-10-31/news/mn-339_1_philip-morris

4. Carmona, Richard. "*The Obesity Crisis in America.*" Statement before the Subcommittee on Education Reform Committee on Education and Workforce, United States House of Representatives. July, 16, 2003. http://www.surgeongeneral.gov/news/testimony/obesity07162003.html

5. Choquet, Helene. Meyre, David. "Genetics of Obesity: What have we Learned?" *Current Genomics*. May 2011; 12(3): 169-179. http://www.ncbi.nlm.nih.gov/pmc/articles/PMC3137002/

6. Smokescam.com. "*American Heart Association*." Integrity in Science: A CSPI Project. http://www.smokescam.com/aha.htm

7. http://playbestfreeonlinegames.com/play-free-online-simpsons-adventures-game/

8. Moss, Michael. *Salt, Sugar and Fat: How the Food Giants Hooked Us*. New York, Random House. 2013.

9. Jefferis, B.G.; Nichols, J.L. Searchlights on Health. Chapter: The Destructive Effects of Cigarette Smoking. 1892. https://www.free-ebooks.net/ebook/Searchlights-on-Health

10. "A Brief History of Tobacco." *CNN.com*. http://edition.cnn.com/US/9705/tobacco/history/

11. World Health Organization *Media Centre* Tobacco. 2014. http://www.who.int/mediacentre/factsheets/fs339/en/

12. Linstrom, Andrew. "40 Gorgeous Vintage Tobacco Advertisements." *wellmedicated.com* February 11, 2009. http://wellmedicated.com/40-gorgeous-vintage-tobacco-advertisements/

13. Garrett, Bridgette. Centers for Disease Control and Prevention. Cigarette Smoking – United States 1965-2008, *Morbidity and Morality Weekly Report (MMWR)*. January 14, 2011; 60(01); 109-113. http://www.cdc.gov/mmwr/preview/mmwrhtml/su6001a24.htm - fig

14. "Tobacco Industry Records." *New York State Education Department Archives*. http://nysa32.nysed.gov/a/research/res_topics_bus_tobacco_adminctr.shtml

15. Tobacco Tactics. "Tobacco Industry Research Committee." December 21, 2012. http://www.tobaccotactics.org/index.php/Tobacco_Industry_Research_Committee

16. "Hollywood 'Paid Fortune to Smoke.'" *BBC News*. September 25, 2008. http://news.bbc.co.uk/2/hi/health/7632963.stm

17. "New Industry Atlas Estimates U.S. $35 Billion Tobacco Industry Profits and Almost 6 Million Annual Deaths." *World Lung Foundation*. March 21, 2012. http://www.worldlungfoundation.org/ht/display/ReleaseDetails/i/20439/pid/6858

18. Wilson, Duff. "Ex-Smoker Wins Against Philip Morris." *New York Times*. November 20, 2009. http://www.nytimes.com/2009/11/21/business/21smoke.html?_r=1&

19. http://en.wikipedia.org/wiki/Michael_R._Taylor *(This information is public knowledge. I cite Wikipedia as my source as it provides a one-stop-shop to reputable sources that verify the technical details. Check it out for yourself!)*

20. Hayes, Jeffrey. 2015. *Bought*. Bobby Sheehan Film. Working Pictures. United States.

21. Bassey, Nnimmo. "Global and National Resistance to GMOs." *Institute for Policy Studies*. May, 15, 2012 http://www.ips-dc.org/global_and_national_resistance_to_gmos/

22. https://www.youtube.com/watch?v=zqaaB6NE1TI

23. Schuck, Peter. *Agent Orange on Trial: Mass Toxic Disasters in the Courts*. Cambridge, Harvard University Press, 1987.

24. Bencko, Vladimir. Foong, Florence. "The History, Toxicity and Adverse Human Health and Environmental Effects Related to the Use of Agent Orange." *Environmental Security Assessment and Management of Obsolete Pesticides in Southeast Europe NATO Science for Peace and Security Series C: Environmental Security*. March 19, 2013: 119-130. http://link.springer.com/chapter/10.1007/978-94-007-6461-3_10

25. Solotaroff, Paul. "In the Belly of the Beast." Rolling Stone. December 10, 2013. http://www.rollingstone.com/feature/belly-beast-meat-factory-farms-animal-activists

26. "Study Finds Link Between Agent Orange, Cancer." *MSNBC*. January 23, 2004. *The Globe and Mail*. "Last Ghost of the Vietnam War." June 12, 2008.

27. Grunwalk, Michael. "Monsanto Hid Decades of Pollution: PCBs Drenched Ala. Town, But No One Was Ever Told." *Washington Post*. January 1, 2002. (Article archived: original text available on *CommonDreams.org*.) http://www.commondreams.org/headlines02/0101-02.htm

28. "Prosecuting American Farmers: Monsanto's Investigations, Coerced Settlements & Lawsuits." Center for Food Safety. *Mindfully.org*. January 12, 2005. http://www.mindfully.org/GE/2005/Monsanto-Prosecuting-Farmers12jan05.htm

29. Richardson, Jill. "rBGH Milk Ruled 'Compositionally Different' in Ohio." *Civil Eats*. October 1, 2010. http://civileats.com/2010/10/01/rbgh-free-claim-ruled-ok-with-no-caveats/

30. Epstein, Samuel. Cummins, Ronnie. Kinsman, John. "Petition Seeking the Withdrawal of the New Drug Application Approval for Posilac—Recombinant Bovine Growth Hormone (rBGH)." *Cancer Prevention Coalition*. February 15, 2007. http://www.preventcancer.com/publications/pdf/Petition_Posilac_feb157.pdf

31. Susan E. Hankinson and others. "Circulating concentrations of insulin-like growth factor I and risk of breast cancer." *Lancet*. May 9, 1998; 351(9113): 1393-1396. http://www.thelancet.com/journals/lancet/article/PIIS0140-6736(97)10384-1/abstract

32. June M. Chan and others, "Plasma Insulin-Like Growth Factor-I and Prostate Cancer Risk: A Prospective Study." *Science*. January 23, 1998; 279: 563-566. http://www.sciencemag.org/content/279/5350/563.full.pdf?sid=546f9420-fb2f-430c-a630-06c82fce45bc

33. Jeff Holly, "Insulin-like growth factor-I and new opportunities for cancer prevention." *Lancet*. May 9, 1998; 351(9113): 1373-1375. http://www.sciencedirect.com/science/article/pii/S0140673605794381

34. Chopra, S. Feeley, M. Lambert, G. Mueller, T. Alexander, I. "rBST (Nutrilac) "Gaps Analysis" Report." *rBST Internal Review Team*. Health Protection Branch, Health Canada. April 21, 1998. http://ucbiotech.org/biotech_info/PDFs/Chopra_rBST_Nutrilac_Gaps_Analysis_Report.pdf

35. "How Does Bt work?" University of California San Diego. *Bacillus thuringiensis*. http://www.bt.ucsd.edu/how_bt_work.html

36. Poulter, Sean. "GM Food Toxins Found in the Blood of 93% of Unborn Babies." *Daily Mail.com*. May, 20, 2011. http://www.dailymail.co.uk/health/article-1388888/GM-food-toxins-blood-93-unborn-babies.html

37. Vendomois, Joel. Roullier, Fracois. Cellier, Dominique. Seralini, Geilles-Eric. "A Comparison of the Effects of Three GM Corn Varieties on Mammalian Health." *International Journal of Biological Sciences*. 2009 5(7): 706-726. http://www.ijbs.com/v05p0706.htm

38. Official Statement provided by Joseph Cummins in Witness Brief for Royal Commission on Genetic Modification, appearing on behalf of GE Free New Zealand in Food and Environment Incorporated. http://www.gefree.org.nz/assets/pdf/joecummins.pdf

39. "About Genetically Engineered Foods." *Center for Food Safety*. http://www.centerforfoodsafety.org/issues/311/ge-foods/about-ge-foods

40. Charles, Dan. "Are Agriculture's Most Popular Insecticides Killing Our Bees?" *NPR.org*. March 25, 2013 http://www.npr.org/blogs/thesalt/2013/03/27/175278607/are-agricultures-most-popular-insecticides-killing-our-bees
41. Hayes, Jeffrey. 2015. *Bought*. Bobby Sheehan Film. Working Pictures. United States.
42. Kaplan, Kim. "Colony Collapse Disorder." United States Department of Agriculture. *Agricultural Research*. May/June 2008. http://ars.usda.gov/is/ar/archive/may08/colony0508.htm
43. Monsanto. "Company History 2007." http://www.monsanto.com/whoweare/pages/monsanto-history.aspx
44. Jolly, David. "Europe Bans Pesticides Thought Harmful to Bees." *New York Times*. April, 29, 2013. http://www.nytimes.com/2013/04/30/business/global/30iht-eubees30.html?_r=2&
45. Smith, Jeffrey. "Genetically Engineered Foods May Cause Rising Food Allergies (Part One)." *Institute for Responsible Technology*. May 7, 2007. http://responsibletechnology.org/genetically-engineered-foods-may-cause-rising-food-allergies-part-one/
46. Smith, Jeffrey. "Genetically Engineered Foods May Cause Rising Food Allergies (Part Two)." *Institute for Responsible Technology*. June 15, 2007. http://responsibletechnology.org/genetically-engineered-foods-may-cause-rising-food-allergies-part-two/
47. "Superweeds: How Biotech Crops Bolster the Pesticide Industry." *Food and Water Watch*. July 1, 2013. https://www.foodandwaterwatch.org/sites/default/files/Superweeds%20Report%20July%202013.pdf
48. Gurian-Sherman, Doug. "Failure to Yield: Evaluating the Performance of Genetically Engineered Crops." *Union of Concerned Scientists*. 2009. http://www.ucsusa.org/sites/default/files/legacy/assets/documents/food_and_agriculture/failure-to-yield.pdf
49. Fagen, John. Antoniou, Michael. Robinson, Claire. "GMO Myths and Truth 2nd Edition." *Earth Open Source*. Great Britain, 2014. http://earthopensource.org/earth-open-source-reports/gmo-myths-and-truths-2nd-edition/
50. Dean, Amy. Armstrong, Jennifer. "Genetically Modified Foods." *American Academy of Environmental Medicine*. May 8, 2009. https://www.aaemonline.org/gmo.php
51. Carman, Judy. Villager, H. Ver Steeg, L. Sneller, V. Robinson, G. Clinch-Jones, K. Haynes, J. Edwards, J. "A Long-Term Toxicology Study on Pigs Fed a Combined Genetically Modified (GM) Soy and GM Corn Maize Diet." June, 11, 2013. http://gmojudycarman.org/relevant-research/
52. The Marshall Protocol Knowledge Base, Autoimmune Research Foundation. "Incidence and Prevalence of Chronic Disease." 2012. http://mpkb.org/home/pathogenesis/epidemiology
53. "GMO Facts." *The Non-GMO Project*. http://www.nongmoproject.org/learn-more
54. Monsanto. "Monsanto Donates Corn and Vegetable Seeds to Haiti." *Improving Agriculture*. January 12, 2010. http://www.monsanto.com/improvingagriculture/pages/haiti-seed-donation.aspx
55. "GMO Seed Refused in Haiti." *Haitain-Truth.Org*. June 25, 2010. http://www.commondreams.org/headlines02/0101-02.htm

56. Swanson, N. Leu, A. Abrahamson, J. Wallet, B. "Genetically Engineered Crops, Glyphosate and the Deterioration of Health in the United States of America." Journal of Organic Systems. 2014; 9(2): 6-37. http://www.organic-systems.org/journal/92/JOS_Volume-9_Number-2_Nov_2014-Swanson-et-al.pdf
57. "Initiative to the Legislature 522 Concerns Labeling of Genetically Engineered Food." Washington State General Election Results. *Office of the Secretary of State*. November 26, 2013. http://results.vote.wa.gov/results/20131105/State-Measures-Initiative-to-the-Legislature-522-Concerns-labeling-of-genetically-engineered-foods.html
58. "Prop 37 Opponents Spending Millions to Oppose Label Law." *Huffington Post*. October 26, 2012. http://www.huffingtonpost.com/2012/10/26/prop-37-opponents_n_2023719.html
59. Goldenberg, Suzanne. "Vermont becomes first US state to require GM labeling for food." *The Guardian*. May, 8, 2014. http://www.theguardian.com/environment/2014/may/08/vermont-first-us-state-gm-labelling-food
60. "Consolidated and Further Continuing Appropriations Act, 2013." March 22, 2013. The 113th Congress of the United States of America. https://www.govtrack.us/congress/bills/113/hr933/text
61. FDA, "Statement of Policy: Foods Derived from New Plant Varieties" (GMO Policy). *Federal Register*. 1992; 57(104): 220. http://www.fda.gov/Food/GuidanceRegulation/GuidanceDocumentsRegulatoryInformation/Biotechnology/ucm096095.htm

Chapter 6—Prescriptions for Pain

1. Barry, John. *The Great Influenza: The Epic Story of the Deadliest Plague in History*. London: Penguin Books, 2004.
2. Racaniello, Vincent. "Swine Flue at Fort Dix." *Virology Blog*. March 16, 2009. http://www.virology.ws/2009/03/16/swine-flu-at-fort-dix/
3. Mike Wallace. "The Swine Flu Fraud of 1976." *60 Minutes*. https://www.youtube.com/watch?v=8elE7Ct1jWw - t=20
4. Mercola. *"Triclosan: The Soap Ingredient You Should Never Use – But 75% of Households Do."* August 29, 2012. http://articles.mercola.com/sites/articles/archive/2012/08/29/triclosan-in-personal-care-products.aspx
5. Aiello, AE. Larson, EL. Levy, SB. "Consumer Antibacterial soaps: Effective or Just Risky?" *Clinical Infectious Diseases*. September 1 2007; 45(2):S137-47. http://www.ncbi.nlm.nih.gov/pubmed/17683018
6. Shields, J.W. "Central Lymph Propulsion." *Lymphology*. 1980; 13: 9-17.
7. Singh, M. Das, R. "Zinc for the Common Cold." *Cochrane Database of Systematic Reviews* 2015, Issue 4. Art. No.: CD001364 http://onlinelibrary.wiley.com/doi/10.1002/14651858.CD001364.pub5/abstract
8. Ankri, S. Mirelman, D. "Antimicrobial Properties of Allicin from Garlic." *Microbial Infections*. Feb 1999; 1(2):125-9. http://www.ncbi.nlm.nih.gov/pubmed/10594976
9. Golomb, Beatrice. Evans, Marcella. "Statin Adverse Effects: A review of the Literature and Evidence for a Mitochondrial Mechanism." *American Journal of Cardiovascular Drugs. 2008*; 8(6): 373-418. http://www.ncbi.nlm.nih.gov/pmc/articles/PMC2849981/

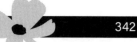

10. Bland, Jeffrey. *The Disease Delusion*. New York: Harper Collins Publishers, 2014.
11. http://www.cnn.com/video/data/2.0/video/showbiz/2013/05/14/early-pkg-jolie-turner.cnn.html
12. Bland, Jeffrey. *The Disease Delusion*. New York: Harper Collins Publishers, 2014.
13. Quigley, Delia. "10 Benefits and Uses for Miso." *Care2.com*. http://www.care2.com/greenliving/10-benefits-and-uses-for-miso.html
14. Challem, Jack. "*The Inflammation Syndrome.*" Hoboken, New Jersey: John Wiley & Sons, 2010.
15. Bancos, S. Bernard, MP. Topham, DJ. Phipps, RP. "Ibuprofen and Other Widely Used Non-Steroidal Anti-Inflammatory Drugs Inhibit Antibody Production in Human Cells." *Cellular Immunology*. 2009; 258(1): 18-28. http://www.ncbi.nlm.nih.gov/pubmed/19345936
16. Titchen, Thirza. Cranswick, Noel. Beggs, Sean. "Adverse Drug Reactions to NSAID drugs, COX-2 inhibitors and Paracetamol in Pediatric Hospital." *British Journal of Clinical Pharmacology*. June 2005; 59(6): 718-723. http://www.ncbi.nlm.nih.gov/pmc/articles/PMC1884871/
17. Bjordal, J. "NSAIDS in Osteoarthritis; Irreplaceable or Troublesome Guidelines?" *British Journal of Sports Medicine*. April 2006; 40(4): 285-286. http://www.ncbi.nlm.nih.gov/pmc/articles/PMC2577511/
18. Christensen, Stephen. "High Blood Pressure and NSAIDS." *Livestrong.com*. February 08, 2014. http://www.livestrong.com/article/1004672-high-blood-pressure-nsaids/
19. Peura, David. Goldkind, Lawrence. "Balancing the Gastrointestinal Benefits and Risks of Nonselective NSAIDS." *Arthritis Research and Therapy*. 2005; 7(4): S7-S13. http://www.biomedcentral.com/content/pdf/ar1793.pdf
20. Feenstra, Johan. Heerdink, Eibert, Grobbee, Diederick. Stricker, Bruno. "Association of Nonsteroidal Anti-Inflammatory Drugs with First Occurrence of Heart Failure and with Relapsing Heart Failure." *JAMA Internal Medicine*. February 11, 2002; 162(3). http://archinte.jamanetwork.com/article.aspx?articleid=210967 - ioi10002t3
21. Christensen, Stephen. "High Blood Pressure and NSAIDs." *Livestrong.com*. http://www.livestrong.com/article/1004672-high-blood-pressure-nsaids/
22. Henry, David. Page, John. Whyte, Ian. Nanra, Ranjit. Hall, Christopher. "Consumption of Non-Steroidal Anti-Inflammatory Drugs and the Development of Functional Renal Impairment in Elderly Subjects." *British Journal of Clinical Pharmacology*. Jul 1997; 44(1): 85-90. http://www.ncbi.nlm.nih.gov/pmc/articles/PMC2042806/
23. Salman, S. Sherif, B. Al-Zohyri, A. "Effects of Some Non Steroidial Anti-Inflammatory Drugs on Ovulation in Women with Mild Musculoskelatal Pain." Annals of the Rheumatic Diseases: The Eular Journal. 2015; 74: 117-118. http://ard.bmj.com/content/74/Suppl_2/117.3.abstract
24. "Rebound Headaches." *WebMD*. http://www.webmd.com/migraines-headaches/guide/rebound-headaches
25. Bancos, S. Bernard, MP. Topham, DJ. Phipps, RP. "Ibuprofen and Other Widely Used Non-Steroidal Anti-Inflammatory Drugs Inhibit Antibody Production in Human Cells." *Cellular Immunology*. 2009; 258(1): 18-28. http://www.ncbi.nlm.nih.gov/pubmed/19345936

26. Yamura, Katsunori. Ogawa, Kohei. Yonekawa, Taeko. Nakumura, Tomonori. Yano, Shingo. Ueno, Koichi. "Inhibition of the Antibody Production by Acetaminophen Independent of Liver Injury in Mice." *Biological and Pharmaceutical Bulletin.* 2002; 25(2): 201-205. https://www.jstage.jst.go.jp/article/bpb/25/2/25_2_201/_pdf

27. Micheli, L. Cerretani, D. Fiaschi, A. Giorgi, G. Romeo, M. Runci, F. "Effect of Acetaminophen on Glutathione Levels in Rat Testis and Lung." *Environmental Health Persective.* 1994 November; 102(9): 63-64. http://www.ncbi.nlm.nih.gov/pmc/articles/PMC1566779/

28. Farquhar, H. Stewart, A. Mitchell, E. Crane, J. Eyers, S. Weatherall, M. Beasley, R. "The Role of Paracetamol in the Pathogenisis of Asthma." *Clinical And Experimental Allergy: Journal of the British Society for Allergy and Cinical Immunology.* 2010 January 40(1): 32-41. http://www.ncbi.nlm.nih.gov/pubmed/20205695

29. Gonzalez-Barcala, Francisco. Pertega, Sonia. Castro, Theresa. Sampedro, Manuel. Lastres, Juan. Gonzalez, Miguel. Bamonde, Luciano. Garnelo, Luciano. Valdes, Luis. Carreira, Jose. Moure, Jose. Silvarrey, Angel. "Exposure to Paracetamol and Asthma Symptoms." *The European Journal of Public Health.* May 29, 2012: 706-710. http://eurpub.oxfordjournals.org/content/23/4/706

30. Gonzalez-Barcala, Francisco. Pertega, Sonia. Castro, Theresa. Sampedro, Manuel. Lastres, Juan. Gonzalez, Miguel. Bamonde, Luciano. Garnelo, Luciano. Valdes, Luis. Carreira, Jose. Moure, Jose. Silvarrey, Angel. "Exposure to Paracetamol and Asthma Symptoms." *The European Journal of Public Health.* May 29, 2012. http://eurpub.oxfordjournals.org/content/23/4/706

31. ClinicalTrials.gov Identifier: NCT00594867 "The Effects of Aspirin and Acetaminophen on the Stomach of Healthy Volunteers." *University of Illinois in Chicago.* January 4, 2008. http://clinicaltrials.gov/show/NCT00594867

32. University of Texas at Austin. "Mouth bacteria can change it's diet." *mBio, American Society for Microbiology.* August 12, 2014. http://medicalxpress.com/news/2014-08-mouth-bacteria-diet-supercomputers-reveal.html

33. Sjolund, M. Wreiber, K. Andersson, DI. Blaser, MJ. Engstrand, L. "Long-term Persistance of Resistant Enterococcus Species After Antibiotics to Eradicate Heliobacter Pylori." *Annals of Internal Medicine Journal.* September 16 2003; 139(6) 483-7. http://annals.org/article.aspx?articleid=716789

34. Burkholder, Paul. McVeigh, Ilda. "Synthesis of Vitamins By Intestinal Bacteria." *Osborn Botanical Laboratory.* Yale University. May 23, 1942. http://www.pnas.org/content/28/7/285?ijkey=931998456351a78f5d633e70cbc46b08369e0414&keytype2=tf_ipsecsha

35. Sears, Cynthia. "A Dynamic Partnership: Celebrating our Gut Flora." *Anaerobe.* October 2005; 11(5): 247-251. http://www.ncbi.nlm.nih.gov/pubmed/16701579

36. Cummings, J.H.; MacFarlane, G.T. (1997). "Role of intestinal bacteria in nutrient metabolism." *Clinical Nutrition.* 16: 3–9. http://www.ncbi.nlm.nih.gov/pubmed/9406136

37. Algareer, A. Alyahya, A. Andersson, L. "The effect of clove and benzocaine versus placebo as topical anesthetics." *Journal of Conservative Dentistry.* November 2006; 34(10): 747-50. http://www.ncbi.nlm.nih.gov/pubmed/16530911

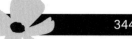

38. Ankri, S. Mirelman, D. "Antimicrobial Properties of Allicin from Garlic." *Microbial Infections.* February 1999; 1(2): 125-9. http://www.ncbi.nlm.nih.gov/pubmed/10594976

39. Pichichero, Michael. "Acute Otitis Media: Part I. Improving Diagnostic Accuracy." *American Family Physician.* April 1, 2000; 61(7): 2051-2056. http://www.aafp.org/afp/2000/0401/p2051.html

40. Bezakova, N. Damoiseaux, R. Hoes, A. Schilder, A. Rovers, M. "Recurrence up to 3.5 years after antibiotic treatment of acute otitis media in very young Dutch children: Survey of trial participants." *British Medical Journal.* 2009; 339:b2525. http://www.bmj.com/content/bmj/338/bmj.b2525.full.pdf

41. Ward, M. "Patient Information: Fever in Children (Beyond the Basics)." *Up To Date.* August 31, 2015. http://www.uptodate.com/contents/fever-in-children-beyond-the-basics - H12

42. Zdenek, Pelikan. "The Role of Nasal Allergy in Chronic Secretory Otis Media." *Allergy Research Foundation.* November 2007; 99(5): 401-407. http://www.annallergy.org/article/S1081-1206(10)60563-7/pdf

43. Weissman, Robert. "Letter to Hospitals: Stop Allowing Formula Companies to Distribute Formula Samples to New Moms." *Public Citizen: Protecting Health, Safety and Democracy.* March 30, 2012. http://citizen.org/Page.aspx?pid=5382

44. Roth, Erich. "Nonnutritive Effects of Glutamine1." *Journal of Nutrition.* October 2008; 138: 2025S-2031S. http://jn.nutrition.org/content/138/10/2025S.short

45. "N-Acetylcysteine." *WebMd.* http://www.webmd.com/vitamins-supplements/ingredientmono-1018-N-ACETYL CYSTEINE.aspx?activeIngredientId=1018&activeIngredientName=N-ACETYL CYSTEINE

46. "SAMe." *WebMD.* http://www.webmd.com/vitamins-supplements/ingredientmono-786-s-adenosyl methionine (same).aspx?activeingredientid=786&activeingredientname=s-adenosyl methionine (same)

47. "Chickenpox: The Disease and the Vaccine Fact Sheet." *National Vaccine Information Center.* http://www.nvic.org/vaccines-and-diseases/Chickenpox/chickenpoxfacts.aspx

48. Ohashi, Y. Ushida, K. "Health-beneficial effects of probiotics: It's mode of action." *Animal Science Journal.* 2009; 80: 361-371. https://www.uni-hohenheim.de/fileadmin/einrichtungen/hebrew-university/Literature/Ohashi-Ushida-ASciJ2009.pdf

49. Hall, Sarah. "Half of probiotic liquids fail bacteria health test." *The Guardian.* August 2006. http://www.theguardian.com/science/2006/aug/08/food.foodanddrink

50. "Could Probiotics Help Alleviate Your Functional Gastrointestinal Symptoms?" International Foundation for Functional Gastrointestinal Disorders. December 13, 2014. http://www.iffgd.org/site/manage-your-health/diet-treatments/probiotics

51. "Top 10 Probiotics Supplements." *Labdoor, Inc.,* 2015. http://labdoor.com

Chapter 7—The Great Debate: Organic Food

1. Herman-Giddens, Marica. Steffes, Jennifer. Harris, Donna. Slora, Eric. Hussey, Michael. Dowshen, Steven. Wasserman, Richard. Serwint, Janet. Smitherman, Lynn. Reiter, Edward. "Secondary Sexual Characteristics in Boys: Data From the Pediatric Research in Office Settings Network." *Journal of the American Academy of Pediatrics*. Oct 20, 2012. doi: 10.1542/peds.2011-3291. http://pediatrics.aappublications.org/content/130/5/e1058
2. Biro, Frank. Greenspan, Louise. Galvez, Maida. "Puberty in Girls of the 21st Century." *Journal of Pediatric & Adolescent Gynecology*. October 2012; 25(5): 289-294. http://www.jpagonline.org/article/S1083-3188(12)00092-7/abstract
3. Solotaroff, Paul. "In the Belly of the Beast." *Rolling Stone*. December 10, 2013. http://feature.rollingstone.com/feature/belly-beast-meat-factory-farms-animal-activists
4. "McDonalds 4 Year of Cheeseburger Video" http://youtu.be/4IGtDPG4UfI
5. "Farm Subsidies." *Environmental Working Group*. 2012. http://farm.ewg.org
6. "34 States Shut Out of Organic Farm Program By Congress and White House." *National Sustainable Agriculture Coalition*. January 24, 2013. http://sustainableagriculture.net/blog/organic-farms-lose-assistance/
7. "The Trouble with Sunscreen Chemicals." *Environmental Working Group*. http://www.ewg.org/2015sunscreen/report/the-trouble-with-sunscreen-chemicals/
8. Howard, Philip (2016). "Organic Processing Industry Structure." *Michigan State University*. "https://msu.edu/~howardp/organicindustry.html
9. Howard, Philip. "Consolidation in the North American Organic Food Processing Sector, 1997-2007." *International Journal of Sociology of Agriculture and Food*. June 2008; 16(1): 13-30.http://www.ijsaf.org/archive/16/1/howard.pdf
10. "Electronic Code of Federal Regulations." U.S. Government Publishing Offices. 2016. http://www.ecfr.gov/cgi-bin/text-idx?c=ecfr&SID=9874504b6f1025eb0e6b67cadf9d3b40&rgn=div6&view=text&node=7:3.1.1.9.32.7&idno=7
11. Howard, Philip (2016). "Concentration and Power in the Food System: Who Controls What We Eat?" New York, NY. Bloomsbury Academic. http://www.cornucopia.org/2016/04/weekend-reading-concentration-and-power-in-the-food-system/

Chapter 8—The Dairy Dilemma

1. Manning, Jeff. "Got Milk? Marketing by Association." *Associations Now: The Center for Association Leadership*. July, 2006. http://www.asaecenter.org/Resources/ANowDetail.cfm?ItemNumber=18644
2. American Academy of Orthopaedic Surgeons. Position Statement. http://www.aaos.org/about/papers/position/1113.asp

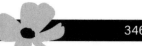

3. Bischoff-Ferrari HA, Dawson-Hughes B, Baron JA, et al. "Calcium intake and hip fracture risk in men and women: a meta-analysis of prospective cohort studies and randomized controlled trials." *American Journal of Clinical Nutrition.* 2007; 86: 1780–90. http://www.ncbi.nlm.nih.gov/pubmed/18065599?dopt=Citation

4. Tucker KL, Morita K, Qiao N, Hannan MT, Cupples LA, Kiel DP. "Colas, but not other carbonated beverages, are associated with low bone mineral density in older women: the Framingham Osteoporosis Study." *American Journal of Clinical Nutrition.* 2006; 84: 936–42. http://www.ncbi.nlm.nih.gov/pubmed/17023723?dopt=Citation

5. Statement by Connie Weaver, Ph.D., of Purdue University, at the Physicians Committee for Responsible Medicine's Summit on the Dietary Guidelines 2000, Georgetown University Medical Center, September, 1998.

6. "Epidemiology." *International Osteoporosis Foundation.* http://www.iofbonehealth.org/epidemiology

7. Center for Disease Control. "Trends in Oral Health Status: United States, 1988-1994 and 1999-2004." *Vital and Health Statistics.* Series 11, Number 248. April, 2007. http://www.cdc.gov/nchs/data/series/sr_11/sr11_248.pdf

8. https://en.wikipedia.org/wiki/List_of_countries_by_milk_consumption_per_capita - cite_note-2

9. "Tomas dispenses dental treatment in the bush of South Sudan." *Field Exchange 8.* November 1999. p.29. http://www.ennonline.net/fex/8/tomas

10. "Healthy Eating Plate & Healthy Eating Pyramid." Harvard School of Public Health. *The Nutrition Source.* http://www.hsph.harvard.edu/nutritionsource/healthy-eating-plate/

11. "Calcium and Milk: What's Best for Your Bones and Health?" Harvard School of Public Health. *The Nutrition Source.* http://www.hsph.harvard.edu/nutritionsource/calcium-full-story/

12. http://www.foodallergy.org/allergens/milk-allergy

13. Swallow, Dallas. "Genetics of Lactase Persistence and Lactose Intolerance." *Annual Review of Genetics.* December 2003; 37: 197-219. http://www.annualreviews.org/doi/abs/10.1146/annurev.genet.37.110801.143820

14. "Signs of Diary Intolerance." *The Food Intolerance Institute of Australia.* January 27, 2013. http://www.foodintol.com/dairy-intolerance/symptoms.

15. Weaver, Connie. Plawecki, Karen. "Dietary Calcium: Adequacy of a Vegetarian Diet." *American Journal of Clinical Nutrition.* 1994; 59: 1238S-41S http://ajcn.nutrition.org/content/59/5/1238S.full.pdf

16. "Chapter 3: Lactose Content of Milk and Milk Products." *American Journal of Clinical Nutrition.* October, 1998; 48(4): 1099-1104. http://ajcn.nutrition.org/content/48/4/1099.full.pdf+html

17. Kunz, C; Lonnerdal, B (1990). "Human-milk proteins: analysis of casein and casein subunits..." *American Journal of Clinical Nutrition.* January 14, 2011; 51(1): 37–46. http://ajcn.nutrition.org/content/51/1/37.full.pdf+html

18. Gina Shaw. MD. "Dairy Products." http://www.vibrancyuk.com/dairy.html

19. "Alert: Protein Drinks" *Consumer Reports Magazine.* July 2010. http://www.consumerreports.org/cro/magazine-archive/2010/july/food/protein-drinks/overview/index.htm

20. Solotaroff, Paul. "In the Belly of the Beast." *Rolling Stone*. December 10, 2013. http://www.rollingstone.com/feature/belly-beast-meat-factory-farms-animal-activists
21. Tavernise, Sabrina. "Farm Use of Antibiotics Defies Scrutiny." *The New York Times.* September 3, 2012. http://www.nytimes.com/2012/09/04/health/use-of-antibiotics-in-animals-raised-for-food-defies-scrutiny.html?pagewanted=all&_r=2&
22. Weise, Elizabeth. "Got milk? Only if it comes from a cow, group argues." *USA Today*, 4/29/2010. http://usatoday30.usatoday.com/news/health/2010-04-29-1Amilkwars29_ST_N.htm
23. Ragalie-Carr, Jean. Miller, Gregory. "NDC Comments on the 2015 Dietary Guidelines Advisory Committee: Milk Alternatives." *National Dairy Counsel*. September 1, 2014. http://www.nationaldairycouncil.org/SiteCollectionDocuments/publiccomments/NDC DGAC Comments Milk Alternatives 9 1 14 FINAL.PDF
24. http://www.choosemyplate.gov/dairy-nutrients-health
25. Greger, Michael. How Not to Die. Discover the Foods Scientifically Proven to Prevent and Reverse Disease. New York: Flatiron, 2015. Print. http://nutritionfacts.org
26. Barnard, N. Scialli, A. Bertron, P. Hurlick, D. Edmondset, K. Acceptability of a Therapeutic Low-Fat, Vegan Diet in Premenopausal Women.Journal of Nutrition Education and Behavior. 2000; 32(6): 314-9. http://www.sciencedirect.com/science/article/pii/S0022318200705905
27. Greger, Michael. How Not to Die. Discover the Foods Scientifically Proven to Prevent and Reverse Disease. New York: Flatiron, 2015. Print. http://nutritionfacts.org

CHAPTER 9—ALLEGORY OF ASTHMA AND ALLERGIES

1. Challem, Jack. *The Inflammation Syndrome*. Hoboken, New Jersey. John Wiley & Sons, Inc. 2010. (p) 1-10.
2. Food Allergy Research and Education. "*Facts and Statistics.*" http://www.foodallergy.org/facts-and-stats
3. Null, Gary. *The Complete Encyclopedia of Natural Healing*. New York, New York. Kensington Publishing Corp. 1998. (p) 44-55.
4. Challem, Jack. *The Inflammation Syndrome*. Hoboken, New Jersey. John Wiley & Sons, Inc. 2010. (p) 35-46.

CHAPTER 10—THE GUT-BRAIN CONNECTION

1. "The Gut-Brain Connection." *Harvard Health Publications*. Harvard Medical School. http://www.health.harvard.edu/healthbeat/the-gut-brain-connection

2. Wright, Steve. Reasoner, Jordan. "Leaky Gut Syndrome in Plain English—And How to Fix It." *SCD Lifestyle*. http://scdlifestyle.com/2010/03/the-scd-diet-and-leaky-gut-syndrome/
3. Challem, Jack. *The Inflammation Syndrome*. Hobeken, New Jersey: John Wiley & Sons, Inc., 2010. p64-65.
4. Wolfe, F. Clauw, D. Fitzcharles, M. Goldenberg, D. Katz, R. Mease, P. Russell, A. Russell, I. Winfield, J. Yunus, M. "The American College of Rheumatology Preliminary Diagnostic Criteria for Fibromyalgia and Measurement of Symptom Severity." *Arthritis Care & Research*. May 2010; 62(5): 600-610. http://onlinelibrary.wiley.com/doi/10.1002/acr.20140/abstract
5. StopLeakyGut.com. *"Healing a Leaky Gut Naturally."*
6. Sturniolo, GC. Di Leo, V. Ferronato, A. D'Odorico, A. D'Inca, R. "Zinc Supplementation Tightens "Leaky Gut" in Chron's Disease." *Inflammatory Bowel Disease*. May 2001; 7(2): 98-8. http://www.ncbi.nlm.nih.gov/pubmed/11383597
7. Chase, Brad. "Warning-If You Have Chrons and Are Taking Meds, Read This." *Progressive Health*. http://www.progressivehealth.com/certain-medications-may-be-causing-your-crohns.htm

Chapter 11—Western Diet Feeds Western Medicine

1. "About Cholesterol." *American Heart Association*. July 2014. http://www.heart.org/HEARTORG/Conditions/Cholesterol/AboutCholesterol/About-Cholesterol_UCM_001220_Article.jsp
2. Tuso, P. Ismail, M. Ha, B. Bartolotto, C. "Nutritional Update for Physicians." Plant-Based Diets." *The Permanente Journal*. 2013; 17(2): 61-66. http://www.ncbi.nlm.nih.gov/pmc/articles/PMC3662288/
3. Kanis, John. Johnell, Olof. De Laet, Chris. Oden, Anders. Ogelsby, Alan. "International Variations in Hip Fracture Probabilities: Implications and Risk Assessment." *Journal of Bone and Mineral Research*. July 2002; 17 (7): 1237-1244. http://onlinelibrary.wiley.com/doi/10.1359/jbmr.2002.17.7.1237/full
4. Munoz, K. Krebs-Smith, S. Ballard-Barbash. Cleveland, Linda. "Food Intakes of US Children and Adolescents Compared with Recommendations." *Pediatrics*. September 1997; 100 (3): 323-329. http://www.ncbi.nlm.nih.gov/pubmed/9282700
5. Greger, Michael. "Treating Asthma and Eczema with Plant-Based Diets." *Nutrition Facts.org*. April 23, 2014; 18. http://nutritionfacts.org/video/treating-asthma-and-eczema-with-plant-based-diets/
6. Greger, Michael. "Preventing Allergies in Adulthood." *Nutrition Facts.org*. January 2012; 7. http://nutritionfacts.org/video/preventing-allergies-in-adulthood/
7. Adams, Kelly. Kohlmeier, Martin. Zeisel, Steven. "Nutrtion Education in U.S. Medical Schools: Latest Update of a National Survey." *Journal of the Association of American Medical Colleges*. September 2010; 85 (9): 1537-1542. http://journals.lww.com/academicmedicine/Abstract/2010/09000/Nutrition_Education_in_U_S__Medical_Schools_.30.aspx

8. Campell, T. Colin. Campbell II, Thomas. *The China Study*. Dallas, Texas: BenBella Books, Inc. 2006. p230.
9. Kennedy, David. Wightman, Emma. "Herbal Extracts and Phytochemicals: Plant Secondary Metabolites and the Enhancement of Human Brain Function." *Advances in Nutrition: An International Review Journal*. 2011; 2: 32-50. http://advances.nutrition.org/content/2/1/32.full
10. Mercola, MD. "Statin Nation: The Great Cholesterol Cover-Up." *Mercola.com*. May, 2013. http://articles.mercola.com/sites/articles/archive/2013/05/11/statin-nation.aspx
11. Celik, Ahmet. Davutoglu, Vedat. Sarica, Kemal. Erturhan, Sakip. Ozer, Orhan. Sari, Ibrahim. Yilmaz, Mustafa. Baltaci, Yasemin. Akcay, Murat. Al, Behcet. Yuce, Murat. Yilmaz, Necat. "Relationship Between Renal Stone Formation, Mitral Annular Calcification and Bone Resorption Markers." *Annals of Saudi Medicine*. Jul-Aug 2010; 30(4): 301-305. http://www.ncbi.nlm.nih.gov/pmc/articles/PMC2931782/
12. McCartney, Paul. *Glass Walls*. https://youtu.be/p_UpyY2MIOc
13. Robbins, John. *The Food Revolution*. San Francisco, California: Conari Press. 2011.
14. Steinfeld, H. et al. 2006. "Livestock's Long Shadow: Environmental Issues and Options." *Livestock, Environment and Development, FAO, Rome*. pp 391.
15. Campell, T. Colin. Campbell II, Thomas. *The China Study*. Dallas, Texas: BenBella Books, Inc. 2006. p230.
16. Washington, Harriet. "Flacking for Big Pharma." *The American Scholar*. Summer 2001. https://theamericanscholar.org/flacking-for-big-pharma/ - .VfbEtniFbAM
17. Oz, Mehmet. "Soy: The Good, the Bad and the Best." *The Dr. Oz Show*. December 11, 2012. http://www.doctoroz.com/article/soy-good-bad-and-best
18. Challem, Jack. "Soy Isoflavones for Women's Health: Is Soy a Viable Alternative to Traditional Estrogen Hormone Replacement?" *Chiro.org*. 1998. http://www.chiro.org/nutrition/FULL/Soy_Isoflavones_for_Womens_Health.shtml

Chapter 12—Seeds of Health

1. Saul, Andrew. "A Timeline of Vitamin Medicine." *DoctorYourself.com*. http://www.doctoryourself.com/timeline.html
2. Hoffer, Abram and Andrew Saul. *The Vitamin Cure for Alcoholism*. Columbus, OH: Basic Health Publications, Inc. 2009. 51-76. Print.
3. *"Nutrient Recommendations: Dietary Reference Intakes (DRI)."* National Institutes of Health, U.S. Department of Health and Human Services. https://ods.od.nih.gov/Health_Information/Dietary_Reference_Intakes.aspx
4. Cheraskin, E. "Antioxidants in Health and Disease: The Big Picture." *Journal of Orthomolecular Medicine*. 1995: 10(2):89-96. http://orthomolecular.org/library/jom/1995/pdf/1995-v10n02-p089.pdf
5. Watson WA, Litovitz TL, Klein-Schwartz W, Rodgers GC Jr, Youniss J, Reid N, Rouse WG, Rembert RS, Borys D. "2003 Annual Report of the American Association of Poison Control Centers Toxic Exposure Surveillance System." *American Journal of Emergency Medicine*. 2004 Sep; 22(5): 335-404.

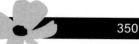

6. Hoffer, A. Janson, M. Levy, T. Dean, C. Foster, H. Paterson, E. Saul, A. "Report of the Independent Vitamin Safety Review Panel." *Orthomolecular Medicine News Service.* May 23, 2006. http://orthomolecular.org/resources/omns/v02n05.shtml
7. "Acetaminophen." *RxMed.* http://www.rxmed.com/b.main/b2.pharmaceutical/b2.1.monographs/CPS- Monographs/CPS- (General Monographs- A)/ABENOL.html
8. "Preventable Adverse Drug Reactions: A Focus on Drug Interactions." U.S. Food and Drug Administration, 2014. http://www.fda.gov/Drugs/DevelopmentApprovalProcess/DevelopmentResources/DrugInteractionsLabeling/ucm110632.htm
9. Hoffer, Abram, and Andrew W. Saul. *Orthomolecular Medicine For Everyone: Megavitamin Therapeutics for Families and Physicians.* Laguna Beach, CA: Basic Health 2008. 56-57. Print. (see associated website @ http://www.doctoryourself.com/effectiveness.html)
10. Sarasua, S. Savitz, D. "Cured and Broiled Meat Consumption in Relation to Childhood Cancer: Denver, Colorado." *Cancer Causes & Control.* 1994; 5(2): 141-8.
11. Block, G. Jensen, C. Norkus, E. Tapashi, D. Wong, L. McManus, J. Hudes, M. "Usage Patterns, Health, and Nutritional Status of Long-Term Multiple Dietary Supplement Users: A cross-sectional Study." *Nutrition Journal.* 2007; 6:30. http://www.ncbi.nlm.nih.gov/pubmed/8167261/
12. Cathcart, Robert. "The Third Face of Vitamin C." *Journal of Orthomolecular Medicine.* 1992 7(4): 197-200. http://orthomolecular.org/library/jom/1992/pdf/1992-v07n04-p197.pdf
13. Schernhammer, E. Kang, J. Chan, A. Michaud, D. Skinner, H. Giovannnuci, E. Colditz, G. Fuchs, C. "A Prospective Study of Aspirin Use and The Risk of Pancreatic Cancer in Women." *Journal of National Cancer Institute.* 2004; 96(1): 22-28. http://jnci.oxfordjournals.org/content/96/1/22.full?sid=f84864fc-178a-415d-ae17-a7bc652a2804
14. Lujian, P. Xiangde, L. Qian, L. Tengqian, T. Zhanyu, Y. "Vitamin E Intake and Pancreatic Cancer Risk: A Meta-Analysis of Observational Studies." *Medical Science Monitor.* 2015; 21:1249-1255. http://www.ncbi.nlm.nih.gov/pmc/articles/PMC4428318/
15. "Top 10 Probiotics Supplements." Labdoor, Inc., 2015. http://labdoor.com
16. Colditz, Graham. Stampfer, Meir. Willett, Walter. "Diet and Lung Cancer: A Review of the Epidemiologic Evidence in Humans." *JAMA Internal Medicine.* January, 1987; 147(1). http://archinte.jamanetwork.com/article.aspx?articleid=607672

Chapter 13—Kid Food Kills

1. Mello, Michelle. Studdert, David. Brennan, Troyen. "Obesity—The New Frontier of Public Health Law." *The New England Journal of Medicine* 2006; 354: 2601-2610. http://www.nejm.org/doi/full/10.1056/NEJMhpr060227
2. Voiland, Adam. Haupt, Angela. "10 Things the Food Industry Doesn't Want You to Know." *U.S. News and World Report.* March, 30, 2012. http://health.usnews.com/health-news/articles/2012/03/30/things-the-food-industry-doesnt-want-you-to-know
3. Freedman DS, Kettel L, Serdula MK, Dietz WH, Srinivasan SR, Berenson GS. "The Relation of Childhood BMI to Adult Adiposity: The Bogalusa Heart Study." *Pediactrics.* 2005;115:22–27. http://www.ncbi.nlm.nih.gov/pubmed/15629977

4. Olshansky, S. Passaro, D. Hershow, R. Layden, J. Carnes, B. Brody, J. Hayflick, L. Butler, R. Allison, D. Ludwig, D. "A Potential Decline in Life Expectancy in The United States in the 21st Century." *New England Journal of Medicine.* 2550; 352:1138-1145, March 17, 2005. http://www.nejm.org/doi/full/10.1056/NEJMsr043743 - t=article
5. Associated Press. "Batter-Coated French Fries Now a Fresh Vegetable on USDA List." *USA Today.* June, 15, 2004. http://usatoday30.usatoday.com/news/nation/2004-06-15-fries_x.htm

CHAPTER 14—AFFORD THE BEST ON A BUDGET OF LESS

1. Cherry, Kendra. "10 Facts About Memory." *About Education Psychology.* http://psychology.about.com/od/memory/ss/ten-facts-about-memory_8.htm
2. "Health Benefits of Coconut Oil." *Organic Facts.* https://www.organicfacts.net/health-benefits/oils/health-benefits-of-coconut-oil.html
3. http://www.mosquitosolutions.com/iastateu.html
4. Fluoride Action Network: Fluoride & the Brain. http://fluoridealert.org/issues/health/brain/
5. Fluoride Action Network, National Research Council Findings 2006 . http://fluoridealert.org/researchers/nrc/findings/
6. http://www.cdc.gov/cancer/dcpc/data/women.htm
7. "Antiperspirants,/Deodorants and Breast Cancer." *National Cancer Institute.* http://www.cancer.gov/about-cancer/causes-prevention/risk/myths/antiperspirants-fact-sheet
8. Mirick, D. Davis, S. Thomas, D. "Antiperspirant Use and the Risk of Breast Cancer. *Journal of the National Cancer Institute.* 2002 October 16; 94(20): 1578-80. http://www.ncbi.nlm.nih.gov/pubmed/12381712
9. McGrath, K. "An Earlier Age of Breast Cancer Diagnosis Related to More Frequent Use of Antiperspirants/Deodorants and Underarm Shaving." *European Journal of Cancer Prevention.* December 2003; 12(6): 479-85. http://www.ncbi.nlm.nih.gov/pubmed/?term=McGrath+2003+breast+cancer+antiperspirant
10. "Cancer's Global Footprint. An Interactive Map." *Pulitzer Center.* http://globalcancermap.com
11. Darbre, PD. Aljarrah, A. Miller, WR, Coldham, NG. Sauer, MJ. Pope, GS. "Concentrations of Parabens in Human Breast Tumours." *Journal of Applied Toxicology*, 2004 Jan-Feb; 24(1): 5-13. http://www.ncbi.nlm.nih.gov/pubmed/14745841
12. Hall, Kathy. "Cosmetics, Parabens and Cancer: What are the Facts?" *Quality Health.* June 7, 2012. http://www.qualityhealth.com/cancer-articles/cosmetics-parabens-cancer-what-facts
13. Scientific Committee on Consumer Safety. "Opinion on the safety of aluminum in cosmetic products." *European Commission.* June 18, 2014. http://ec.europa.eu/health/scientific_committees/consumer_safety/docs/sccs_o_153.pdf

14. Kawahara, Masahiro. Kato-Negishi, Midori. "Link between Aluminum and the Pathogenesis of Alzheimer's Disease: The Integration of the Aluminum and the Amyloid Cascade Hypothesis." *International Journal of Alzheimer's Disease.* 2011; 2011: 276393. http://www.ncbi.nlm.nih.gov/pmc/articles/PMC3056430/
15. Riggins, Kimberly. "What are the Benefits of Raw Shea Butter?" *Livestrong.com*. January 30, 2014. http://www.livestrong.com/article/324195-what-are-the-benefits-of-raw-shea-butter/
16. "Beeswax." *WebMD.* http://www.webmd.com/vitamins-supplements/ingredientmono-305-BEESWAX.aspx?activeIngredientId=305&activeIngredientName=BEESWAX
17. "Charcoal, Activated." *The American Society of Health-System Pharmacists.* April 2014. http://www.drugs.com/monograph/charcoal-activated.html
18. "The Ominous Truth Behind Cosmetic Beauty Claims." *Mercola.com*. August 14, 2010. http://articles.mercola.com/sites/articles/archive/2010/08/14/red-alert-on-cosmetic-products-will-they-cause-a-health-disaster-like-asbestos-did.aspx
19. "FDA Authority Over Cosmetics." http://www.fda.gov/cosmetics/guidanceregulation/lawsregulations/ucm074162.htm
20. Mercola. "If You Wear Make-Up, Your body Could be Absorbing Up to 5lbs of Chemicals Per Year." *Organic Consumers Association.* June 22, 2007. https://www.organicconsumers.org/news/if-you-wear-make-your-body-could-be-absorbing-5-lbs-chemicals-year
21. Environmental Working Group. "Natural Products Contain Carcinogenic Contaminant." March 14, 2008. http://www.ewg.org/enviroblog/2008/03/natural-products-contain-carcinogenic-contaminant
22. Mercola. "Deadly and Dangerous Shampoos, Toothpastes and Detergents: Could 16,000 Studies be Wrong About SLS?" *Mercola.com.* July 13, 2010. http://articles.mercola.com/sites/articles/archive/2010/07/13/sodium-lauryl-sulfate.aspx - _edn1
23. Kowalsky, Susan. "The Potential Implications of SLS and SLES on Human Health. *Natural Health Information Center.* http://www.natural-health-information-centre.com/sls-health-implications.html
24. Chassaing, Benoit. Koren, Omry. Goodrich, Julia. Poole, Angela. Srinivasan, Shanthi. Ley, Ruth. Gewirtz, Andrew. "Dietary emulsifiers impact the mouse gut microbiota promoting colits and metabolic syndrome." *Nature.* March 5, 2015; 519: 92-96. http://www.nature.com/nature/journal/v519/n7541/full/nature14232.html
25. Barr, L. Metaxas, G. Harbach, C. Savoy, L. Darbre, P. "Measurement of Paraben Concentrations in Human Breast Tissue at Serial Locations Across the Breast from Axilla to Sternum." *Journal of Applied Toxicology.* Jan 12, 2012. DOI: 10.1002/jat.1786. http://onlinelibrary.wiley.com/doi/10.1002/jat.1786/abstract;jsessionid=D715345619D8FCC958CF30A4C10424A3.d01t04
26. Hall, Kathy. "Cosmetics, Parabens and Cancer: What are the Facts?" *Quality Health.* June 7, 2012. http://www.qualityhealth.com/cancer-articles/cosmetics-parabens-cancer-what-facts
27. Calafat, A. Kuklenyik, Z. Reidy, J. Caudill, S. Ekong, J. Needham, L. "Urinary Concentrations of Biphenol A and 4-Nonylphenol in a Human Reference Population." *Environmental Health Perspectives.* April 2005; 113(4): 391-395. http://www.ncbi.nlm.nih.gov/pmc/articles/PMC1278476/

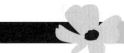

28. "Fourth National Report on Human Exposure to Environmental Chemicals." *Centers for Disease Control.* 2015.http://www.cdc.gov/biomonitoring/pdf/FourthReport_UpdatedTables_Feb2015.pdf
29. Blum, A. Balan, S. Scheringer, M. Trier, X. Goldenman, G. Cousins, I. Diamond, M. Fletcher, T. Higgins, C. Lindeman, A. Peaslee, G. Voogt, P. Wang, Z. Weber, R. "The Madrid Statement on Poly- and Perfluoroalkyl Substances (PFASs)." *Environmental Health Perspectives.* May 2015; 123 (5): A107-A111. http://ehp.niehs.nih.gov/1509934/ - tab1
30. "Ingredients." *International Fragrance Association.* 2011. http://www.ifraorg.org/en-us/ingredients - .U9qfRoBdVss
31. Sigurdson, Tina. "Expert Panel Confirms that Fragrance Ingredient can Cause Cancer." *Environmental Working Group.* August 7, 2014. http://www.ewg.org/enviroblog/2014/08/expert-panel-confirms-fragrance-ingredient-can-cause-cancer
32. Mercola. *"Triclosan: The Soap Ingredient You Should Never Use – But 75% of Households Do."* August 29, 2012. http://articles.mercola.com/sites/articles/archive/2012/08/29/triclosan-in-personal-care-products.aspx
33. Calafat, Antonia. Ye, Xiaoyun. Wong, Lee-Yang. Reidy, John. Needham, Larry. "Urinary Concentrations of Triclosan in the U.S. Population: 2003-2004." *Environmental Health Perspectives*, March 2008; 116(3): 303-307. http://www.ncbi.nlm.nih.gov/pmc/articles/PMC2265044/
34. Aiello, A. Larson, E. Levy, S. "Consumer Antibacterial Soaps: Effective or Just Risky?" *Clinical Infectious Diseases.* September 2007; 45(2): S137-47. http://www.ncbi.nlm.nih.gov/pubmed/17683018
35. Andersen, K. Storrs, F. "Skin Irritation Caused by Propylene Glycols." *Hautarzt.* January 1982; 33(1): 12-4. http://www.ncbi.nlm.nih.gov/pubmed/7085276
36. "Toxic Substances Portal – Propylene Glycol." *Agency for Toxic Substances & Disease Registry*. http://www.atsdr.cdc.gov/toxprofiles/TP.asp?id=1122&tid=240
37. "Review of the Formaldehyde Assessment in the National Toxicology Program 12th Report on Carcinogens." *Board on Environmental Studies and Toxicology.* 2014. http://www.nap.edu/openbook.php?record_id=18948&page=R1
38. Klement, Rainer. Kammerer, Ulrike. "Is there a role for carbohydrate restriction in treatment and prevention of cancer?" *Nutrition and Metabolism.* 2011; 8 (75). http://nutritionandmetabolism.biomedcentral.com/articles/10.1186/1743-7075-8-75

CHAPTER 14B—INVEST THE REST

1. Kroger-Ohlsen, M. Trugvason, T. Skribsted, L. Michaelsen, K. "Release of Iron into Foods Cooked in Iron Pot: Effect of pH, Salt, and Organic Acids." *Journal of Food Science.* July 20, 2006. DOI: 10.1111/j.1365-2621.2002.tb09582.x. http://onlinelibrary.wiley.com/doi/10.1111/j.1365-2621.2002.tb09582.x/abstract
2. "20 Reasons You Should Drink Lemon Water in the Morning." *Living Traditionally*. January 31, 2014. http://livingtraditionally.com/20-reasons-drink-lemon-water-mornings/

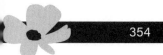

3. Vallejo, F. Tomas-Barberan, F. Garcia-Viguera. "Phenolic Compound Contes in Edible Parts of Broccoli Inflorescences After Domestic Cooking." *Journal of the Science of Food and Agriculture.* November 2003; 83(14): 1511-1516. http://onlinelibrary.wiley.com/doi/10.1002/jsfa.1585/abstract

4. Lee, Lita. *"Microwaves and Microwave Ovens."* May 14, 2001. http://www.litalee.com/documents/Microwaves And Microwave Ovens.pdf

5. European Parliament. "The Physiological and Environmental Effects of Non-Ionising Electromagnetic Radiation." *STOA (Scientific and Technological Options Assessment).* March 2001. http://www.goodhealthinfo.net/radiation/health_efx_western.htm

6. "Microwave Oven and Microwave Cooking Overview." *Powerwatch.* http://www.powerwatch.org.uk/rf/microwaves.asp

7. Institute of Medicine (US) Committee on Sleep Medicine and Research. "Sleep Disorders and Sleep Deprivation: An Unmet Public Health Problem." *National Academies Press* (US). 2006. http://www.ncbi.nlm.nih.gov/books/NBK19958/

8. Jones, Maggie. "How Little Sleep Can You Get Away With?" *New York Times.* April 15, 2011. http://www.nytimes.com/2011/04/17/magazine/mag-17Sleep-t.html?_r=0

CHAPTER 15—CREATE YOUR OWN BRAND OF HEALTH AND HAPPINESS

1. Krystal, John. Webb, Elizabeth. Cooney, Ned. Kranzler, Henry. Charney, Dennis. "Specificity of Ethanollike Effects Elicited by Seroteonergic and Noradrenergic Mechanisms." *JAMA Psychiatry.* 1994;51 (11): 898-911. http://archpsyc.jamanetwork.com/article.aspx?articleid=496839

2. Covey, Stephen. *"The 7 Habits of Highly Effective People."* New York: Simon & Schuster, 1985. Print.

ENDNOTES

Acknowledgments

The big, little (and mostly self-imposed) obstacles in my life have fueled my passion for this book. Crisis always comes before triumph—or there would be nothing to triumph over. There are many people that have helped me overcome my obstacles. I am so very grateful for the angels in my life.

I was posting a lot of vegan food pictures to Facebook when a friend encouraged me to start a blog. The suggestion came on a cold winter day when I was feeling very low. I figured that since I felt like crap anyway, why not plant a seed? The challenge lifted my spirits and the seed blossomed into this book. Thanks Heather.

Waking up Vegan began with simple recipes and silly commentary. My first attempt to write with style was a post called, "My Gardening Fantasy Comes True." My first husband saw talent. He encouraged me to develop the skill. He also "shared" the post on Facebook (which doubled the traffic to my website). We coined the phenomenon as the "Chad bump." Thanks Chad.

Tony invited me to work for his on-line magazine, *Spaces Quarterly*. He educated me on the nuances of "doing it right." I learned the importance of SEO (search engine optimization), 3rd party editing, social media and professional images. I also learned patience (in theory). He took the book's cover pictures and made the videos for my website. Thanks Tony.

When I decided to write a book, I had no idea where to start. The reality was a far-fetched dream. An emotional exchange with my teenage son put me to the test. "Mom, you keep saying you are writing a book. Where is this book? No one cares if you write a book. It doesn't make you more or less important. Write it if you want. Just stop *talking* about writing it." Great advice. Thanks Zac.

Kim volunteered to read my first draft. She had many great suggestions. I made revisions. I passed out a few more copies. My father, Missy, Patti, and Nicole skipped the "good job" kudos and pointed out the flaws. My dad insisted on more imagery and less words. Patti and Nicole wanted side bar content and recipes. Missy was frustrated by my apparent disconnect with the "real" world and demanded solutions for moms that work outside the home. They all agreed several stories were too personal for a new audience. "This is supposed to be a fun book on food. I want the recipe for cashew cream, not a recap of how you escaped from a psyche ward." (Maybe I'll share that story in my next book.) My friends helped me identify the needs and feelings of my target audience. Thanks friends.

Heather manages my website, helps with social media, creates the images, does the layouts, cover design and more. She transformed my 95,000-Word document into a 3-dimensional, image-filled publication. She talks me off the ledge, laughs at my jokes and responds to my demands with, "I don't work here! Wait. Yes, I do. You owe me money." That and more! Thanks, Heather.

Finding a professional editor was the final step of the process (said no published author ever). Karen connected me with Lori in Chicago, who did an initial manuscript evaluation. She complimented my talents for observation and interpretation. But she found the book too focused on *my* story. The reader must be able to see *their* story. Faced with the decision to proceed as it was just to say it was done, or go back to the beginning and do it right, I hired her. Over the next year, she wrote missives, assigned homework, coached and encouraged. She taught me the necessary evil of "killing the darlings." I said a tearful goodbye to alliterations, clichés, purple prose, wordy passive sentences, tangents and "–ly" words. Her tutelage changed the book and the course of my life. Thanks, Lori.

My husband believed this book would be written before I had the nerve to take my dream seriously. He dries my tears, extracts me from rabbit holes, and steadies me when I'm off balance—which is often. My refusal to wear a helmet at all times makes him uneasy because I'm quite accident prone. As a medical doctor, he holds my research to the highest standard. He challenges my sources and debates my conclusions, which forces me to triple-check my facts. He advises me on sections that call for more research or simplified instruction. The pride in his eyes motivates me to raise the bar. Love you, baby.

My kids have been so very supportive and respectful of this project. They leave me sticky notes like, "Mom, you make a difference," and sneak up when I am too engrossed to notice and rub my shoulders. Their tender gestures bring tears to my eyes. Zachary, Kyle, Anna and Kate--you are my heart.

I said I wanted to write a book. Had I known what that meant, I may not have started. But the journey has been fabulous. As I publish *Life Off the Label: A Handbook to Create Your Own Brand of Health and Happiness*, I'm outlining my next endeavor. New material appears daily. Thanks Life!